TRENDS IN DIABETES RESEARCH

TRENDS IN DIABETES RESEARCH

ASHLEY M. FORD
EDITOR

Nova Biomedical Books
New York

For permission to use material from this book please contact us:
Telephone 631-231-7269; Fax 631-231-8175
Web Site: http://www.novapublishers.com

Library of Congress Cataloging-in-Publication Data
Available upon request.

ISBN 1-59454-796-3

Published by Nova Science Publishers, Inc. ✢New York

Contents

Preface

In Chapter I, cardiovascular disease (CVD) is the most prevalent and detrimental complication of diabetes mellitus, accounting for aproximately 80% of chronic complication hospitalizations suffered by this patients. The incidence of CVD among diabetic patients is so high that diabetes mellitus is currently defined as a cardiovascular disease equivalent. Furthermore, the prognosis of diabetic patients after a cardiac event is significantly worse than that observed in non-diabetics. Therefore, primary and secondary preventive measures have a critical importance in this population subgroup.

There is substantial evidence that the efficacy of pharmacological therapies for primary and secondary cardiovascular prevention is much higher in diabetic patients than in nondiabetics. This chapter reviews the evidences of the efficacy of pharmacological prevention therapies in diabetic patients to support an aggressive pharmacological preventive strategy for them. An intesified multifactorial treatment aproach involving multiple risk factors like hypertension or dyslipidemia should be recommended. Every diabetic patient without known cardiovascular disease should receive treatment with angiotensina-converting enzyme inhibitors and statins, and in high-risk individuals, with low-dose aspirin.

There is consistent evidence that the benefits of secondary cardiovascular prevention with β-blockers, angiotensin converting enzyme inhibitors and statins is higher among diabetic patients than in non-diabetics. In our view, unless formal contraindications are present, diabetic patients with ischemic heart disease, particularly those with previous myocardial infarction, should receive always treatment with aspirin, β-blockers, angiotensin converting enzyme inhibitors and statins, regardless of lipid levels, left ventricular systolic function or the presence of congestive heart failure.

Despite the strong evidence that supports an aggressive pharmacological cardiovascular prevention treatment for diabetic patients, a number of registries throughout the world consistently reveal a significant underuse of these therapies. There is a need to develop strategies aimed to expand the degree of education about the importance of cardiovascular prevention in diabetics, to increase the use of proven useful preventive interventions, and to narrow the gap between clinical practice and the recommendations of guidelines among physicians involved in the management of these patients, particularly primary care physicians.

Chapter II presents a global epidemic of type 2 Diabetes exists and in the near future it may be closely associated with an epidemic of cardiovascular disease. Both diabetes mellitus and cardiovascular disease are major problems and among the diabetic population, the two problems taken together constitute a “double jeopardy”.

Control of hyperglycaemia became an important target as proven by studies like the Diabetes Control Complications Study and the United Kingdom Prospective Diabetes Study (UKPDS).

At first review of some of the available oral antidiabetic agents with a focus on Sulphonylureas and the recently documented selectivity as regards their mechanism of action on the potassium ATP channels that completely mimicked the pre-conditioning phenomena, moreover, blocking these channels with some of the sulphonylurea compounds abolished this protective effect.

Metformin is currently, the most extensively used oral antidiabetic agent worldwide. Its use as monotherapy offers several advantages : improvement of insulin sensitivity and blood lipid profile. Based on UKPDS, metformin monotherapy in overweight diabetic subjects was the only arm of the study showing a significant reduction in cardiovascular events and overall mortality.

Thiazolidinediones are a relatively new class of agents that enhance insulin sensitivity in the liver, adipose tissue and muscles without affecting insulin secretion. There are still some controversial issues about the benefits of Thiazolidinediones on vascular function that might reduce cardiovascular risk.

There are on-going studies on the role of conventional and intensive insulin therapy in type 2 diabetes mellitus and its possible effect on cardiovascular disease and mortality. Recently the “Diabetes mellitus, Insulin Glucose Infusion in Acute Myocardial Infarction Study Group (DIGAMI-2)” in contrast to the DIGAMI-1 study showed no beneficial effect of insulin treatment in myocardial infarction patients. Patients on oral antidiabetic agents including Sulphonylureas had similar prognosis to those on insulin therapy.

There is some speculation on the role of intensive insulin therapy in stabilizing macrovascular disease or preventing progression in those already at risk.

The large-scale clinical trials in type 2 diabetes mellitus support the fact that lowering blood glucose significantly lowers the risk of diabetic complications. Quality of life studies performed as part of the UKPDS showed that allocation to different treatment did not in itself have an effect on quality of life.

The risks and benefits of a HbA1c goal of < 7% are currently being tested in an ongoing study Action to Control Cardiovascular Risk in Diabetes (ACCORD) which will show the efficacy of reducing cardiovascular risk factors in preventing or slowing cardiovascular disease. The American Diabetes Association recommends that targets of management should include blood pressure control, treatment of dyslipidaemia, aspirin therapy and cessation of smoking. Emphasis should be put on reducing cardiovascular risk factors as a main goal in addition to treating hyperglycaemia in subjects with type 2 diabetes mellitus.

In chapter IV, diabetes mellitus is associated with an increased prevalence of cardiovascular disease. Enhanced oxidative stress has been implicated in impaired vasomotor responsiveness in diabetes. Recent evidence suggests that reactive oxygen species (ROS) induced by hyperglycemia play an essential role in altered activity of potassium (K^+)

channels, a target of endothelium-dependent hyperpolarizing factors (EDHFs). The enhanced oxidative stress may occur prior to the development of frank diabetes, such as insulin resistance. This review focuses on the mechanism of ROS production in hyperglycemia and insulin resistance and describes the consequences on hyperpolarization-mediated vasodilation.

Several pathways have been proposed as mechanisms for hyperglycemia-induced-superoxide overproduction, including activation of polyol pathway, activation of the diacylglycerol-protein kinase C pathway, upregulation of NADPH oxidase and mitochondrial generation of ROS. The resulting excess production of superoxide has been implicated in the impaired dilator responses to K_{ATP} channel openers in aorta, mesenteric and cerebral arteries of streptozotosin-induced diabetic rats and in coronary arterioles from patients with diabetes. This may have important implications in ischemia-mediated vasodilation. The effect of ROS on K_v channel function has been examined in xenopus oocytes where shaker and shaw channel were expressed. Reduced K^+ currents were observed in most shaker channels. Incubation of small rat coronary arteries in high glucose for 24 hours increases both superoxide and peroxynitrite generation, which greatly reduces K_v channel activity and functional responses, both of which can be partially restored by antioxidant treatment. In contrast to K_{ATP} and K_v channels, Ca^{2+}-activated K^+ channels are refractory to superoxide providing a compensatory mechanism for reduced dilator response to activation of other K^+ channels. However, in conditions where peroxynitrite is increased, K_{Ca} channel function is inhibited. In this circumstance, compensatory dilator mechanism acting through hyperpolarization may fail.

Insulin resistance, a condition where insulin-induced glucose uptake is reduced, is considered to be a precursor to the development of type II diabetes mellitus. In hyperinsulinemia, impaired vasodilator responses are observed in variety of vascular beds of obesity animals even in normoglycemia or mild hyperglycemia. Reduced K^+ channel function, such as K_{Ca} and K_{ATP} channels, may be a mechanism responsible for the impaired vascular reactivity in insulin resistance. Treatment with antioxidants such as superoxide dismutase restores the dilator response in obese animals supporting an inhibitory role of ROS in vasomotor function in the insulin resistant state.

In summary, determining the effect of ROS on K^+ channel mediated dilation is important for understanding the pathophysiology of vascular dysfunction in diabetes and insulin resistance and may suggest new therapies to improve tissue perfusion.

Chapter V informs about, that treatment for childhood Acute Lymphoblastic Leukaemia (ALL) improved dramatically during the second half of the twentieth century, with four-year survival rates of up to 60% being recorded. Extramedullary relapse in the central nervous system (CNS) required the introduction of cranial irradiation and intrathecal methotrexate. The second most common extramedullary site to show ALL relapse is the testis. The development of more intensive treatment protocols has reduced the incidence of testicular relapse, but relapse in the testis may still occur 13 years after initial treatment. However the pathogenesis of testicular leukaemia remains unclear. It is not known whether malignant lymphoblasts survive long-term in the testicular interstitium, or spread into the testis from subclinical leukaemic involvement on the bone marrow. Animal models, and some clinical data, may provide a sanctuary site from chemotherapeutic agents. In addition, the local micro-environment in the testis may provide cytokines and growth factors which support the survival and proliferation of the malignant lymphoblasts. This review summarises the current state of our understanding of which of these factors may be important in the testis, and of the known effects on ALL cells.

Chapter VI presents transplantation of insulin producing cells in diabetic patients requires technologies to transplant tissues in the absence of immunosuppression since the side effect of immunosuppression can never be an acceptable alternative for insulin therapy. Much effort has been put into the development of immunomodulating technologies to transplant genetically or otherwise modified islet tissue in order to decrease the immunogenicity of the islet tissue. A number of these approaches have been shown to be effective in small rodents and to allow for life-long survival of islet grafts[1,2]. In spite of some successes it has not yet come to clinical application. Another approach is immunoisolation of tissue by encapsulation of pancreatic islets to protect the tissue from the host immune system by an artificial membrane. Basically, there are three major approaches of encapsulation. These include intravascular macrocapsules, which are anastomosed to the vascular system as AV shunt, extravascular macrocapsules, which are mostly diffusion chambers transplanted at different sites, and extravascular microcapsules transplanted in the peritoneal cavity. All systems have been shown to be successful in preclinical studies. These studies also showed that not all approaches meet the technical or physiological requirements for application in men. The extravascular approach provides advantages over the intravascular systems since it is associated with fewer complications such as thrombosis and infection. Microcapsules, due to their spatial characteristics, offer better diffusion capacity than macrocapsules. Recent progress in biocompatibility of microcapsules has brought this technology near clinical application. Critical issues such as limitations in the functional performance and survival are being discussed. The latest results show that both issues can be solved by transplantation of microencapsulated islets near blood vessels in prevascularized solid supports. Also, latest insights will be presented into the composition of the membranes for immuoisolating devices and the associated biocompatibility.

In chapter VII we investigated the effect of chronic administration of highly purified eicosapentaenoic acid ethyl ester (EPA-E), an n-3 polyunsaturated fatty acid, on alloxan (ALL) induced diabetic Wistar rats. After four weeks of ALL (55 mg/kg, I.V.) administration, the diabetic animals were randomly divided into three groups. 1. Diabetic control, 2. EPA-E treated diabetic rats and 3. Verapamil treated diabetic rats. EPA-E and Verapamil were administered to the diabetic rats daily for three months. Age matched normal rats served as normal controls. During this study, plasma glucose, glycosylated hemoglobin, plasma triglycerides, cholesterol, LDL and HDL cholesterol. A significant increase in the plasma glucose, glycosylated hemoglobin, plasma triglycerides, cholesterol, and LDL and HDL ratio in diabetic control over normal control were noticed. EPA-E treatment significantly prevented the above parameters better than Verapamil. At the end of experiment, ECG, gravimetric ratio and myocardial enzyme markers were studied. In diabetic control group, diabetic cardiomyopathy was characterized by elevated CPK, gravimetric ratio, ST/R ratio in the ECG and bradycardia. EPA-E treatment significantly prevented the above parameters better than Verapamil. EPA-E may be considered as one of the treatment modalities for diabetic cardiomyopathy.

In: Trends in Diabetes Research
Editor: Ashley M. Ford, pp. 1-22
ISBN: 1-59454-796-3

Chapter I

Prevention of Ischemic Heart Disease in Patients with Diabetes Mellitus

Hector Bueno
Hospital General Universitario "Gregorio Marañón", Department of Cardiology, Dr Esquerdo, 46, 28007, Madrid, Spain; hecbueno@jet.es

Abstract

Cardiovascular disease (CVD) is the most prevalent and detrimental complication of diabetes mellitus, accounting for aproximately 80% of chronic complication hospitalizations suffered by this patients. The incidence of CVD among diabetic patients is so high that diabetes mellitus is currently defined as a cardiovascular disease equivalent. Furthermore, the prognosis of diabetic patients after a cardiac event is significantly worse than that observed in non-diabetics. Therefore, primary and secondary preventive measures have a critical importance in this population subgroup.

There is substantial evidence that the efficacy of pharmacological therapies for primary and secondary cardiovascular prevention is much higher in diabetic patients than in nondiabetics. This chapter reviews the evidences of the efficacy of pharmacological prevention therapies in diabetic patients to support an aggressive pharmacological preventive strategy for them. An intesified multifactorial treatment aproach involving multiple risk factors like hypertension or dyslipidemia should be recommended. Every diabetic patient without known cardiovascular disease should receive treatment with angiotensina-converting enzyme inhibitors and statins, and in high-risk individuals, with low-dose aspirin.

There is consistent evidence that the benefits of secondary cardiovascular prevention with β-blockers, angiotensin converting enzyme inhibitors and statins is higher among diabetic patients than in non-diabetics. In our view, unless formal contraindications are present, diabetic patients with ischemic heart disease, particularly those with previous myocardial infarction, should receive always treatment with aspirin, β-blockers, angiotensin converting enzyme inhibitors and statins, regardless of lipid levels, left ventricular systolic function or the presence of congestive heart failure.

Despite the strong evidence that supports an aggressive pharmacological cardiovascular prevention treatment for diabetic patients, a number of registries throughout the world consistently reveal a significant underuse of these therapies. There is a need to develop strategies aimed to expand the degree of education about the importance of cardiovascular prevention in diabetics, to increase the use of proven useful preventive interventions, and to narrow the gap between clinical practice and the recommendations of guidelines among physicians involved in the management of these patients, particularly primary care physicians.

Key words: Diabetes. Ischemic heart disease. Myocardial infarction. Primary prevention. Secondary prevention.

Diabetic patients have a markedly increased risk of cardiovascular disease compared with non diabetic individuals, particularly of ischemic heart disease. Approximately 50 to 75% of deaths in patients with diabetes are attributable to cardiovascular disease. In fact, the prognosis of diabetic patients without established ischemic heart disease is similar to that of non-diabetics with previous myocardial infarction. [1] This significant effect of diabetes on morbidity and mortality has resulted in diabetes being described as a coronary heart disease risk equivalent.[2-5] Furthermore, diabetic patients who develop clinical ischemic heart disease have a significantly lower survival rate than do patients without diabetes. This implies that preventive interventions for asymptomatic diabetic individuals are especially important, particularly measures to control the metabolic syndrome and those focused in other cardiovascular risk factors that are frequently associated. Primary prevention measures must include lifestyle changes (healthy diet, avoidance of overweight, increase in physical activity, and the absolute cessation of smoking).[6-9] Once non-pharmacological measures have been introduced, pharmacological treatment for the prevention of the development of cardiovascular diseases must be considered (Table 1). Several recommendations for the control of all these risk factors in diabetic patients have been released by scientific societies, although its implementation is still far away from optimal.

Table 1. Therapeutic Goals For Preventive Treatment In Diabetic Patients Without Cardiovascular Disease

Glycemic control	Hb $A_{1C} \leq 6.1\%$ Pre-prandial glycemia < 110 mg/dl Post-prandial glycemia < 135 mg/dl
Stop smoking all forms of tobacco	
Avoiding overweight	
Blood pressure control	BP < 130/80 mmHg
Plasma lipids	Total cholesterol < 175 mg/dl LDL-cholesterol < 100 mg/dl Triglycerides < 150 mg/dl

Pharmacological Treatment of Diabetic Patients without Cardiovascular Disease (Primary Prevention)

Glycemic Control

The pathophysiology of type 2 diabetes is characterized by metabolic abnormalities beginning several years before the onset of overt hyperglycemia. Insulin resistance and compensatory hyperinsulinemia are the main causes of this process. Furthermore, insulin resistance not only produces hyperglycemia but is associated to a series of abnormalities that have been called the metabolic syndrome (central obesity, hypertriglyceridemia, low levels of HDL-cholesterol, hypertension and abnormal fibrinolysis), which is responsible at least in part of the increased incidence of cardiovascular diseases in diabetic patients.

There is convincing evidence from randomized controlled trials that good metabolic control prevents microvascular complications in patients with type 1 and type 2 diabetes. Glycemic control, evaluated by glycosylated hemoglobin levels, has been shown to predict cardiac events and mortality in patients with diabetes,[10] and even in those without diabetes who have levels at the upper end of the normal range.[11] Although it is clear that strict glycemic control improves microvascular disease, its effect on macrovascular disease is not so obvious. An analysis of the UKPDS data by glycemic control showed a significantly lower incidence of cardiovascular events in patients whose levels of glycosylated hemoglobin were below 7%. A recent meta-analysis estimated in 13% (95% CI, 1% to 26%) the risk reduction in cardiovascular events (total mortality, cardiovascular mortality, non-lethal myocardial infarction, and stroke) associated with pharmacological interventions to strictly control glycemia in diabetic patients.[12] However, several pharmacological interventions directed to improve glycemic control have failed to demonstrate a reduction in the risk of cardiovascular events.[13,14] In one of the most important of these studies, UKPDS (*UK Prospective Diabetes Study*), the intensive treatment of hyperglycemia with a sulfonylurea or insulin in 2,729 patients with recently diagnosed type 2 diabetes mellitus only produced a non-significant reduction in the incidence of acute myocardial infarction (16%; $p = 0.052$), which was more marked among the 342 obese diabetics treated with metformin (39%; $p = 0.01$).[13] So, metformin is one of the few drugs that has been shown to decrease cardiovascular events in patients in patients with type 2 diabetes to date. Although metformin has a small effect as a peripheral insulin sensitizer, its main mechanism is inhibiting hepatic gluconeogenesis. It has been suggested that the use of drugs that directly improve insulin sensitivity, such as thiazolidinediones, may have direct vascular effects beyond glycemic control. Ongoing clinical trials such as ACCORD (*Action to Cardiovascular Control Risk in Diabetes*), DREAM (*Diabetes Reduction Approaches with Ramipril and Rosiglitazone Medications*) or ADOPT (*A Diabetes Outcome Progression Trial*) will evaluate their cardiovascular protective effect in diabetic patients. A recent multicenter study, the STOP-NIDDM trial, randomized 1,429 patients with impaired glucose tolerance to receive acarbose 100 mg three times a day or placebo. After a three year follow-up, treatment with acarbose was associated with a 49% relative risk reduction in the incidence of cardiovascular events (a combined end-point including coronary heart disease, cardiovascular death, congestive heart failure, cerebrovascular events and peripheral vascular disease). Acarbose was also associated with a 34% relative risk reduction in the incidence of new cases of hypertension, even after adjustment for major risk factors.[15]

Therefore, multifactorial interventions directed to obtain a strict control of glycemia are essential in the prevention of diabetic microvascular complications, however they will not completely prevent the development of macrovascular disease.

Lipid Lowering Therapy

Dyslipidemia is a typical feature in diabetic patients. Among individuals with diabetes mellitus, 97% have at least one lipid abnormality and, as demonstrated the MRFIT (*Multiple Risk Factor Intervention Trial*) study, a two to threefold increase in cardiovascular risk for each lipid level (Figure 1).[16] The most common pattern of dyslipidemia in diabetics is hypertriglyceridemia and low HDL cholesterol levels. LDL concentrations do not usually differ in diabetics and non-diabetics, but non-HDL cholesterol (VLDL + LDL) levels are usually high in diabetics. In addition, type 2 diabetic patients typically have a preponderance of smaller, oxidized and denser LDL particles, which possibly increases atherogenicity even if the absolute concentration of LDL cholesterol is not significantly increased. Finally, it has to be considered that glycemic control usually improves lipid levels in the diabetic patient, but it does not always optimize the lipid profile.

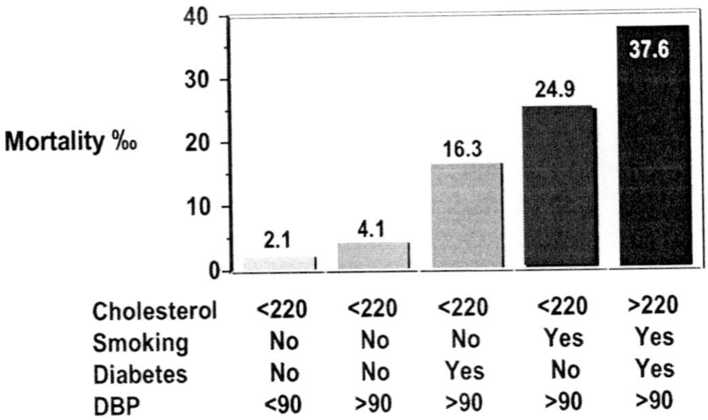

Figure 1. Cardiovascular risk assesment according to the number of risk factors. (adapted from the Multiple Risk Factor Intervention Trial). DBP: dyastolic blood pressure.

Most of the information we have regarding primary pharmacological prevention in patients with diabetes mellitus comes from *post hoc* analyses of small subgroups of diabetic patients enrolled in some of the large primary prevention clinical trials. The AFCAPS/TexCAPS (*Air Force/Texas Coronary Atherosclerosis Prevention Study*) was designed to assess whether treatment with lovastatin for at least 5 years could reduce the incidence of first major coronary events (non-lethal acute myocardial infarction, unstable angina, or sudden death) in individuals without known cardiovascular disease, intermediate levels of total and LDL-cholesterol, and low HDL-cholesterol. Six percent of the patients were diabetic (n= 394). They showed a greater reduction in the incidence of coronary events (43%) compared with the whole group (37%), although the difference did not reach statistical significance.[17] In the Helsinki Heart Study, treatment with gemfibrozil was also associated with a non-significant reduction in the incidence of ischemic heart disease in diabetics.[18]

The first study that prospectively demonstrated the efficacy of a lipid lowering drug in reducing morbidity and mortality in diabetics was HPS (*Heart Protection Study*). In this trial, 20,536 patients at high risk of coronary artery disease and no clear indication for cholesterol-lowering therapy were randomized to receive simvastatin 40 mg, antioxidant vitamins, both or placebo. Simvastatin therapy was associated with a significant 12% overall mortality reduction (12.9% versus 14.6%) and a 17% reduction in cardiovascular mortality (7.7% versus 9.2%). A 24% reduction (19.9% versus 25.4%) in the incidence of acute cardiovascular events (coronary events, stroke, and coronary revascularization) was also observed. This study recruited 5,963 patients with type 1 or type 2 diabetes, approximately 4,000 of them without known cardiac or peripheral arterial disease. The relative reduction in the risk of cardiovascular events in this subgroup was similar to that observed in high-risk patients, regardless of patient's age, sex or cholesterol level.[19]

The Steno-2 trial, compared the effect of a targeted, intensified, multifactorial intervention with that of conventional treatment on modifiable risk factors for cardiovascular disease (hyperglycemia, hypertension, and dyslipidemia) in patients with type 2 diabetes and microalbuminuria, which included treatment with atorvastatin. This study showed a significant reduction not only in the risk of microvascular events but also in cardiovascular risk.[20] Currently, there is a number of ongoing trials designed to confirm the benefit on cardiovascular risk of different lipid lowering agents in diabetic patients without evidence of ischemic heart disease, such as ASPEN (*Atorvastatin Study for the Prevention of coronary heart disease End-points in NIDDM*) and FIELD (*Fenofibrate Intervention and Event Lowering in Diabetes*) study.

Although the published evidence is scarce, there is a high degree of consensus in the recommendations of the main scientific societies clinical guidelines. The current recommendations for the treatment of hyperlipidemia of the American Diabetes Association, American Heart Association and the third report of the National Cholesterol Education Program (NCEP III) establish a common therapeutic goal of LDL-cholesterol <100 mg/dl for all diabetics, recommending non-pharmacological measures such as behavioral counseling, physical activity, weight control and dietary measures for patients with values beyond that level.[3-5] The undisputed LDL-cholesterol threshold to begin pharmacological treatment in diabetic patients without known cardiovascular disease is 130 mg/dl,[3,4] whereas in patients with c-LDL values between 100 and 129 mg/dl, the decision should be based on a global cardiovascular risk assessment (Table 2).[3,5]

No specific treatment goals are defined for HDL-cholesterol or triglycerides, but their concentrations are used as markers of increased risk. HDL-cholesterol >40 mg/dl in men, >46 mg/dl in women, or triglycerides >150 mg/dl are markers of an increased cardiovascular risk and can be used to guide the choice of drug therapy.

The priorities in the treatment of dyslipidemias in diabetics must be: *a)* to reduce high LDL levels; *b)* to raise HDL levels, and *c)* to reduce triglyceride levels.[4] Pharmacological treatment should begin with moderate doses of statins as the first choice. The use of fibrates or bile acid sequestrants in combined treatment is recommended only when monotherapy fails to control dyslipidemia.[3-5] The benefit of treating hypertriglyceridemia is not well known. However, drug therapy is recommended for severe hypertriglyceridemia (>400 mg/dl) in the absence of other risk factors and for moderate hypertriglyceridemia (>200 mg/dl) in patients with other risk factors. Statins are the drugs of choice when high LDL-cholesterol levels are associated, and fibrates when only triglyceride levels are elevated (Table 2).[4]

Table 2. Current Indications of Pharmacological Treatment In DIABETIC Patients Without Cardiovascular Disease

	Condition	Indication	Drugs	Observations
Antihypertensive therapy				
	BP > 135 / 80 mmHg	Always	ACEI, ARB Diuretic, BB, ACEI, ARB or CCB	If + Proteinuria If – Proteinuria
Lipid-lowering therapy				
	c-LDL ≥130 mg/dl	Always	Statin	
	c-LDL 100 to 129 mg/dl	10-year risk > 5%	Statin	
	Triglycerides >400 mg/dl	Always	Statin Fibrate	If c-LDL >100 mg/dl If c-LDL normal
	Triglycerides 200-400 mg/dl	>1 CVRF	Statin Fibrate	If c-LDL >100 mg/dl If c-LDL normal
Antithrombotic therapy				
	Age >55	>1 CVRF	Aspirin 75-150 mg/day	Class IIA

ACEI: angiotensin-converting enzyme inhibitors. ARB: angiotensin II receptor blockers. BB: beta-blockers. CCB: calcium channel blockers. c-LDL: cholesterol low density lipoproteins. CVRF: cardiovascular risk factor.

Blood Pressure Control

Hypertension is a an extremely common comorbid condition in diabetes. The incidence of hypertension is approximately twice as frequent in patients with diabetes than in normal individuals.[21] A recent registry performed in Spain revealed that 75% of diabetic patients are also hypertensive.[22] On the other hand, metabolic abnormalities are more frequent in hypertensive patients. These data suggest that there is an association between hypertension and diabetes mellitus, a pernicious coexistence strongly linked to cardiovascular disease, stroke, progression of renal disease and diabetic retinopathy.[23-25]

Pharmacological treatment of hypertension prevents the development of cardiovascular disease in the general population. The decrease in blood pressure in hypertensive individuals is associated with a reduction in mortality and cardiovascular events. Several studies have shown a superior benefit of treating hypertension in diabetic patients compared with non-diabetics. This advantage is observed regardless of the drugs and doses used.[26-28] The question of which agent class is superior for lowering blood pressure is not so important if we consider that the majority of diabetic patients will require two or more drugs to achieve blood pressure control. Randomized controlled trials that have included large diabetic populations, including UKPDS, HOT (*Hypertension Optimal Treatment*), Syst-EUR (*Systolic Hypertension in Europe*), HOPE (*Heart Outcomes Prevention Evaluation Study Investigators*), LIFE (*Losartan Intervention For Endpoint Reduction in Hypertension Study*), SHEP (*Systolic Hypertension in the Elderly Program*), and ALLHAT (*Antihypertensive and Lipid-Lowering treatment to prevent Heart Attack Trial*), have demonstrated that adequate blood pressure control improves cardiovascular outcomes, especially stroke, when aggressive targets are achieved.[29-35]

The studies that compared strategies of different intensity in blood pressure control demonstrated that the maximal benefit is obtained achieving the lowest levels of blood pressure.[27-29] Therefore, regimes directed to obtain tight a blood pressure control are desirable. The HOT study randomly allocated 18,790 hypertensive patients to three progressive strategies of control, based on diastolic blood pressure (<90, <85 and <80 mm Hg, respectively). Among the 1,501 diabetic patients included, a progressive reduction in major cardiovascular episodes was observed as a more accurate control of diastolic blood pressure was reached. In addition, diabetics assigned to the group of more strict control of blood pressure (diastolic pressure <80 mm Hg) had a cardiovascular mortality rate three times lower than that observed in the other two groups.[28] The hypertension control arm of the UKPDS showed a 15% reduction in diabetes-related mortality, 11% in myocardial infarction and 13% in microvascular complications such as retinopathy and nephropathy for each 10 mm Hg decrease in systolic blood pressure. This benefit was obtained even in ranges of blood pressure considered normal.[30]

These findings suggest that blood pressure reduction *per se* improves cardiovascular prognosis in diabetic patients. The benefit is greater as control of blood pressure is tightest. This is the rationale on which the recommendation to set a lower threshold of blood pressure to initiate pharmacological treatment in diabetic patients stands. The current recommendations of the seventh report of the Joint National Committee (JNC-VII) are concordant with the American Diabetes Association guidelines, which recommend a blood pressure level lower than 130/80 mmHg for diabetic patients.[31]

However, it is not clear if the beneficial effect of lowering blood pressure in patients with diabetes mellitus is independent of the antihypertensive agent used. In the ALLHAT study the doxazosine treatment arm was discontinued because it was associated with more than two-fold increase in the incidence of heart failure and a 24% increase in cardiovascular episodes in comparison with the chlorthalidone-treated group, both in diabetic and non-diabetic patients.[32] Chlorthalidone reduced the incidence of myocardial infarction and cardiovascular mortality similarly to lisinopril or amlodipine.

In the ABCD (*Appropriate Blood Pressure Control in Diabetes*) study, in which 470 non-insulin-dependent diabetics with hypertension were randomized to receive treatment with nisoldipine or enalapril, the nisoldipine arm was prematurely discontinued because of the higher incidence of lethal and non-lethal acute myocardial infarction in this group of patients (adjusted RR, 4.2; 95% CI, 1.8%-10.1%).[33,34] A recent meta-analysis suggests that, compared with other antihypertensive drugs, the use of calcium-channel blockers in diabetic patients is associated with a significant increase of 55% in the incidence of myocardial infarction and 44% in major cardiovascular events.[35] However, the ABCD-2 study, published later, showed that in diabetic patients with normal blood pressure levels, nisoldipine is similar to lisinopril in the prevention of stroke or development of albuminuria.[36] The CAPP (*Captopril Prevention Project*) study compared captopril with conventional therapy in 10,985 patients, 572 of them diabetics. Captopril showed no benefit in non-diabetic individuals, but was associated with a 46% reduction in total mortality (95% CI, 4-54%) and 66% in the incidence of acute myocardial infarction (95% CI, 33%-83%) in diabetic patients.[37] The LIFE study compared the treatment with losartan and atenolol during an average of 4.7 years in hypertensive patients with electrocardiographic signs of left ventricular hypertrophy. Among the 1,195 diabetic patients enrolled losartan showed a 27% reduction (95% CI, 5%-43%) in the primary endpoint (cardiovascular death, acute myocardial infarction or stroke) compared with atenolol, mainly due to a 38% reduction (95%CI, 8%-59%) in cardiovascular mortality. In addition, a 40% reduction in total mortality and 43% in the incidence of heart failure was found.[38]

In the Micro-HOPE study,[39] a predefined substudy of the HOPE trial, 3,577 diabetic patients without clinical proteinuria, heart failure, or left ventricular systolic dysfunction were randomly distributed to receive placebo or ramipril 10 mg daily. The treatment group showed a significantly lower incidence of the combined endpoint (25% risk reduction) and of each of its components: myocardial infarction (22%), stroke (33%), and cardiovascular death (37%). A significant reduction in total mortality (24%), heart failure of any degree (20%), and overt nephropathy (24%) was also found. This beneficial effect was observed with a reduction in systolic blood pressure at the end of the study of only 1.9 mm Hg, and 3.3 mm Hg in diastolic pressure. All subgroups of diabetic patients showed some degree of risk reduction, although it was more evident in patients with dietetic control of hyperglycemia, in those with microalbuminuria at the beginning of the study, and in those with previous cardiovascular disease (secondary prevention). The maximal benefit was observed in patients with type 1 diabetes, although the differences did not reach statistical significance because this patient subgroup was very small.[39]

Regarding microvascular complications, a recent meta-analysis confirmed that treatment with ACE inhibitors in type 1 normotensive diabetics with microalbuminuria reduces the progression to macroalbuminuria and increases the probability of regression to normoalbuminuria regardless blood pressure control.[40] More recently, angiotensin receptor blockers such as irbesartan (IRMA II: *Irbesartan in Patients with type II Diabetes and Microalbuminuria Study*, or IDNT: *Irbesartan Diabetic Nephropathy Trial*),[41,42] and losartan (RENAAL: *Reduction of Endpoints in NIDDM with the Angiotensin II Antagonist Losartan*)[43] have demonstrated their ability to reduce the progression of diabetic nefropathy but with no significant effect in terms of mortality or macrovascular complications. The American Diabetes Association recommends ACE inhibitors or angiotensin receptor blockers for diabetic patients with chronic kidney disease, in order to prevent deterioration of glomerular filtration or worsening of albuminuria.

All these findings suggest that drugs that block the renin-angiotensin-aldosterone system may be superior to other antihypertensives for the prevention of renal dysfunction as well as for cardiovascular risk reduction in patients with diabetes mellitus. Therefore, ACE inhibitors must be considered the treatment of choice in all diabetics with a blood pressure above the threshold value (130/80 mm Hg), regardless of the presence of proteinuria. Nevertheless, in the light of the results of the Micro-HOPE study, the indication of ACE inhibitors may be extended to all diabetic patients with other risk factors, regardless of blood pressure levels.

Antithrombotic Therapy

There are several evidences supporting the beneficial effect of aspirin for cardiovascular prevention in diabetics. In primary prevention, the *Physicians' Health Study* investigated the effect of 325 mg of aspirin every other day to reduce cardiovascular mortality in a placebo-controlled randomized trial that studied 22,071 USA male physicians. After a 5 year follow-up period, aspirin did not prove any significant effect on cardiovascular mortality but reduced the risk of myocardial infarction by 44% (95% CI: 30% to 65%). The risk reduction was 61% among the 533 diabetic participants (4.0% versus 10.1%) compared with 40% among non-diabetics (1.2% versus 2.0%). The difference in risk reductions between both groups was not statistically significant, suggesting that the efficacy is at least similar in diabetics as in non-diabetics.[44] The *Early Treatment Diabetic Reninopathy Study* (ETDRS) enrrolled 3,711 diabetics with diabetic retinopathy —30% type 1 diabetes mellitus, and 48% with known cardiovascular disease—, that were randomized to receive a relatively high dose of aspirin (650 mg daily) or placebo. After 5 years of follow-up, the incidence of myocardial infarction decreased by 28% (99% CI: 5% to 45%), from 12.3% in the placebo group to 9.1% in the treated group.[45] The HOT (*Hypertension Optimal Treatment*) trial randomized 18,790 patients with hipertension —less than 10% of them with cardiovascular disease— to receive antihypertensive therapies with three different intensities in the degree of diastolic blood pressure to address the optimal blood pressure therapeutic target. In addition, the HOT trial investigated the benefit of adding 75 mg of aspirin daily, through a parallel placebo-controlled randomization. Aspirin therapy decreased by 36% the incidence of myocardial infarction, but did not influence cardiovascular mortality or the risk of stroke. Quantitatively analyzed, it was estimated that aspirin could prevent 15 myocardial infarctions per 10,000 patients/year in the whole group, with a reduction of 25 myocardial infarctions per 10,000 diabetic patients/year.[28] The results of the 4,961 diabetics without cardiovascular disease included in the placebo-controlled trials investigating antiplatelet therapies performed until 1997 were pooled in the *Antithrombotic Trialists' Collaboration* metanalysis, which confirms the beneficial effect of aspirin therapy, with a 1% absolute and 7% relative reduction (8% standard deviation) in the incidence of major vascular events.[46] The authors pointed out that the lack of statistical significance must not be interpreted as a lack of efficacy but as a lack of difference in effect with that observed in other high risk subgroups, such as those with previous myocardial infarction or stroke, because the 99% confidence interval includes the 25% risk reduction, that observed in the whole population included in the analysis.

The main limitation of chronic aspirin therapy is the increase in bleeding risk. According to the findings of ETDRS and HOT trials, aspirin does not increase the incidence of lethal hemorrhages, stroke, or cerebral or retinal hemorrhage, but it does increase by 80% the rate of major non-lethal hemorrhages and minor bleedings.[28,47]

Based on these evidences, the use of aspirin is recommended in all diabetic patients with concomitant cardiovascular disease and in those without disease but at a high risk. Provided that low doses of aspirin (75-150 mg daily) are associated with a similar or greater efficacy than higher doses[46] and that they should be associated with a lower incidence of bleeding, particularly of a gastric origin, the generalized recommendation is to use low doses of aspirin for cardiovascular prevention therapy. The *Antithrombotic Trialists' Collaboration* metanalysis concludes that "it may be appropriate to consider antiplatelet therapy in diabetic patients who are at substantial risk of a first vascular event (such as those with proteinuria)".[46] The sixth *American College of Chest Physicians* guideline on antithrombotic therapy, establishes a 2A type recommendation for the use of aspirin for primary prevention in men and women over 50 years of age with diabetes mellitus that have no contraindications to its use.[48] The *American Diabetes Association* recommends to consider treatment with aspirin at a dose of 75-325 mg/day in type I or type II diabetics older than 30 years of age at a high cardiovascular risk (with family history of coronary artery disease, any other risk factor, micro o macroalbuminuria or obesity) that do not show contraindications.[49,50] More generically, the *American Heart Association* recommend to use 75–160 mg of aspirin daily for individuals without cardiovascular disease at a high risk of developing it (particularly in those with an estimated risk ≥10% in 10 years).[51] Finally, the *American Diabetes Association* recommend to consider clopidogrel as an alternative to aspirin in non-tolerant patients and as a combined therapy in very high-risk patients.[50]

Pharmacological Treatment of Diabetics with Coronary Artery Disease (Secondary Prevention)

Diabetics who survive an acute coronary event have a much higher incidence of short- and long-term complications and mortality compared with non-diabetics. Consequently, diabetic patients with ischemic heart disease deserve an aggressive strategy of secondary cardiovascular prevention.

Beta-Blocker Therapy

Early oral beta-blocker treatment.[51,53-54] is associated with a better outcome in patients with acute myocardial infarction. However, there is not much information from randomized trials regarding the specific efficacy of long-term beta-blocker therapy in diabetic patients surviving an acute myocardial infarction compared with non-diabetics. On the contrary, several observational studies suggest a much greater benefit in patients with diabetes mellitus, particularly in older patients.[55]

Lipid Lowering Therapy

There is a robust evidence demonstrating the efficacy of lipid lowering therapies for secondary cardiovascular prevention in diabetic patients with known cardiovascular disease. In the LIPID study (*Long-Term Intervention with Pravastatin in Ischaemic Disease*), pravastatin showed a favorable effect on the incidence of death due to coronary artery disease and non-lethal acute myocardial infarction both in diabetic and non-diabetic patients with ischemic heart disease and cholesterol concentrations of 155 to 271 mg/dl.[57] The 4S (*Scandinavian Simvastatin Survival Study*) trial, in which only 202 of 4,444 patients were diabetics (4.5%), the reduction in 5-year death rate was much greater in absolute terms (10.4%) among the diabetic patients than in non-diabetics (3%). The reduction of both non-lethal coronary and other cardiovascular events showed a parallel pattern to that observed for mortality, with the exception of stroke, the only event not significantly reduced in diabetics.[58] The CARE (*Cholesterol and Recurrent Events Trial*) evaluated the effect of pravastatin in 4,159 patients <76 years old with previous myocardial infarction, total cholesterol <240 mg/dl, and LDL-cholesterol <175 mg/dl, 14% of them diabetics. The relative reduction in the cumulative incidence of coronary events (death due to coronary artery disease, non lethal acute myocardial infarction, coronary artery bypass grafting and coronary angioplasty) was similar in diabetics (25%) and non-diabetics (23%). Nevertheless, since the number of events was approximately two times greater in diabetics, the benefit was also greater in absolute terms. Of note, the divergence in the survivals curves in diabetics began to be apparent in the fourth year of treatment.[58] A recent analysis of the *Pravastatin Pooling Project*, focused on the 20% of patients with LDL-cholesterol values <125 mg/dl included in the CARE and LIPID trials, has shown that while 5.5 years of pravastatin therapy was not associated with any beneficial effect in non-diabetic patients, the incidence of coronary events was reduced by 44% (95% CI, 17% to 63%) in diabetics (an absolute reduction of 12%, from 34% to 22%).[59] This analysis showed no significant differences the incidence of cancer in patients treated with pravastatin or placebo.

A reduction in the incidence of adverse episodes in patients with diabetes mellitus has been demonstrated not only with statins. The VA-HIT study (*Veteran Affairs High-Density Lipoprotein Cholesterol Intervention Trial*), which enrolled patients with known coronary artery disease, intermediate LDL-cholesterol levels (<140 mg/dl), and low HDL-cholesterol concentrations (<40 mg/dl), treatment with gemfibrozil 1,200 mg daily produced a 24% relative reduction in the primary endpoint (death due to coronary artery disease, non-lethal acute myocardial infarction or confirmed stroke) in both groups, but the absolute reduction in events was greater in diabetics (8%) than in non diabetics (5%).[60] In a similar way, the Helsinki Heart Study confirmed that gemfibrozil reduces the incidence of coronary events in type 2 diabetic patients.[18]

Current guidelines recommend to begin pharmacological therapy with moderate doses of statins in diabetic patients with macrovascular disease (ischemic heart disease, cerebrovascular disease or peripheral arterial disease) and LDL-cholesterol levels over 100 mg/dl. [4,5] Pharmacological treatment is recommended for triglyceride levels above 150 mg/dl in patients with known cardiovascular disease (Table 2). Statins are recommended as the first choice, particularly when cholesterol levels are elevated. If an adequate control is not obtained, a fibrate should be added, although potential side effects such as hepatic toxicity and rhabdomyolysis must be ruled out during follow up.

Treatment with ACE Inhibitors

One of the most consistently documented beneficial effects in secondary cardiovascular prevention in diabetes mellitus is the reduction in mortality observed with ACE inhibitors in diabetic patients with previous myocardial infarction.[8,61-63] All placebo-controlled randomized trials that have analyzed the influence of diabetes on the efficacy of ACE inhibitors in this context have shown comparable results: a significant mortality reduction in the whole group, based mainly on the reduction in mortality in diabetic patients (Table 3). In addition, long-term therapy with ACE inhibitors decreases the incidence of heart failure [39,61,63] and acute myocardial infarction.[39]

Table 3. Efficacy of Angiotensin-Converting Enzyme Inhibitors for Cardiovascular Secondary Prevention in Diabetic and Non-Diabetic Patients

Study Drug	Group	Follow-up	Mortality Placebo	Mortality ACEI	Absolute reduction	Relative reduction	95% CI
GISSI-3		6 weeks					
Lisinopril	DM		12.4	8.7	3.7	32	14 – 47
	Non-DM		5.9	5.6	0.3	5	-9 – 17
TRACE		26 months					
Trandolapril	DM		61	45	16	36	9 – 55
	Non-DM		39	33	6	18	3 – 31
SMILE*		6 weeks					
Zofenopril	DM		16.5	7.2	9.3	61	16 – 82
	Non-DM		9.0	7.1	1.9	23	-17 – 50
HOPE		5 years					
Ramipril	DM		14.0	10.8	3.2	24	8 – 37
	Total		12.2	10.4	1.8	16	5 – 25

ACEI: angiotensin-converting enzyme inhibitors. CI: confidence interval. DM: diabetic patients. Non-DM: non-diabetic patients.
* Death + severe CHF

Antithrombotic Therapy

The efficacy of aspirin for secondary cardiovascular prevention is very clearly established, with an effect that seems to be maximal at doses of 75-150 mg daily (absolute reduction of 4.3 major vascular events per 100 patients treated).[46] There is no evidence that the clinical efficacy of aspirin may be less in diabetics with cardiovascular disease, therefore as these patients do have a much higher risk of subsequent vascular events than non-diabetics, it seems that the benefit of secondary cardiovascular prevention with aspirin in absolute terms is superior in diabetics than in non-diabetic patients. Regarding the efficacy of other antiplatelet agents, the CAPRIE (*Clopidogrel versus Aspirin in Patients at Risk of Ischemic Events*) trial evaluated the effect of clopidogrel on the incidence of ischemic (cardiovascular death, myocardial infarction, stroke and rehospitalization due to ischemic events) and hemorrhagic events (rehospitalization due to hemorrhage) in patients with known cardiovascular disease, compared with aspirin. A *post-hoc* analysis of this trial estimated that among 3,866 diabetic patients enrolled, treatment with clopidogrel could prevent 21 ischemic or hemorrhagic events a year compared with the treatment with aspirin. This benefit was greater in insulin-treated diabetics (38 events prevented a year). A multivariate analysis adjusting for baseline clinical features selected treatment with clopidogrel as an independent predictor of a lower rate of ischemic-hemorrhagic events compared with aspirin (risk reduction: 13.1%; 95% CI: 1.2% to 23.7%, p=0.032).[64]

Pharmacological Cardiovascular Prevention and Diagnosis of New Onset Diabetes

An interesting aspect of the relation between cardiovascular prevention and diabetes is the finding that several preventive pharmacological interventions used in a non-diabetic population may reduce the incidence of new onset type 2 diabetes mellitus (Figure 2). The ARIC (*Atherosclerosis Risk In Communities*), carried out on 12,550 individuals without diabetes, evaluated the relation between antihypertensive therapy and risk of developing diabetes mellitus in a 6-year follow-up cohort study. It was observed that among all antihypertensive therapies, beta-blockers were the only ones associated with an increased risk of new diagnosis of diabetes mellitus during follow-up (probably due to their ability to reduce insulin sensitivity). However, the main determinant of the risk of developing diabetes was the presence of hypertension, regardless of the treatment received.[65] In the LIFE trial, treatment with losartan was associated with a 25% lower incidence of newly diagnosed diabetes mellitus compared with atenolol, although both groups showed a similar reduction in blood pressure.[66] In the CAPPP study, hypertensive patients who received treatment with captopril had an 14% lower incidence (95% CI, 1% to 26%) of newly diagnosed diabetes mellitus than those individuals who received conventional therapy.[37]

In the HOPE study the incidence of development of new onset diabetes mellitus (diagnosed after the study began) was 30% lower in the patients who received ramipril than in those in the placebo arm.[67] These studies suggest an ethiologic and pathophysiological relationship between hypertension and type 2 diabetes mellitus. Moreover, pharmacological treatment of hypertension may influence the rate of diabetes incidence. While drugs that block the renin-angiotensin-aldosterone system seem to prevent or delay the development of type 2 diabetes mellitus, beta-blockers may accelerate it.

The mechanisms by which ACE inhibitors and angiotensin II receptor antagonists may exert their protective are unknown, but it has been hypothesized that their ability to improve insulin resistance in hypertensive patients may play a role.[68]

Not only antihypertensive agents but also statins have been shown to prevent the appearance of type 2 diabetes mellitus. Thus, in the WOSCOPS (*West Of Scotland Coronary Prevention Study*) trial, the incidence of new onset diabetes mellitus was 32% lower in patients treated with pravastatin than in those who received placebo.[69] The mechanism of this protective effect are not known. It has been speculated that it might be due their anti-inflammatory effect.[70] Insulin resistance has been related to the concentrations of C reactive protein, a mediator of inflammation.[71] The mechanism by which the statins can reduce reactive protein C values[72,73] could be similar to that associated with the reduction of insulin resistance, although other mechanisms have been proposed, such as the improvement in physical activity capacity of patients treated with statins due to the reduction in the incidence of angina associated with their use.[74,75]

These findings open new research pathways about the pathophysiological relationship between cardiovascular risk factors, their prevention and treatment, but also strengthen the evidences supporting an aggressive treatment strategy with these drugs in diabetic patients, regardless of the presence of known cardiovascular disease.

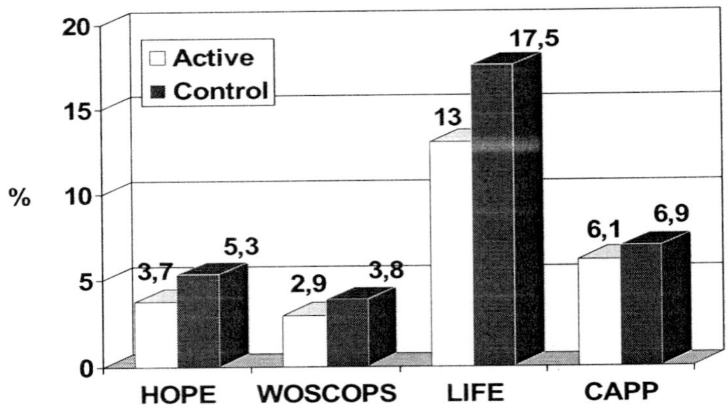

Figure 2. Incidence of new-onset type 2 diabetes mellitus in clinical trials testing pharmacological cardiovascular preventive therapies according to allocated treatment. HOPE (Heart Outcomes Prevention Evaluation): ramipril versus placebo.WOSCOPS (West Of Scotland Coronary Prevention Study): pravastatin versus placebo.LIFE (Losartan Intervention For Endpoint Reduction in Hypertension Study): losartan versus atenolol.CAPP (Captopril Prevention Project): captopril versus conventional antihypertensive treatment (diuretics or beta blockers).

Use of Cardiovascular Prevention Interventions in Diabetic Patients in the Real World

In spite of the strong evidences supporting the fact that a number of pharmacological interventions may improve prognosis in high-risk populations through a reduction in cardiovascular risk, these therapies are frequently underused in diabetic patients. Several registries have evaluated the patterns of use and appropriateness of pharmacological treatment in diabetic patients. All them show that the adherence to evidence-based medicine is generally poor in the community.[76-80]

The RISK-HIA *(Register of Information and Knowledge about Swedish Heart Intensive care Admissions)* registry collected data from 25,633 patients with acute coronary syndromes admitted to 58 coronary care units in Sweden, 5,193 of them (20%) diabetics. During hospitalization, patients with diabetes mellitus received significantly less reperfusion therapy (41% versus 31%, $p<0.001$) or intravenous beta blockers. Thrombolytic therapy was less utilized even after multiple regression analyses. Serious events were, however, more common among the diabetic patients. In parallel, a similar pattern of underutilization of several evidence-based therapies at hospital discharge was found. The use of β-blockers was high in both groups (75% in diabetics, 80% in non-diabetics), but only 25% of diabetic patients were discharged on statin therapy. There was an exception, the use of ACE inhibitors was more common in diabetics.[76]

Underuse of effective therapies is not the only problem observed in diabetics, but lack of achievement of therapeutic goals is also relevant in diabetic patients receiving pharmacological treatment. The EUROASPIRE survey, focused on patients with established coronary artery disease, found that only 54% of diabetic patients were receiving beta blockers and 30% ACE inhibitors. In addition, 49% of patients who were on lipid-lowering therapy still had their cholesterol above 5.5 mmol/l.[77] The L-TAP (*Lipid Treatment Assesment Project*) study showed similar results in patients with diabetes: less than 10% were taking lipid lowering drugs and, among treated patients, almost none of them achieved recommended cholesterol values (only 1% had levels of LDL-cholesterol below 100 mg/dl).[78] These limitations have been found also in primary care. The TranSTAR, a prospective study that recorded blood pressure, lipid levels and pharmacological therapy in 388 consecutive type 2 diabetes patients visited in 326 primary care centers in Spain during October 2001, found that underutilization of preventive measures is common in general practice. The prevalence of hypertension and dyslipidemia in these patients was 58% and 52%, respectively and 10% had known cardiovascular disease. The rate of use of lipid lowering therapies, ACE inhibitors and β-blockers was 57%, 27% and 4%, respectively. During the visits, 86% of hypertensives showed blood pressure values above the current recommendations. Only 8% of the patients who were receiving lipid-lowering agents showed a fully appropriate lipid profile. Among diabetics with cardiovascular disease, the proportion of patients on statins was 36%, 50% on ACE inhibitors and 11% on β-blockers.[79,80]

Despite the fact that aspirin is very efficient for cardiovascular prevention, particularly in very high risk patients such as those with diabetes and cardiovascular disease, and that it is an inexpensive therapy, its use is far from common. A recently published study based on 1,718 answers to an interview sent to the 4,707 adult members of a local diabetic association in

Spain found that the rate of regular aspirin use was 21% in this population, ranging from 53% among those with known cardiovascular disease and 14% in those without. [81] These results are very similar to those obtained in the third *National Health and Nutrition Examination Survey* (NHANES III)[82] and concordant with other studies suggesting that the use of aspirin in diabetic patients with ischemic heart disease is still low (between 37% and 63%).[83,84] It is important to realize that the main determinant of aspirin use for cardiovascular prevention in diabetic patients is being counseled about aspirin use by a physician,[85] so even in groups with low aspirin prescription rates, as much as 80% of patients who received counseling were on aspirin regardless the presence of cardiovascular disease.[81]

Conclusions

Diabetic patients are at a high-risk of future cardiovascular disease, particularly coronary artery disease. Whereas lifestyle and pharmacological interventions directed to optimize glycemic control reduce the incidence of microvascular disease (nephropathy, retinopathy...), their effect on macrovascular disease is limited. Therefore, the use of other proven therapies to reduce cardiovascular risl is warranted in these patients. At the present moment, there is a robust evidence to recommend treatment with statins and ACE inhibitors in all diabetic patients, regardless of their lipid profile and blood pressure levels. Hypertensive diabetics must have strict blood pressure control that should always include an ACE inhibitor (or an angiotensin II receptor blocker when proteinuria is present). In diabetic patients with other risk factors or at a high cardiovascular risk, the association of low dose aspirin should also be weighed.

The risk of new cardiovascular events in diabetic patients with coronary artery disease is very high, but the potential benefit of secondary prevention interventions is also higher than that obtained in the general population. All diabetics with known coronary artery disease —and probably those with carotid artery disease or peripheral artery disease— must receive treatment with aspirin (75-150 mg daily), beta-blockers, ACE inhibitors and statins regardless of their clinical characteristics (lipid profile, blood pressure, left ventricular systolic function, presence of congestive hear failure...) unless formal contraindications are present.

In spite of the magnitude of the benefits achieved in diabetic patients with primary and secondary pharmacological cardiovascular prevention interventions, registries of clinical practice consistently reveal a large gap with guidelines recommendations and a significant underuse of these therapies. This adverse scenario must be viewed as an opportunity for improvement, in which strategies aimed to expand the degree of education about the importance of cardiovascular prevention in diabetics, to increase the use of proven useful preventive interventions, and to narrow the gap between clinical practice and the recommendations of guidelines must be developed. These interventions should be directed to all physicians involved in the management of diabetic patients: endocrinologists, diabetologists, cardiologists, internal medicine physicians, geriatricians, and specially to primary care physicians.

References

[1] Haffner SM, Lehto S, Rönnemaa T, Pyörälä K, Laakso M. Mortality from coronary heart disease in subjects with type 2 diabetes and in nondiabetic subjects with and without prior myocardial infarction. *N. Engl. J. Med.* 1998; 339:229-34.

[2] Grundy SM, Benjamin IJ, Burke GL, Chait A, Eckel RH, Howard BV, et al. Diabetes and cardiovascular disease: A statement for health professionals from the American Heart Association. *Circulation* 1999;100: 1134 –1146.

[3] A Joint Editorial Statement by the American Diabetes Association; the National Heart, Lung, and Blood Institute; the Juvenile Diabetes Foundation International; the National Institute of Diabetes and Digestive and Kidney Diseases; and the American Heart Association. Diabetes Mellitus: A Major Risk Factor for Cardiovascular Disease. *Circulation* 1999;100: 1132-1133.

[4] American Diabetes Association Management of dyslipidemia in adults with diabetes. *Diabetes Care* 2002; 25 (Suppl. 1): S74-S77.

[5] Expert Panel on Detection, Evaluation, and Treatment of High Blood Cholesterol in Adults. Executive Summary of the Third Report of the National Cholesterol Education Program (NCEP) Expert Panel on Detection, Evaluation, and Treatment of High Blood Cholesterol in Adults (Adult Treatment Panel III). *JAMA* 2001; 285:2486-2497.

[6] American Diabetes Association Position Statement: Evidence-based nutrition principles and recommendations for the treatment and prevention of diabetes and related complications. *J. Am. Diet. Assoc.* 2002; 102:109-118.

[7] Tuomilehto J, Lindstrom J, Eriksson JG, Valle TT, Hämäläinen H, Ilanne-Parikka P, et al. Prevention of type 2 diabetes mellitus by changes in lifestyle among subjects with impaired glucose tolerance. *N. Engl. J. Med.* 2001; 344:1343–1350.

[8] Eriksson KF, Lindgarde F. Prevention of type 2 (non-insulin-dependent) diabetes mellitus by diet and physical exercise: the 6-year Malmö feasibility study. *Diabetologia* 1991; 34: 891-8.

[9] American Diabetes Association. Smoking and Diabetes. *Diabetes Care* 2002; 25 (Suppl. 1):S80-S81.

[10] Kuusisto J, Mykkänen L, Pyörälä K, Laakso M. NIDDM and its metabolic control predict coronary heart disease in elderly subjects. *Diabetes* 1994; 43:960–967.

[11] Khaw KT, Wareham N, Luben R, Bingham S, Oakes S, Welch A, Day N. Glycated haemoglobin, diabetes, and mortality in men in Norfolk cohort of European Prospective Investigation of Cancer and Nutrition (EPIC-Norfolk). *BMJ* 2001; 322:15–18.

[12] Huang ES, Meigs JB, Singer DE. The effect of interventions to prevent cardiovascular disease in patients with type 2 diabetes mellitus. *Am. J. Med.* 2001;111: 633– 642.

[13] UK Prospective Diabetes Study (UKPDS) Group. Intensive blood-glucose control with sulphonylureas or insulin compared with conventional treatment and risk of complications in patients with type 2 diabetes (UKPDS 33). *Lancet* 1998; 352:837-53.

[14] Diabetes Control and Complications Trial Research Group. The effect of intensive treatment of diabetes on the development and progression of long-term complications in insulin-dependent diabetes mellitus. *N. Engl. J. Med.* 1993;329: 977–986.

[15] Chiasson JL, Josse RG, Gomis R, Hanefeld M, Karasik A, Laakso M. Acarbose treatment and the risk of cardiovascular disease and hypertension in patients with impaired glucose tolerance. The STOP-NIDDM trial. *JAMA* 2003;290:486-94.

[16] Multiple Risk Factor Intervention Trial Research Group. Multiple Risk Factor Intervention Trial: risk factor changes and mortality. *JAMA* 1982; 248:1465–77.

[17] Downs JR, Clearfield M, Weis S, Whitney E, Shapiro DR, Beere PA, et al. Primary prevention of acute coronary events with lovastatin in men and women with average cholesterol levels. *JAMA* 1998;279:1615–1622.

[18] Koskinen P, Manttari M, Manninen V, Huttunen JK, Heinonen OP, Frick MH. Coronary heart disease incidence in NIDDM patients in the Helsinki Heart Study. *Diabetes Care* 1992;15:820–825.

[19] MRC/BHF Protection Study of cholesterol-lowering with simvastatin in 5963 people with diabetes: a randomised placebo-controlled trial. Heart Protection Study Collaborative Group. *Lancet* 2003; 361:2005-16.

[20] Gaede P., Pernillo V., Larsen N., et al. Multifactorial intervention and cardiovascular disease in patients with type 2 diabetes. *N. Engl. J. Med.* 2003; 348:383-93.

[21] Simonson DC. Etiology and prevalence of hypertension in diabetic patients. *Diabetes Care* 1998; 11: 821-27.

[22] González Juanatey JR, Alegría E, García Acuña JM, et al. Impacto de la diabetes en las enfermedades cardíacas en España. Estudio Cardiotens 1999. *Med. Clin. (Barc)* 2001; 116: 686-91.

[23] Hinderliter AL, Runge MS. Who´s on first? Does hypertension in type 1 diabetes result from nephropathy or metabolic alterations? *Circulation* 2001; 104: 508-510.

[24] Mogensen CE, Osterby R, Hansen KW, et al. Blood pressure elevation versus abnormal albuminuria in the genesis and prediction of renal disease in diabetes. *Diabetes Care* 1992;15:1192–1204.

[25] La Rocca E, Gobbi C, Ciurlino D, et al. Improvement of glucose/insulin metabolism reduces hypertension in insulin-dependent diabetes mellitus recipients of kidney-pancreas transplantation. *Transplantation*. 1998;65: 390–393.

[26] Curb JD, Pressel SL, Cutler JA, Savage PJ, Applegate WB, Black H, et al. Effect of diuretic-based anti-hypertensive treatment on cardiovascular risk in older diabetic patients with systolic hypertension. *JAMA* 1996;276: 1886-92.

[27] Tuomilehto J, Rastenyte D, Birkenhäger WH, Thijs L, Antikainen R, Bulpitt CJ, et al. Effects of calcium-channel blockade in older patients with diabetes and systolic hypertension. *N. Engl. J. Med.* 1999;340:677-684.

[28] Hansson L, Zanchetti A, Carruthers SG, Dahlof B, Elmfeldt D, Julius S, et al. Effects of intensive blood-pressure lowering and low-dose aspirin in patients with hypertension: principal results of the Hypertension Optimal Treatment (HOT) randomised trial. HOT Study Group. *Lancet* 1998; 351:1755-62.

[29] Hansson L, Lindholm LH, Ekborn T, Dahlof B, Lanke J, Scherstén B, et al. Randomised trials of old and new antihypertensive drugs in elderly patients: cardiovascular mortality and morbidity. The Swedish Trial in Old Patients with Hypertension-2 study. *Lancet* 1999;354:1751-1756.

[30] UK Prospective Diabetes Study Group. Tight blood pressure control and risk of macrovascular and microvascular complications in type 2 diabetes: UKPDS 38. *Br. Med. J.* 1998; 317:703-713.

[31] The Seventh Report of the Joint National Committee on Prevention, Detection, Evaluation, and Treatment of High Blood Pressure. Bethesda, Md: National Institutes of Health, National Heart, Lung, and Blood Institute, National High Blood Pressure Education Program. *Hypertension* 2003; 42: 1206-1252.

[32] The ALLHAT Officers and Coordinators for the ALLHAT Collaborative Research Group. Major cardiovascular events in hypertensive patients randomized to doxazosine vs chlortalidone. The Antihypertensive and Lipid-Lowering treatment to prevent Heart Attack Trial (ALLHAT). *JAMA* 2000; 283;1967-75.

[33] Estacio RO, Jeffers BW, Hiatt WR, Biggerstaff SL, Gifford N, Schrier RW. The effect of nisoldipine as compared with enalapril on cardiovascular outcomes in patients with non-insulin-dependent diabetes and hypertension. *N. Engl. J. Med.* 1998;338:645-52.

[34] Schrier RW, Estacio RO. Additional follow-up from the ABCD Trial in patients with type 2 diabetes and hypertension. *N. Engl. J. Med.* 2000;342:1969.

[35] Pahor M, Psaty BM, Alderman MH, Applegate WB, Williamson JD, Cavazzini C, et al. Health outcomes associated with calcium antagonists compared with other first-line antihypertensive therapies: a meta-analysis of randomised controlled trials. *Lancet* 2000; 356:1949–54.

[36] Schrier RW, Estacio RO, Esler A, Mehler P. Effects of aggressive blood pressure control in normotensive type 2 diabetic patients on albuminuria, retinopathy and strokes. *Kidney Int.* 2002;61:1086–1097.

[37] Hansson L, Lindholm LH, Niskanen L, Lanke J, Hedner T, Niklason A, et al. Effect of angiotensin-converting-enzyme inhibition compared with conventional therapy on cardiovascular morbidity and mortality in hypertension: the Captopril Prevention Project (CAPPP) randomised trial. *Lancet* 1999;353:611-6.

[38] Lindholm LH, Ibsen H, Dahlöf B, Devereux RB, Beevers G, de Faire U, et al. Cardiovascular morbidity and mortality in patients with diabetes in the Losartan Intervention For Endpoint reduction in hypertension study (LIFE): a randomised trial against atenolol. *Lancet* 2002;359: 1004–10.

[39] Heart Outcomes Prevention Evaluation (HOPE) Study Investigators. Effects of ramipril on cardiovascular and microvascular outcomes in people with diabetes mellitus: results of the HOPE study and MICRO-HOPE substudy. *Lancet* 2000;355:253–59.

[40] The ACE Inhibitors in Diabetic Nephropathy Trialist Group. Should all patients with type 1 diabetes mellitus and microalbuminuria receive angiotensin-converting enzyme inhibitors? A meta-analysis of individual patient data. *Ann. Intern. Med.* 2001;134:370-379.

[41] Parving H-H, Lehnert H, Brochner-Mortensen J, Gomis R, Andersen S, Arner P. The effect of irbesartan on the development of diabetic nephropathy in patients with type 2 diabetes. *N. Engl. J. Med.* 2001;345:870-878.

[42] Lewis EJ, Hunsicker LG, Clarke WR, Berl T, Pohl MA, Lewis JB, et al. Renoprotective effect of the angiotensin-receptor antagonist irbesartan in patients with nephropathy due to type 2 diabetes. *N. Engl. J. Med.* 2001;345:851-60.

[43] Brenner BM, Cooper ME, de Zeeuw D, Keane WF, Mitch WE, Parving H-H, et al. Effects of losartan on renal and cardiovascular outcomes in patients with type 2 diabetes and nephropathy. *N. Engl. J. Med.* 2001;345:861-869.

[44] Steering Committee of the Physicians' Health Study Research Group. Final report on the aspirin component of the ongoing Physicians' Health Study. *N. Engl. J. Med.* 1989; 321:129-135.

[45] ETDRS Investigators. Aspirin effects on mortality and morbidity in patients with diabetes mellitus. *JAMA* 1992; 268:1292-1300.

[46] Antithrombotic Trialists' Collaboration. Collaborative meta-analysis of randomised trials of antiplatelet therapy for prevention of death, myocardial infarction, and stroke in high risk patients. *Br. Med. J.* 2002;324:71-86.

[47] Chew EY, Klein ML, Murphy RP, Remaley NA, Ferris FL. Early Treatment Diabetic Retinopathy Study Research Group. Effects of aspirin on vitreous/preretinal hemorrhage in patients with diabetes mellitus. *Arch. Ophthalmol.* 1995;113:52-55.

[48] Cairns JA, Théroux P, Lewis HD Jr., Ezekowitz M, Meade TW. Antithrombotic Agents in Coronary Artery Disease. *Chest.* 2001;119: 228S–252S.

[49] American Diabetes Association. Aspirin Therapy in Diabetes. *Diabetes Care* 2003;25 (suppl.1): S87-S88.

[50] American Diabetes Association. Standards of medical care for patients with diabetes mellitus. *Diabetes Care* 2003; 26 (Suppl. 1): S33-S50.

[51] Pearson TA, Blair SN, Daniels SR, Eckel RH, Fair JM, Fortmann SP, et al. AHA Guidelines for primary prevention of cardiovascular disease and stroke: 2002 Update. Consensus panel guide to comprehensive risk reduction for adult patients without coronary or other atherosclerotic vascular diseases. *Circulation* 2002; 106:388-91

[52] ISIS-2 (Second International Study of Infarct Survival) Collaborative Group. Randomised trial of intravenous streptokinase, oral aspirin, both, or neither among 17,187 cases of suspected acute myocardial infarction: ISIS-2. *Lancet* 1988; 2:349-60.

[53] Malmberg K, Herlitz J, Hjalmarson A, Rydén L. Effects of metoprolol on mortality and late infarction in diabetics with suspected acute myocardial infarction. Retrospective data from two large studies. *Eur. Heart J.* 1989;10: 423– 8.

[54] Gundersen T, Kjekshus J. Timolol treatment after myocardial infarction in diabetic patients. *Diabetes Care* 1983;6:285–90.

[55] Chen J, Marciniak TA, Radford M, Wang Y, Krumholz HM. Beta-Blocker Therapy for Secondary Prevention of Myocardial Infarction in Elderly Diabetic Patients. Results From the National Cooperative Cardiovascular Project. *J. Am. Coll. Cardiol.* 1999; 34: 388-94.

[56] The Long-Term Intervention with Pravastatin in Ischaemic Disease (LIPID) Study Group. Prevention of cardiovascular events and death with pravastatin in patients with coronary heart disease and a broad range of initial cholesterol levels. *N. Engl. J. Med.* 1998;339:1349-1357

[57] Pyörälä K, Pedersen TR, Kjekshus J, Faergeman O, Olsson AG, Thorgeirsson G, for the Scandinavian Simvastatin Survival Study (4S) Group. Cholesterol lowering with simvastatin improves prognosis of diabetic patients with coronary heart disease: a

subgroup analysis of the Scandinavian Simvastatin Survival Study (4S). *Diabetes Care* 1997;20:614 –620.

[58] Goldberg RB, Mellies MJ, Sacks FM, Moyé LA, Howard BV, Howard WJ, el al. Cardiovascular events and their reduction with pravastatin in diabetic and glucose-intolerant myocardial infarction survivors with average cholesterol levels subgroup analyses in the cholesterol and recurrent events (CARE) Trial. *Circulation* 1998; 98:2513-19.

[59] Sacks FM, Tonkin AM, Craven T, Pfeffer MA, Shepherd J, Keech A, et al. Coronary heart disease in patients with low LDL-cholesterol benefit of pravastatin in diabetics and enhanced role for HDL-cholesterol and triglycerides as risk factors. *Circulation* 2002;105:1424-1428.

[60] Rubins HB, Obins SJ, Collins D, Fye CL, Anderson JW, Elam MB, et al. Gemfibrozil for the secondary prevention of coronary heart disease in men with low levels of high-density lipoprotein cholesterol. *N. Engl. J. Med.* 1999;341:410-8.

[61] Zuanetti G, Latini R, Maggioni AP, Franzosi MG, Santoro L, Tognoni G, for the GISSI 3 Investigators. Effect of the ACE inhibitor lisinopril on mortality in diabetic patients with acute myocardial infarction. Data from the GISSI-3 Study. *Circulation* 1997;96:4239-4245.

[62] Gustafsson I, Torp-Pedersen C, Køber L, Gustafsson F, Hildebrandt P. Effect of the angiotensin-converting enzyme inhibitor trandolapril on mortality and morbidity in diabetic patients with left ventricular dysfunction after acute myocardial infarction. Trace Study Group. *J. Am. Coll. Cardiol.* 1999;34:83-89.

[63] Ambrosioni E, Borghi C, Magnani B, for the Survival of Myocardial Infarction Long-Term Evaluation (SMILE) Study Investigators. The effect of the angiotensin-converting–enzyme inhibitor zofenopril on mortality and morbidity after anterior myocardial infarction. *N. Engl. J. Med.* 1995;332:80-85.

[64] Bhatt DL, Marso SP, Hirsch AT, Ringleb PA, Hacke W, Topol EJ. Amplified benefit of clopidogrel versus aspirin in patients with diabetes mellitus. *Am. J. Cardiol.* 2002; 90: 625– 628.

[65] Gress TW, Nieto FJ, Hahar E, Wofford MR, Brancati FL, for the Atherosclerosis Risk In Communities Study. Hypertension and antihypertensive therapy as risk factors for type 2 diabetes mellitus. *N. Engl. J. Med* 2000;342:905-12.

[66] Lindholm LH, Ibsen H, Borch-Jonsen K, Hetch Olsen M, Wachtell K, Dahlöf B et al. The LIFE study group. Risk of new-onset diabetes in the Losartan Intervention For Endpoint reduction in hypertension study. *J. Hypertens.* 2002; 20: 1879-1886.

[67] The Heart Outcomes Prevention Evaluation Study Investigators. Effects of an angiotensin-converting-enzyme inhibitor, ramipril, on cardiovascular events in high-risk patients. *N. Engl. J. Med.* 2000;342:145-153.

[68] Mykkänen L, Kuusisto J, Pyörälä K, Laakso M, Haffner SM. Increased risk of non-insulin-dependent diabetes mellitus in elderly hypertensive subjects. *J. Hypertens.* 1994;12:1425–1432.

[69] Freeman DJ, Norrie J, Sattar N, Neely DG, Cobbe SM, Ford I, et al. Pravastatin and the development of diabetes mellitus: evidence for a protective treatment effect in the West of Scotland Coronary Prevention Study. *Circulation* 2001;103:357–362.

[70] Haffner SM. Do interventions to reduce coronary heart disease reduce the incidence of type 2 diabetes? A possible role for inflammatory factors. *Circulation* 2001;103:346-7.

[71] Schmidt MI, Duncan BB, Sharrett AR, Lindberg G, Savage PJ, Offenbacher S, et al. Markers of inflammation and prediction of diabetes mellitus in adults (Atherosclerosis Risk in Communities study): a cohort study. *Lance*t 1999;353:1649 –1652.

[72] Ridker PM, Hennekens CH, Buring JE, Rifai N. C-reactive proteins and other markers of inflammation in the prediction of cardiovascular disease in women. *N. Engl. J. Med.* 2000;342:836 –843.

[73] Ridker PM, Rifai N, Pfeffer MA, Sacks F, Braunwald E. Long-term effects of pravastatin on plasma concentrations of C-reactive protein: the Cholesterol and Recurrent Events (CARE) Investigators. *Circulation* 1999;100:230 –235.

[74] Ur E, Shlossberg A. Do statins reduce the risk for diabetes by improving exercise capacity? *Circulation* 2001;104:E104-E105.

[75] Ross SD, Allen IE, Connelly JE, Korenblat BM, Smith ME, Bishop D, et al. Clinical outcomes in statin treatment trials: a meta-analysis. *Arch. Intern. Med.* 1999;159:1793–1802.

[76] Norhammar A, Malmberg K, Rydén L. Underutilisation of evidence-based treatment partially explains for the unfavourable prognosis in diabetic patients with acute myocardial infarction. *Eur. Heart. J.* 2003;24:838-44.

[77] Pearson TA, Laurora I, Chu H, Kafonek S. The lipid treatment assessment project (L-TAP): a multicenter survey to evaluate the percentages of dyslipemic patients receiving lipid-lowering therapy and achieving low-density lipoprotein cholesterol goals. *Arch. Intern. Med.* 2000; 160:459-67.

[78] EUROASPIRE Study Group. A European Society of Cardiology survey of secondary prevention of coronary heart disease: principal results. *Eur. Heart. J.* 1997; 18: 1569±82.

[79] Sarnago Cebada F, Bueno H, Gambús G. Grupo TranSTAR. ¿Cómo se utilizan las medidas de prevención cardiovascular basadas en el control lipídico en la población diabética española? *Rev. Esp. Cardiol.* 2003; 56 (Suppl 2): 160-161 (Abstr).

[80] Sarnago Cebada F, Bueno H, Gambús G. Grupo TranSTAR. Inadecuado control de la tensión arterial en la población diabética española. Resultados del estudio TranSTAR. *Rev. Esp. Cardiol.* 2003; 56 (Suppl 2): 163-164 (Abstr).

[81] Esmatjes E, Castell C, Franch J, Puigoriol E, Hernáez R. Consumo de ácido acetil salicílico en pacientes con diabetes mellitus. *Med. Clin (Barc)* 2004;122: 96-98.

[82] Rolka DB, Fagot-Campagna A, Narayan V. Aspirin Use Among Adults With Diabetes. Estimates from the Third National Health and Nutrition Examination Survey. *Diabetes Care* 2001;24:197-201.

[83] Wood DM, Plehwe WE, Colman PG. Aspirin usage in a large teaching hospital diabetes clinic setting. *Diabet Med.* 1999:16:605–608.

[84] Krumholz HM, Chen YT, Wang Y, Radford MJ. Aspirin and angiotensin-converting enzyme inhibitors among elderly survivors of hospitalization for an acute myocardial infarction. *Arch. Intern. Med.* 2001;161:538–544.

[85] Krein Sl, Vijan S, Pogach LM, Hogan MM, Kerr EA. Aspirin use and counseling about aspirin among patients with diabetes. *Diabetes Care* 2002;25:965–970.

In: Trends in Diabetes Research
Editor: Ashley M. Ford, pp. 23-35

ISBN: 1-59454-796-3

Chapter II

Reducing Cardiovascular Disease Risk Through Management of Hyperglycaemia: Prospects and Pitfalls

N. A. Abdella [1]
Departments of Medicine, Faculty of Medicine
Kuwait University, Kuwait

Abstract

A global epidemic of type 2 Diabetes exists and in the near future it may be closely associated with an epidemic of cardiovascular disease. Both diabetes mellitus and cardiovascular disease are major problems and among the diabetic population, the two problems taken together constitute a "double jeopardy".
Control of hyperglycaemia became an important target as proven by studies like the Diabetes Control Complications Study and the United Kingdom Prospective Diabetes Study (UKPDS).
At first review of some of the available oral antidiabetic agents with a focus on Sulphonylureas and the recently documented selectivity as regards their mechanism of action on the potassium ATP channels that completely mimicked the pre-conditioning phenomena, moreover, blocking these channels with some of the sulphonylurea compounds abolished this protective effect.
Metformin is currently, the most extensively used oral antidiabetic agent worldwide. Its use as monotherapy offers several advantages : improvement of insulin sensitivity and blood lipid profile. Based on UKPDS, metformin monotherapy in overweight diabetic subjects was the only arm of the study showing a significant reduction in cardiovascular events and overall mortality.

[1] Corresponding Author: Dr. Nabila Abdella, Department of Medicine, Faculty of Medicine Kuwait University, Kuwait.Telephone: 965 531 9596 Fax : 965 533 8907Email : nabdella12@yahoo.com

Thiazolidinediones are a relatively new class of agents that enhance insulin sensitivity in the liver, adipose tissue and muscles without affecting insulin secretion. There are still some controversial issues about the benefits of Thiazolidinediones on vascular function that might reduce cardiovascular risk.
There are on-going studies on the role of conventional and intensive insulin therapy in type 2 diabetes mellitus and its possible effect on cardiovascular disease and mortality. Recently the "Diabetes mellitus, Insulin Glucose Infusion in Acute Myocardial Infarction Study Group (DIGAMI-2)" in contrast to the DIGAMI-1 study showed no beneficial effect of insulin treatment in myocardial infarction patients. Patients on oral antidiabetic agents including Sulphonylureas had similar prognosis to those on insulin therapy.
There is some speculation on the role of intensive insulin therapy in stabilizing macrovascular disease or preventing progression in those already at risk.
The large-scale clinical trials in type 2 diabetes mellitus support the fact that lowering blood glucose significantly lowers the risk of diabetic complications. Quality of life studies performed as part of the UKPDS showed that allocation to different treatment did not in itself have an effect on quality of life.
The risks and benefits of a HbA1c goal of $< 7\%$ are currently being tested in an ongoing study Action to Control Cardiovascular Risk in Diabetes (ACCORD) which will show the efficacy of reducing cardiovascular risk factors in preventing or slowing cardiovascular disease. The American Diabetes Association recommends that targets of management should include blood pressure control, treatment of dyslipidaemia, aspirin therapy and cessation of smoking. Emphasis should be put on reducing cardiovascular risk factors as a main goal in addition to treating hyperglycaemia in subjects with type 2 diabetes mellitus.

Introduction

Type 2 Diabetes (DM) is a modern age epidemic that exists and in the near future it may be closely associated with an epidemic of cardiovascular disease (CVD). In the last decade the number of people with diabetes have risen sharply and a continued increase is projected, which will lead to a global prevalence of diabetes in excess of 220 million by 2010 [1]. Increases in both type 1 and type 2 DM have been observed in all societies studied in the last 30 years [2]. Type 2 DM accounts for most of the current and forecasted figures. In developing countries Type 2 DM is occurring with increasing frequency in younger people [3,4]. Of particular concern is the worldwide emergence of type 2 DM in the very young, including children and also adolescents [5]. This downward shift in the age at which DM develops has serious implications for the development of complications, in particular CVD which is more likely to develop at an earlier age. Both DM and CVD are major problems and among the diabetic population the two problems taken together constitute a "double jeopardy". The complex link between DM and CVD is based on a combination of insulin resistance state, hyperglycaemia and dyslipidaemia. Dysfunction of the endothelial cell monolayer leads to increased vascular tone and permeability and a prothrombotic environment. The poor outcome of CVD among diabetic compared to non-diabetic put an important focus on Type 2 DM treatment in relation to CVD and its outcome.

Control of hyperglycaemia became an important target as proven by studies like the Diabetic Control Complications study (DCCT) [6] and the United Kingdom Prospective

Diabetes Study (UKPDS) [7]. The majority of studies that have evaluated the link between blood glucose levels and mortality among the population of people with DM find a positive, significant association [8].

Many prospective observational studies have found associations between hyperglycaemia and coronary artery disease [9]; stroke [10]; peripheral vascular disease [11] and lower extremity amputations [12]. Measures of glycaemia by fasting plasma glucose and HbA1C have been independently associated with death from macrovascular disease [13].

Having defined the magnitude of the problem of Type 2 DM and its close relationship to CVD disease there is definite evidence of the role of glycaemia control in prevention of diabetes – related macrovascular complications. It is clear that long term glycaemic control, best reflected by HbA1C levels, is an important factor in microvascular complications, as is already well established and also in myocardial infarction and cerebro vascular accident [6,7].

Therefore, antidiabetic treatment should be aimed at obtaining the best possible metabolic control.

- How then to achieve control of hyperglycaemia with groups of drugs with minimal effect on cardiovascular risks among the diabetic subjects?
- Does Sulphonylurea treatment of Type 2 DM contribute to the cardiovascular risk?

Historically, the concern about the safety of Sulphonylureas (SUs) dates back to 1970 when the UGDP [14] concluded that tolbutamide treatment caused increased cardiovascular mortality, a study which at the time led to curtailment of oral antidiabetic treatment in the USA, but was received with skepticism in Europe. Later criticism of its methodology reduced the impact of the study. However, the question of the safety of SUs in type 2 diabetic patients with CHD has been reopened because of new experimental data. SUs has been prescribed by three generations of diabetologists. SUs provided alternative therapy to insulin for type 2 diabetes. However, despite their relatively long use it is only recently that the mechanism of action of this therapeutic class of drugs at molecular level has been clearly understood. SUs stimulate insulin secretion in type 2 diabetic patients by blocking ATP-sensitive K^{+}_{ATP} channels in the pancreatic β-cell membrane by binding to the SU receptor (SUR1) subunit of the channel. K^{+}_{ATP} channels are also present in a range of extrapancreatic tissues, but may contain alternative types of SUR subunit (SUR2A in heart and SUR2B in smooth muscle) The SU sensitivity of K^{+}_{ATP} channels varies with the type of SUR subunit: thus, gliclazide and tolbutamide potently block the β-cell (SUR1), but not the cardiac (SUR2A) or smooth muscle (SUR2B) types of K^{+}_{ATP} channel. In contrast, glibenclamide and glimepiride block all three types of K^{+}_{ATP} channel with similar potency. Therefore, administration of SU compound such as glibenclamide that has a K^{+}_{ATP} -channel-blocking effect should be expected to increase ischaemic damage and abolish the protective action of channel openers.

It is known from, in vitro, as well as in vivo studies that activation of K^{+}_{ATP} channels constitutes an important cardioprotective mechanism against ischemic damage. Since the discovery of K^{+}_{ATP} channels in the heart, numerous investigators have evaluated their role in cardiac adaptation to ischaemic insults. The high levels of ATP in the normal cardiomyocyte probably keep most K^{+}_{ATP} channels in the closed state [15], but these are opened when the level is lowered thereby leading to multiple changes in cardiac metabolism, electrical activity and mechanical function, which results from ischemia. Soon after the onset of ischaemia, activation of outward flow of K+ currents through the K^{+}_{ATP} channels results in earlier repolarization of the myocyte and shortening of the action potential, which leads to a reduction of calcium influx through voltage-gated calcium channels [16-19]. The resulting decrease in contractility protects the ischaemic cardiomyocyte by reducing its oxygen demand. In addition, opened arterial wall K^{+}_{ATP} channels during ischaemia decrease the vascular resistance, thus increasing coronary blood flow [20,21]. Another consequence of ischaemia is intracellular accumulation of adenosine derived from the breakdown of ATP, which may leak out from cells and activate plasma membrane-A1 receptors in an autocrine manner, thus leading to opening of K^{+}_{ATP} channels [22, 23]. Adenosine has been suggested to be a major cardioprotective agent; it seems to mediate its effect through a variety of mechanisms, including direct vasodilatory and anti-arrhythmic actions, attenuation of the heart response to sympathetic stimuli, inhibition of platelet aggregation, and reduction of free radical formation [24-26]. The latter may be especially important in the protection against post-infarct reperfusion injury, believed to be caused by the burst of free radicals on reoxygenation.

Brief episodes of ischaemia render the heart more resistant to subsequent ischemic events, with marked reduction in infarct size and contractile dysfunction [27,28]. This phenomenon called 'ischaemic preconditioning', operates in most species including man [29, 30]. Activation of K^{+}_{ATP} channels completely mimicked the preconditioning, moreover, blocking the channels with antagonists such as glibenclamide abolished the protective effect of preconditioning [31, 32]. Adenosine also seems to be important for preconditioning: short-term infusion of adenosine reduced the extent of myocardial necrosis in dogs with the same efficiency as preconditioning, the effect being mediated through a K^{+}_{ATP} channel related mechanism, blocked by glibenclamide pretreatment [33,34]. Preconditioning is not limited to the heart, it is probably a major protective mechanism in many other tissues.

The other effects of SUs on cardiovascular risk factors should be taken into consideration, namely lowering lipid levels. It has been shown that SUs lowers plasma total cholesterol, total triglyceride, VLDL cholesterol, LDL cholesterol and apolipoprotein B [35]. In some [36] but not all studies [37] HDL cholesterol was lower in patients treated with insulin, despite comparable glycaemic control. Most of these investigations were conducted with gliclazide. In addition, gliclazide has been shown to inhibit thrombus formation, improve fibrinolysis and reduce platelet adherence and aggregation [38].

The UKPDS study [7] recruited 3,867 newly diagnosed type 2 diabetic patients into a multi-centre randomized controlled trial that sought to compare the effects of intensive blood glucose control (with SUs or insulin) with conventional treatment (diet) on risk of microvascular or macrovascular complications in diabetes. A total of 1,138 patients and 2,729 patients were, respectively, assigned conventional and intensive treatment in 23 centers in the UK. The study end-points were: diabetes-related death and all-cause mortality. The results suggested that intensive blood glucose control significantly decreased the risk of microvascular, but not macrovascular disease in patients with type 2 diabetes. There was no particular adverse cardiovascular risk with SUs or insulin. It would therefore appear that the potential advantage of SUs in modulating hyperglycaemia far outweighs any theoretical risk from a postulated increased liability to macrovascular disease.

Recently the GUIDE – Study (Glucose control in type 2 diabetes: Diamicron MR versus Glimepiride) [39] showed almost identical efficacy of both drugs in improving diabetes long term control, irrespective of the patients previous antidiabetic treatment (ie diet alone or metformin or α-glucosidase inhibitors). The safety of Diamicron MR (Gliclazide MR) was significantly better demonstrating about 50% less hypoglycaemic episodes in comparison with Glimepiride.

More recently the UKPDS investigators looked at case fatality in DM. Results clearly show that there is no difference in terms of myocardial infarction case fatality between those taking SUs (alone or in combination) and those not taking SUs.

This is a very important and reassuring finding, bearing in mind the millions of patients treated for years with SUs. Some previous publications [14] suggested that patients treated with SUs had a higher MI fatality than those not taking SUs, which created a number of difficulties in therapeutic decision making.

Metformin

This is currently the most extensively used oral agent for type 2 diabetes worldwide. Metformin has a variety of metabolic effects; it acts partly by improving insulin action and partly by effects that are not directly insulin dependent. Reduction of excessive hepatic glucose production is thought to be the principal mode of action. At the cellular level, metformin can improve insulin sensitivity by increasing the insulin stimulated tyrosine kinase signaling activity of the insulin receptor. Signaling is also increased through the enhanced activity of a range of post-receptor insulin-signaling pathways. Monotherapy with Metformin offers several advantages such as improvement of insulin sensitivity and blood lipid profile, thus plasma concentrations of triglycerides, free fatty acids and low density LDL-cholesterol tend to fall, while high density HDL– cholesterol tends to rise.

Based on the UKPDS [40] patients who started antidiabetic therapy with Metformin showed a reduced risk of myocardial infarction of 39% after 10 years. In addition to effects on body weight and lipid profile, several others potentially vasoprotective effects, including increased fibrinolysis and a reduced plasminogen activator inhibitor 1 (PAI-1) concentration has been reported. As monotherapy or in combination with other antidiabetic agents or insulin, Metformin, offers great benefits to diabetic subjects with CHD but precaution should be taken in gross congestive cardiac failure in addition to renal function impairment.

Metformin monotherapy in overweight diabetic subjects was the only arm of the UKPDS study [40] showing a significant reduction in CV events and overall mortality.

Thiazolidinediones

Thiazolidinediones (TZD) are a relatively new class of agents that enhance insulin sensitivity in the liver, adipose tissue and muscles without affecting insulin secretion. Their site of action is believed to be mediated through selective activation of peroxisome proliferators-activated receptor gamma (PPAR Gamma), a nuclear receptor that plays an important role in adipogenesis [41]. The efficacy of TZD has been shown in multiple clinical trials [42, 43]. Obese and hyperinsulinaemic individuals are more likely to respond than those who have insufficient insulin. A significant disadvantage of the combination of TZDs and SUs is the associated weight gain that can be as high as 6.5 kg after one year of therapy. When TZDs are used as monotherapy a modest increase in body weight is observed [44].

As regards TZD effects related to CVD both LDL and HDL cholesterol tend to increase and serum triglyceride level may decrease with pioglitazone but not with rosiglitazone. While rosiglitazone has a pure PPAR gamma agonist activity, pioglitazone has in addition some PPAR alpha activity that may account for its effect on lowering serum triglyceride level.

TZDs are not recommended in patients with New York Heart Association (NYHA) class III or IV congestive heart failure as TZDs can lead to fluid retention and subsequent plasma volume expansion [45,46].

There are still some controversial issues about the benefits of TZDs on vascular function, which might reduce cardiovascular risk, as well as on the production of some inflammatory cytokines and its effects on transforming monocytes to macrophages in the vascular wall. The precautions related to heart disease, oedema, anemia and liver function include intermittent monitoring.

Exogenous Insulin Administration and Cardiovascular Risk in Type 2 Diabetes Mellitus

A progressive β-cell failure is a characteristic feature of type 2 DM based on the evidence in Type 1 DM treatment. Early epidemiological studies [8,9] reported insulin as an independent risk factor for cardiovascular disease. The 5-year follow-up analysis of the Helsinki Policemen Study [47] supported the hypothesis that high circulating level of insulin is related although probably indirectly to an increased incidence of complications of atherosclerosis such as myocardial infarction and angina pectoris. A current controversial issue is whether intensive insulin treatment of diabetes decreases the risk for cardiovascular complications by lowering glucose levels or increases the risk by postulated direct atherogenic effects of high circulating levels of exogenous insulin.

A growing number of investigators believe that the high circulating serum insulin level is simply a marker for the insulin-resistant state and therefore does not have a direct role in the pathogenesis of atherosclerosis. Although some in vitro experiments and animal models of atheroma formation have shown that high insulin level leads to accelerated plaque formation [48,49], clinical evidence does not exist as yet. A substantial amount of indirect data suggests that hyperglycaemia may have a causal role in atheroma formation [50,51] and may have a prothrombic effect on the coagulation cascade [52]. Improved glycaemic control has been shown to lower low-density lipoprotein cholesterol levels [53,54], which theoretically should lower the risk of developing CHD for patients with diabetes. Prospective epidemiologic studies [55] that had analyzed the relationship between the fasting blood glucose level or $HbA1_c$ level and the risk of CHD showed a linear association between worsening glycaemic control and an increased risk of CHD, although Singer et al. disagreed [13]. In the most compelling study, the Wisconsin Epidemiological Study of Diabetic Retinopathy, investigators analyzed cause-specific mortality over a 10-year period and found that death due to CHD was much more common in patients with worse glycaemic control (relative risk, 1.10 for each 1% increase in HbA1c; 95% confidence interval, 1.07-1.17) [56] than in others. In 3 randomized controlled trials of glycaemic control in type 2 diabetes, a sufficient number of cardiovascular events were recorded to make meaningful comparisons between treatment groups [57,58,59]. Too few events were recorded in the Kumamoto study [57] because of the exclusion of patients with hypertension, hypercholesterolemia and obesity. In the University Group Diabetes Program (UGDP) [58], no significant difference was found in the rate of myocardial infarction between the intensive and conventional treatment groups (20.6 vs. 20.2%, respectively, p=1.00), despite a much higher prevalence of cardiaovascular risk factors in the intensive treatment group. A shorter study, 'Diabetes mellitus, Insulin Glucose Infusion in Acute Myocardial Infarction Study Group (DIGAMI-1) [59], tested the hypothesis that intensive metabolic treatment with insulin glucose infusion followed by multidose insulin treatment in patients with diabetes mellitus and acute myocardial infarction improved the prognosis. The authors concluded that insulin treatment in diabetic patients with acute myocardial infarction improved long term survival by nearly a third, and the effect seemed to last for at least 3.5 years. Much more importantly, the absolute reduction in mortality was 11%, implying one saved life for 9 patients treated according to the insulin glucose infusion protocol. The reduction in mortality was most apparent in patients without previous insulin treatment and at a low cardiovascular risk. In contrast to the DIGAMI-1 study, in the DIGAMI-2 study, there was no beneficial effect of insulin treatment in myocardial infarction patients. Patients on oral antidiabetics, including SUs, had a similar prognosis to those on insulin treatment. But it was again confirmed that glucose level is a strong independent predictor of long-term mortality in patients with type 2 diabetes following myocardial infarction [60]

When all major CV and peripheral vascular events were combined in the DCCT, intensive therapy was found to reduce the risk of macrovascular disease by 41% (from 0.8 to 0.5 events per 100 patient-year), but the difference was not significant [61]. In addition, intensive therapy was associated with small but significant reductions in the development of hypercholesterolaemia and hypertriglyceridaemia [61]. Lawson et al [62] reviewed randomized controlled trials of intensive insulin therapy (IIT) in type 1 DM, the meta analysis demonstrated that IIT significantly decreased the total number of macrovascular events but had no significant effect on the number of subjects developing macrovascular disease or on macrovascular mortality. The authors speculate that IIT may stabilize macrovascular disease or prevent progression in those already already at risk. Although the authors conclude that long term prospective studies are needed to confirm these data and fully understand the effect of IIT on macrovascular disease in individuals with type 1 DM they also appropriately point out that future trials of IIT versus conventional therapy would seem to be unethical in patients with type 1 DM, given the positive effects of IIT on microvascular complications. Thus, the answer to this question may never to be more definitely answered.

Conclusions

The benefits of intensive glycaemic management do not come without risks. Essentially all of the studies of intensive therapy in type 1 DM for the prevention of microvascular and neuropathic complications demonstrated an increase of hypoglycaemia associated with intensive treatment.

The meta analysis by Egger et al [63] identified 26 deaths among patients with type 1 diabetes, 15 among those receiving intensive therapy and 11 among those receiving conventional therapy (OR 1.40, 95% CI 0.65-3.01). This analysis confirmed a non significant reduction in cardio-vascular mortality among intensive treated patients (OR 0.42, 95% CI 0.13-1.40).

Similar to the DCCT [64,65] results, the UKPDS [66] showed that intensive therapy included an increased risk of hypoglycaemia and increase in both weight, particularly among patients randomized to insulin. Weight gain was no greater in the metformin group than in the diet-controlled group. Quality of life studies performed as part of the UKPDS showed that allocation to different treatment did not in itself have an effect on quality of life.

A common problem in clinical practice is that monotherapy with oral agents either fails initially or fails over time. This important clinical observation was confirmed in the UKPDS. In order to achieve an optimal outcome, multiple drug therapy or a combination of oral agents and insulin is often needed. An important question that needs to be explored is whether triple oral therapy when used to avoid insulin use in particular in the elderly diabetic subject has any potential advantages over insulin therapy alone. When using such a regimen, one should consider the high cost of therapy and possible increased adverse events as a result of drug interactions. This latter concern is very legitimate when dealing with a frail population with multiple coexisting medical conditions and where polypharmacy is common. Further studies are needed to evaluate the advantages and disadvantages of triple or quadruple oral therapy and its impact on the quality of life when compared with insulin monotherapy.

The large scale trials in type 2 DM, UKPDS [66],The Stockholm Diabetes Intervention Study (SDIS) [67], the Steno type 2 randomized study [68] support the fact that lowering blood glucose is an effective mean to lower the risk of diabetic complications. The UKPDS [66] and the Kumamoto study [57] show beyond doubt a significant risk reduction for microvascular complications with improved glycaemic control. The UKPDS [66] results show that intensive blood glucose control was associated with a risk reduction of CVD but that the p value was 0.052. While this result is on the margin of statistical significance, the clinical significance is likely to be high; in part because the degree of risk reduction is so closely in line with what would have been expected from observational studies. The risk reduction associated with Metformin for CVD was very impressive possibly reflecting benefits from Metformin beyond those strictly related to glucose lowering.

The problem of defining the goals of glycaemic control is still under study as more stringent goals (i.e; a normal $HbA_1C<6\%$) can be considered in individual patients based on epidemiological analysis that suggest that there is no lower limit of Hb A_1C at which further lowering does not reduce risk of complications, at the risk of increased hypoglycaemia. The risks and benefits of a HbA_1C goal of <6% are currently being tested in an on going study ACCORD (Action to Control Cardiovascular Risk in Diabetes) [69].

Elevated post challenge (2-h OGTT) glucose has been associated with increased CV risk independent of fasting plasma glucose in some epidemiological studies. There are now pharmacological agents (for example Repaglinide) that primarily modify postprandial glucose and thereby reduce HbA_1C in parallel.

However, the effect of post prandial glycaemic control on micro or macrovascular complications has not been studied. Having discussed earlier the risks and benefits of therapy in its different form with particular re-assurance from the literature on prescribing SUs to type 2 diabetic subjects with CVD and the UKPDS results with Metformin in conclusion the focus should be on global management of cardiovascular risk factors among the diabetic population.

Studies have shown the efficacy of reducing cardiovascular risk factors in preventing or slowing CVD. Based on the American Diabetes Association recommendations management should also include blood pressure control [70], treatment of dyslipidaemia [71] aspirin therapy [72] and cessation of smoking [73].

Emphasis should be put on reducing cardiovascular risk factors as a main goal in addition to treating hyperglycaemia in subjects with type 2 DM.

References

[1] Amos AF, McCarty DJ, Zimmet P: The rising global burden of diabetes and its complications: estimates and projections to the year 2010. *Diabet Med* 1997; 14(Suppl 5): S7-85.

[2] Gruber W, Leese B, Songer T, Williams R (eds) : The economics of diabetes and diabetes care. *IDF and WHO*1997; Brussels, Belgium.

[3] King H, Aubert RE, Herman WH: Global burden of diabetes, 1995-2025: prevalence, numerical estimates and projections. *Diabetes Care*1998; 21: 9.

[4] Onkano P, Vaananen S, Karvonen M, Tuomilehto J: Worldwide increase in incidence of type 1 diabetes – the analysis of the data on published incidence trends. *Diabetologia* 1999; 42: 1395-1403.

[5] Fagot-Campagna A : Emergence of type 2 diabetes mellitus in children: epidemiological evidence. *J. Paediatr. Endocrin. Metab.* 2000; 13: 1395-1402.

[6] The Diabetes Control and Complications : Trial Research Group: The effect of intensive treatment of diabetes on the development and progression of long term complications in insulin-dependent diabetes mellitus. *N. Engl. J. Med.* 1993; 329: 977-986.

[7] UK Prospective Diabetes Study (UKPDS) Group: Intensive blood glucose control with sulphonylurea or insulin compared with conventional treatment and risk of complications in patients with type 2 diabetes (UKPDS 33). *The Lancet* 1998; 352: 837-865.

[8] Eschwege E, Richard JL, Thibult N, et al: Coronary heart disease mortality in relation with diabetes blood glucose and plasma insulin levels: The Paris Prospective Study, ten years later. *Horm. Metab. Res.* (Suppl) 1985; 41-46.

[9] Welborne TA, Wearne K : Coronary heart disease and Cardiovascular mortality in Busselton with reference to glucose and insulin concentrations. *Diabetes Care* 1979; 2: 154-160.

[10] Nielsen NV, Ditzel J : Prevalence of macro- and Microvascular disease as related to glycosylated hemoglobin in type 1 and 2 diabetic subjects: an epidemiologic study in Denmark.. *Horm. Metab. Res.* (Suppl.)1985; 15:19-23.

[11] Adler A, Stevens R, Neil H, Holman R, Turner R: Hyperglycaemia and other potentially modificable risk factors for peripheral vascular disease in type 2 diabetes. *Diabetic Medicine* 1999; 16:16.

[12] Lehto S, Ronnemaa T, Pyörälä K, Laakso M: Risk factors predicting lower extremity amputations in patients with NIDDM. *Diabetes Care* 1996; 19:607-612.

[13] Singer DE, Nathan DM, Anderson KM, Wilson PW, Evans JC : Association of HbA1c with prevalent cardiovascular disease in the original cohort of the Framingham Heart Study. *Diabetes* 1992; 41: 202-208.

[14] University Group Diabetes Program: A study of the effects of hypoglycemic agents on vascular complications in patients with adult- onset diabetes. V1. Supplementary report on non fatal events treated with tolbutamide. *Diabetes* 1976; 25:1129-1152.

[15] Noma A: ATP-regulated K^{+}_{ATP} channels in cardiac muscle. *Nature* 1983; 305: 147-148.

[16] McPherson C, Pierce G, Cole W : Ischemic cardioprotection by ATP-sensitive K^{+} channels involves high energy phosphate preservation. *Am. J. Physiol.* 1993; 265: H1809-H1818.

[17] Lee C : Gating mechanisms of ATP sensitive potassium channels:implication in reperfusion injury and preconditioning. *Cardiovasc. Res.* 1994; 28: 729-734.

[18] Gross GJ, Yao Z, Pieper GM, Auchampach JA : The ATP-regulated potassium channel in ischemia-reperfusion injury. *Ann. N. Y. Acad. Sci.* 1994; 723: 71-81.

[19] Sanguinetti MC : Modulation of potassium channels by antiarrhythmic and hypertensive drugs. *Hypertension*1992; 19:228-236.

[20] Brayden JE : Hyperpolarization and relaxation of resistance arteries in response to adenosine diphosphate. *Circ. Res.* 1991;69:1415-1420.

[21] Daut J, Maier-Rudolph W, von Beckerath N, Mehrke G, Gunther K, Goedel-Meinen L: Hypoxic dilatation of coronary arteries is mediated by ATP-sensitive potassium channels. *Science* 1990; 247:1341-1344.

[22] Auchampach JA, Gross GJ: Adenosine A1 receptors, K_{ATP} channels and ischemic preconditioning in dogs. *Am. J. Physiol.* 1993; 264: H1327-H1336.

[23] Kirsch GE, Codina J, Birnbaumer L, Brown AM : Coupling of ATP-Sensitive K^{+} channels to A1 receptors by G proteins in rat ventricular myocytes. *Am. J. Phsiol.* 1990; 259:H820-H826.

[24] Wainwright CL, Parrat JR : An antiarrhythmic effect of adenosine during myocardial ischemia and reperfusion. *Eur. J. Pharmacol.* 1988 ; 145: 183-194.

[25] Belardinelli L, Linden J, Berne RM : The cardiac effects of adenosine. *Prog.Cardiovasc. Dis.* 1989; 32: 73-97.

[26] Smits P, Lenders JWM, Willemsen JJ, Thien T : Adenosine attenuates the response to sympathetic stimuli in man. *Hypertension* 1991; 18: 216-223.

[27] Murray CE, Jennings RB, Reimer KA : Preconditioning with ischemia : a delay of lethal cell injury in ischemic myocardium. *Circulation* 1986; 74:1124-1136.

[28] Fralix TA, Steenbergen C, London RE, Murphy E : Glibenclamide does not abolish the protective effect of preconditioning on stunning in the isolated perfused rat heart. *Cardiovasc. Res.* 1993; 27: 630-637.

[29] Schulz R, Rose J, Heusch G : Involvement of activation of ATP-dependent potassium channels in ischemic preconditioning in swine. *Am. J. Physiol.* 1994; 267:H1341-H1352.

[30] Tomai F, Crea F, Gaspardone A, et al : Ischemic preconditioning during coronary angioplasty is prevented by glibenclamide, a selective ATP-sensitive K+ channel blocker. *Circulation* 1994; 90: 700-705.

[31] Gross G, Auchampach J : Blockade of ATP- sensitive potassium channels prevents myocardial preconditioning in dogs. *Circ. Res.* 1992; 70:223-233.

[32] Kubota I, Yamaki M, Shibata T, Ikeno E, Hosoya Y, Tomoike H : Role of ATP-sensitive K^+ channels on ECG ST segment elevation during a bout of myocardial ischemia. A study on epicardial mapping in dogs. *Circulation* 1993; 88: 1845-1851.

[33] Downey JM, Liu GS, Thornton JD: Adenosine and anti-infarct effects of preconditioning. *Cardiovasc. Res.* 1993; 27:3-8.

[34] Yao Z, Gross GJ : A comparison of adenosine-induced cardioprotection and ischemic preconditioning in dogs. Efficacy, time course, and role of K_{ATP} channels. *Circulation* 1994 ; 89:1229-1236.

[35] Taskinen MR, Beltz WF, Harper I, et al : Effects of NIDDM on very low-density lipoprotein triglyceride and apolipoprotein B metabolism : studies before and after sulfonylurea therapy. *Diabetes* 1986; 35:1268-1277.

[36] Calvert GD, Graham JJ, Mannik T, Wise PH, Yeates RA : Effects of therapy on plasma high-density-lipoprotein-cholesterol concentration in diabetes mellitus. *Lancet* 1978;2:66-68.

[37] Huupponen RK, Viikari JS, Saarimaa H : Correlation of serum lipids with diabetes control in sulfonylurea-treated diabetic patients. *Diabetes Care* 1984; 7:575-578.

[38] Colwell JA : Pathophysiology of vascular disease in diabetes: effects of gliclazide. *Am. J. Med* .1991;90 (suppl 6A): 505-545.

[39] Schernthaner G, Grimaldi A, Di Mario U, Drzewoski J, Kempler P, Kvapil M, Novials A, Rottiers R, Rutten GE, Shaw KM: GUIDE study: double-blind comparison of once-daily gliclazide MR and glimepiride in type 2 diabetic patients. *Eur. J. Clin. Invest.* 2004;34(8):535-542.

[40] UKPDS Group: Effect of intensive blood glucose control with metformin on complications in overweight patients with type 2 diabetes (UKPDS 34). *Lancet* 1998; 352: 854-865.

[41] Day C : Thiazolidinediones: a new class of antidiabetic drug. *Diabetic Med* 1999; 16:1-14.

[42] Evans AJ, Krentz AJ : Recent developments and emerging therapies for type 2 diabetes mellitus. In: Krentz AJ, Ed. Drug treatment of type 2 diabetes. *Auckland: Adis International*, 2000; 1-22.

[43] Howlett HCS, Bailey CJ : A risk-benefit assessment of metformin in type 2 diabetes mellitus. In: Krentz AJ, Ed. Drug treatment of type 2 diabetes. *Auckland: Adis International*, 2000; 61-76.
[44] Murphy E, Nolan JJ: Insulin sensitizer drugs. *Exp. Opin. Invest. Drugs* 2000; 9:1347-1361.
[45] Schoonjans K, Auwerx J: Thiazolidinediones: an update. *Lancet* 2000; 355:1008-1010.
[46] Spiegelman BM : PPARγ: adipogenic regulator and Thiazolidinedione receptor. *Diabetes* 1998; 47:507-514.
[47] Pyörälä K, Savolainen E, Kaukola S, Haapakoski J : Plasma insulin as coronary heart disease risk factor: relationship to other risk factors and predictive value over 9.5 year follow up of the Helsinki Policeman Study population. *Acta Med. Scand.* 1985;(Suppl): 38-52.
[48] Sato Y, Shiraishi S, Oshida Y, Ishiguro T, Sakamoto N: Experimental atherosclerosis-like lesions induced by hyperinsulinism in Wistar rats. *Diabetes* 1989; 38: 91-96.
[49] Stout RW, Bierman EL, Ross R : Effect of insulin on the proliferation of cultured primate arterial smooth muscle cells. *Circ. Res.*1975; 36: 319-327.
[50] Bruno G, Cavallo-Perin P, Bargero G, Borra M, D'Errico N, Pagano G : Association of fibrinogen and glycemic control and albumin excretion rate in patients with non-insulin-dependent diabetes mellitus. *Ann. Intern. Med.* 1996;125: 653-657
[51] Yegin A, Ozben T, Yegin H : Glycation of lipoproteins and accelerated atherosclerosis in non-insulin-dependent diabetes mellitus. *Int. J. Clin. Lab. Res.* 1995; 25: 157-161.
[52] Colwell JA: Vascular thrombosis in type 2 diabetes mellitus. *Diabetes* 1993; 42:8-11.
[53] Taskinen MR, Kuusi T, Helve E, Nikkila EA, Yki JH : Insulin therapy induces antiatherogenic changes of serum lipoproteins in non-insulin-dependent diabetes. *Arteriosclerosis* 1988; 8: 168-177.
[54] Agardh CD, Nilsson EP, Schersten B: Improvement of the plasma lipoprotein pattern after institution of insulin treatment in diabetes mellitus. *Diabetes Care* 1982; 5: 322-325.
[55] Gall MA, Borch-Jonhnsen K, Hougaard P, Nielsen FS, Parving HH : Albuminuria and poor glycemic control predict mortality in NIDDM. *Diabetes* 1995;44: 1303-1309.
[56] Moss SE, Klein R, Klein BE, Meuer SM : The association of glycemia and cause-specific mortality in a diabetic population. *Arch. Intern. Med.* 1994; 154: 2473-2479.
[57] Ohkubo Y, Kishikawa H, Araki E, et al: Intensive insulin therapy prevents the progression of diabetic microvascular complications in Japanese patients with non-insulin –dependent diabetes mellitus: a randomized prospective 6-year study. *Diabetes Res. Clin. Pract.* 1995; 28: 103-117.
[58] Kilo C, Miller JP, Williamson JR: The Achilles heel of the University Group Diabetes Program. *JAMA* 1980; 243: 450-457.
[59] Malmberg K: Prospective randomized study of intensive insulin treatment on long term survival after acute myocardial infarction in patients with diabetes mellitus. *BMJ* 1997; 314: 1512-1515.
[60] Mogensen CE : Interesting positive news about Sulfonylureas, especially gliclazide, from the EASD congress in Munich(2004). *Int. J. Metab.* 2004;7:29.

[61] The Diabetes Control and Complications Trial Research Group: The effect of intensive treatment of diabetes on the development and progression of long term complications in insulin-dependent diabetes mellitus. *N. Engl. J. Med.* 1993;329:977-986.

[62] Lawson ML, Tsui E, Gerstein HC, Zinman B: Effect of intensive therapy on early macrovascular disease in young individuals with type 1 diabetes – a systematic review and meta-analysis. *Diabetes Care* 1999; 22(2): B35-B39.

[63] Egger M, Smith GD, Stettler C, Diem P : Risk of adverse effects of intensified treatment in insulin-dependent diabetes mellitus: a meta-analysis. *Diabetic Med.* 1997;14: 919-928.

[64] The Diabetes Control and Complications Trial Research Group: Influence of intensive diabetes treatment on quality-of-life outcomes in the The Diabetes Control and Complications Trial . *Diabetes Care* 1996; 19: 195-203.

[65] The Diabetes Control and Complications Trial Research Group: The absence of a glycemic threshold for the development of long-term complications: the perspective of the The Diabetes Control and Complications Trial . *Diabetes* 1996; 45: 1289-1298

[66] American Diabetes Association : Implications of the United Kingdom Prospective Diabetes Study. *Diabetes Care* 2002; (Suppl 1): 28-32.

[67] Reichard P, Berglund B, Britz A, Cars I, Nilsson BY, Rosenqvist U: Intensified conventional insulin treatment retards the microvascular complications of insulin-dependent diabetes mellitus (IDDM): the Stockholm Diabetes Intervention Study (SDIS) after five years. *J .Intern. Med* .1991; 230: 101-108.

[68] Gaede P, Vedel P, Parving HH, Pedersen O: Intensified multifactorial intervention in patients with type 2 diabetes mellitus and microalbuminuria: the Steno type 2 randomised study. *Lancet* 1999; 353(9153): 617-622.

[69] Halimi S, Charpentier G, Grimaldi A, Grenier JL, Baut F, Germain B, MagnetteJ: Effect on compliance, acceptability of blood glucose self-monitoring and (1c) of a self-monitoring system developed according to patients wishes ACCORD study. *Diabetes Metab.* 2001; 6: 681-687.

[70] American Diabetes Association : Hypertension management in adults with Diabetes. *Diabetes Care*(Middle East edn.) 2004; (Suppl 1): 65-67.

[71] American Diabetes Association : Dyslipidemia management in adults with Diabetes. *Diabetes Care*(Middle East edn.) 2004; (Suppl 1): 68-71.

[72] American Diabetes Association : Aspirin Therapy in Diabetes. *Diabetes Care* (Middle East edn.) 2004; (Suppl 1): 72-73.

[73] American Diabetes Association : Smoking and Diabetes. *Diabetes Care*(Middle East edn.) 2004; (Suppl 1): 74-75.

In: Trends in Diabetes Research
Editor: Ashley M. Ford, pp. 37-69
ISBN: 1-59454-796-3

Chapter III

Genetics of the Dysmetabolic Syndrome

Martin Ridderstråle and Leif Groop*
Department of Clinical Sciences, Wallenberg Laboratory,
Lund University, Malmö, Sweden

Definition of the Dysmetabolic Syndrome

The metabolic, or rather, *dysmetabolic* syndrome (DMS) is a heterogeneous condition originally recognized due to the clustering of several risk factors for cardiovascular morbidity and mortality (Figure 1). These risk factors include insulin resistance, obesity, hypertension, dyslipidemia, hypercoaguability, microalbuminuria and more recently endothelial dysfunction and chronic inflammation [1].

In light of the heterogeneity of the syndrome and the largely unknown underlying pathophysiology and not least etiology, there has been, and still is, some controversy as to its definition. In accordance with a WHO proposal a person with type 2 diabetes or impaired glucose (IGT) is diagnosed with concomitant DMS when two of the criteria for obesity, dyslipidemia, hypertension and microalbuminuria listed below are fulfilled. A person with normal glucose tolerance (NGT) has DMS when two of the criteria are fulfilled in addition to being insulin resistant. Insulin resistance is defined as lowest quartile of insulin sensitivity (by golden standard insulin stimulated glucose uptake during hyperinsulinemic euglycemic clamp) or highest quartile of surrogate measures of insulin resistance such as fasting insulin or homeostasis model of assessment (HOMA) insulin resistance index in the studied population [2,3].The defining criteria are: 1) hypertension defined as antihypertensive treatment and/or blood pressure >140/90 mm Hg (>160/90 in the original definition); 2) dyslipidemia defined as an elevated plasma triglyceride level (≥1.7 mmol/l)

* Address: Leif Groop Department of Clinical Sciences University Hospital MAS Lund University S-205 02 Malmö, Sweden Phone: +46-(0)40-337217 Fax: +46-(0)40-337042 E-mail: Leif.Groop@med.lu.se

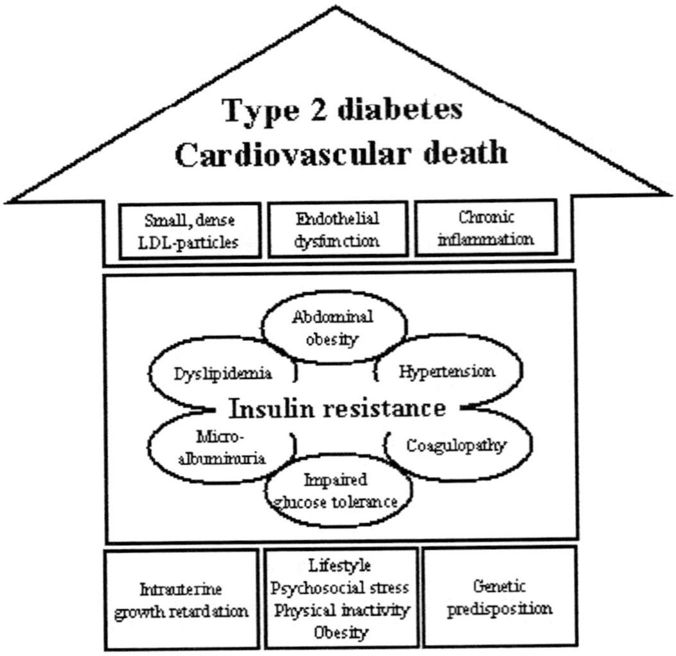

Figure 1. The house we built with welfare: Schematic representation of the underlying mechanisms, components and adverse outcome of the dysmetabolic syndrome.

and/or low HDL cholesterol concentration (<0.9 mmol/l in males and <1.0 mmol/l in females); 3) obesity defined as a body mass index (BMI) ≥30 m^2 and/or a waist-to-hip ratio (WHR) >0.90 in males and >0.85 in females; and 4) microalbuminuria (overnight urinary albumin excretion rate ≥20μg/min.). The European Group for the Study of Insulin Resistance does not recognize microalbuminuria as a component of the syndrome and have thus suggested a somewhat different definition of what they denote the *insulin resistance syndrome* [4]. More recently the US National Cholesterol Education Program (NCEP) have suggested a simpler and perhaps more clinically oriented definition [5]. The reader is directed to recent reviews on the definitions of the syndrome and their possible clinical implications [6,7].

Applying the WHO definition to the population from the Botnia study in Finland and Sweden, a large family based study on the genetics and mechanisms of diabetes which to date comprises more than ten thousand subjects [8], about 10% of subjects with normal glucose tolerance (NGT; defined by an oral glucose tolerance test), 40% of persons with impaired glucose tolerance (IGT) and 85% of patients with type 2 diabetes would have the dysmetabolic syndrome [9]. The prevalence of the syndrome is also age-dependent and more prevalent in males than in females. Importantly, the presence of DMS was associated with a 3-fold increased risk of coronary heart disease, myocardial infarction and stroke and consequently, reduced survival (Figure 2).

In subjects IGT or impaired fasting glucose (IFG, i.e. a fasting blood glucose concentration 5.6 –6.0 mmol/l or plasma glucose concentration 7.1–7.7 mmol/l) the presence of DMS was associated with reduced survival particularly due to increased cardiovascular mortality. Ultimately, this raises the critical question whether IGT and/or IFG associated with DMS should be considered as a high-risk condition requiring treatment, especially in light of several recent successful intervention studies including both life-style and pharmacological agents [10-12].

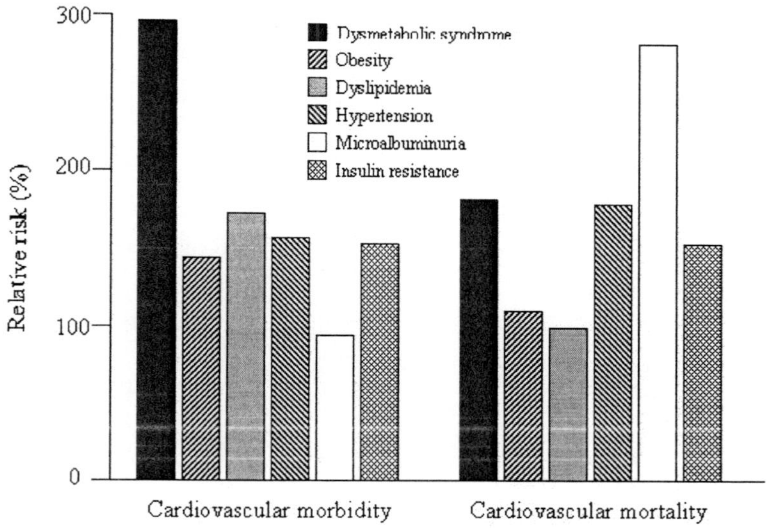

Figure 2. Increased risks for cardiovascular morbidity and mortality associated with the dysmetabolic syndrome and components (2401 patients in the Botnia study (209 deaths). Adapted from Isomaa B, et al. (2001). Diabetes Care 24:683-689 (Ref 9).

Inheritance of the Dysmetabolic Syndrome

Insulin resistance clusters in families and nearly half (45%) of first-degree relatives of patients with type 2 diabetes are insulin resistant compared with 20% of subjects without a family-history of diabetes [8,13,14]. Although insulin resistance is an early detectable defect in subjects at increased risk of developing type 2 diabetes, obesity, and particularly abdominal obesity, usually precedes insulin resistance in these individuals. About 40% of the variation in body fat can be attributed to genetic factors [15,16]. The genetic influence is even more impressing for abdominal obesity. For example, genes are considered to explain 60% of the variance in abdominal fat in postmenopausal women [17,18]. The inheritance of type 2 diabetes thus seems to favor fat accumulation in the intra-abdominal region. First-degree relatives of patients with type 2 diabetes have an increased waist-hip ratio compared with their spouses without a family-history of diabetes, and this increase in abdominal fat is seen without a significant increase in total body fat. Importantly, the redistribution of fat to the abdominal region is seen at completely normal glucose tolerance [8]. Intraabdominal fat has been shown to be metabolically very active with a high rate of free fatty acid (FFA) turnover and relatively resistant to the effect of insulin in abdominally obese [19]. By contrast, the beta-3-adrenergic receptor of visceral fat is more sensitive to stimulation by catecholamines [20]. This will ensure a large supply of FFA to the portal vein for further transport to the liver and other tissues such as skeletal muscle where it can be used for energy consumption or stored as intracellular triglycerides. Additionally, lipolysis in subcutaneous fat is more sensitive to the inhibitory effect of insulin, which will favor re-esterification of FFA to triglycerides [21].

Abdominal Obesity and Insulin Resistance

There is a strong inverse correlation between insulin sensitivity and the amount of intraabdominal fat measured by computed tomography or waist circumference [22]. Abdominal fat tissue could provide a signal for the chain of events leading to skeletal muscle insulin resistance. Two such candidate signals are the adipocyte hormones leptin, and another tumor necrosis factor-α (TNF-α) [23,24]. A change in the sensitivity of intraabdominal and subcutaneous fat tissue lipolysis to catecholamines or insulin could result in increased lipolysis in abdominal fat and increased re-esterification in subcutaneous fat. An increased supply of FFA, in turn, result in increased FFA uptake and re-esterification in muscle. In fact, increased intramyocellular triglyceride concentrations have been reported in insulin resistant obese individuals and correlate with the rate of insulin-stimulated glucose metabolism [25]. An increased FFA turnover within the muscle could through activation of the FFA/glucose cycle (Randle cycle) lead to impaired insulin-stimulated glycogen synthesis [26].

Thrifty Genotype and Thrifty Phenotype

Why does DMS develop in individuals switching from a rural to an urban lifestyle? In 1962 the thrifty gene hypothesis was put forward Neel [27]. It proposes that individuals living in a harsh environment with unstable food supply would maximize their probability of survival if they could maximize storage of surplus energy. Genetic selection would favor energy conserving genotypes in such environments and storage of energy as fat rather than glycogen would ensure energy during longer periods of starvation. Support for this hypothesis comes from a study in the *ob* and *db* mice [28]. Homozygous animals of these strains develop obesity and diabetes. Heterozygous animals with the same body weight as the wild type mice survived longer during total fasting than the insulin-sensitive wild type mice. The sand rat is another example of such an insulin-resistant thrifty genotype with a metabolism aimed at storing energy to ensure survival during long periods of fasting in the desert. When this energy storing genotype is exposed to the abundance of food typical for the Western society, it will develop glucose intolerance [29]. It can be assumed that thrifty genes predispose to DMS. Such putative genes could be expected to influence not only lipolysis, fuel oxidation and skeletal muscle glucose metabolism, but also eating behavior, choice of foods, exercise habits and energy consumption.

An alternative explanation, the so-called thrifty phenotype hypothesis, has also been proposed [30]. It suggests that the occurrence of DMS is programmed *in utero*. Intrauterine malnutrition would lead to a low birth weight and increased risk of developing DMS later in life. Although these findings have been replicated in several studies, it has also been shown that the risk for DMS due to low birth weight is increased particularly in subjects with a family history of DMS, suggesting that a low birth weight could be a phenotype of a thrifty gene [31]. In support of this, children with a glucokinase defect and thereby a decrease in serum insulin concentrations, have a low birth weight [32]. This was particularly apparent in children of diabetic mothers, since these children would be expected to have a high birth weight as a consequence of high glucose passing the placenta during pregnancy, thereby stimulating the fetal pancreas to produce increasing amounts of anabolic insulin.

Search for Thrifty Genes

Two major approaches are being used in the search for thrifty genes, or genes predisposing to (abdominal) obesity. The *candidate gene approach* aims at the identification of genes based upon information of their function. While this approach has been successful in a number of monogenic disorders with known biochemical defects (e.g. phenylketonuria), our knowledge about the underlying defects causing DMS is limited. It is therefore not surprising that the candidate gene approach has not been very successful for the identification of thrifty genes.

The *random gene search*, also referred to as *positional cloning*, assumes no knowledge of the underlying defects. Instead, positional cloning aims at localizing the disease gene on the basis of its position in the genome. If a chromosomal region has been linked to the disease, the next step would be the search for attractive candidate genes in the region, or to narrow the region by linkage disequilibrium mapping. This approach has been successful in a number of monogenic disorders where the relationship between genotype and penetrance of the phenotype is more straightforward than for abdominal obesity, e.g. diastrophic dysplasia [33]. For DMS the situation will be more complicated. Although it has been proposed that an autosomal recessive locus would account for 51% of the variance in visceral fat in one study [34], we can assume that common variants in a number of genes will increase susceptibility to DMS and that these genes will act in concert with a number of environmental factors.

An important factor to keep in mind when studying these potential candidate genes is that the phenotype under study as well as the population will actually decide what genes we will be able to pick up. For example, consider four different populations that are commonly under study; lean vs. obese and NGT vs. type 2 diabetes. When the combined geneticist-physician, or *phenotician*, dissects these populations further he will find that although most lean subjects display NGT, some are even type 2 diabetic. Most type 2 diabetics are overweight and some are even obese but most obese subject are not type 2 diabetic. In fact, many obese will be NGT (Figure 3).

There are also problems that are inherent to the methods that need to be taken into consideration. Most case control studies are so underpowered that it is more surprising that they show association than that they do not. In fact, if the risk of developing type 2 diabetes due to the peroxisome proliferator-activated receptor-gamma (PPARγ) Pro12Ala polymorphism was to have been picked up in a case control study it would have required the inclusion of over 30.000 subjects (see below). The final proof that a gene or genetic variant exerts a significant biological effect is often sought in animal models.

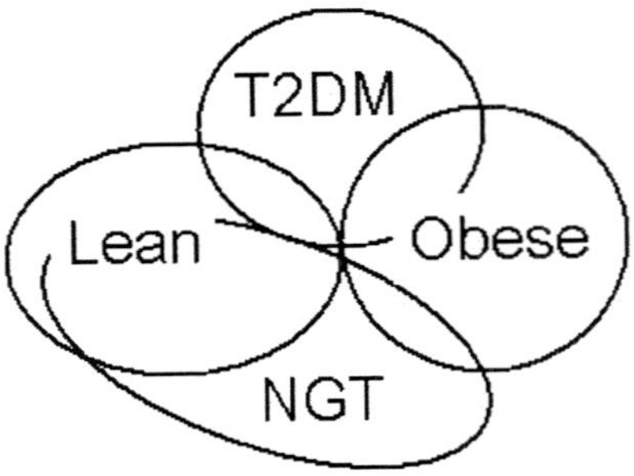

Figure 3. Schematic representation of a complex polygenic inherited disease.

However, these investigations are only likely to answer the questions they were designed for under certain assumptions such as genetic background and environment. All the same, there are several good examples of the successful use of these methods in the current literature, certainly when considering a combination of several techniques.

Candidate Genes for the Dysmetabolic Syndrome

The thrifty gene hypothesis proposes that efficient storage of energy could have been associated with survival advantage during the evolution [13,27]. Efficient storage of energy must include storage of fat and weight gain. Given the scenario presented earlier, obesity genes could predispose to DMS and thereby to type 2 diabetes. Despite large fluctuations in food intake and energy expenditure, body fat is tightly regulated in humans. A powerful feedback system (also referred to as the *lipostat hypothesis*) between fat and a satiety/energy expenditure center in the hypothalamus has been postulated, since damage to this region causes morbid obesity.

Leptin and the Leptin Receptor

Data generated from obese animal models has expanded our knowledge of the interactions between brain and fat. They have also revealed some spectacular examples of monogenic obesity but on the whole not contributed much to explain common obesity. The ob/ob mouse become obese and insulin resistant when fed a fat diet. When joined with a normal mouse in parabiosis experiments, the ob/ob mouse eats less and gains less weight. This finding postulated that the ob/ob mouse lacks a satiety signal, which is supplied by the normal animal, the ob protein. In corresponding experiments joining a normal mouse with the db/db mouse, the normal mouse dies of starvation. The db/db mouse appeared to have a defect in the action of the ob protein, a receptor defect, resulting in high levels of ob protein that could signal in normal mice [35]. This field of research has moved into a new exciting era with the discovery of the ob-gene, which codes for a novel protein expressed in fat, *leptin* [23]. The human homologue is located on chromosome 7. A mutation in the leptin gene results in complete absence of the protein in the ob/ob mouse. Treatment of the ob/ob mouse with leptin resulted in marked weight loss [36]. But man is not mouse, and obese humans actually have elevated rather than decreased levels of leptin [37]. In fact, the leptin levels show a strong positive correlation with the total fat mass [38]. In this regard, humans resemble the db/db mouse in which the mRNA for leptin is increased in fat tissue [39]. One human exception has been reported. Two morbidly obese children from consanguineous parents had very low circulating leptin levels due to a frameshift mutation involving a deletion of a single guanine nucleotide in codon 133 of the leptin gene [40]. Whereas some progress in treatment of these children with leptin has been reported, treatment of obese subjects without mutations the leptin gene has been less successful.

The human counterpart of the db-gene, the leptin receptor gene (*LEPR*), has subsequently been cloned and mapped to the short arm of human chromosome 1 [41]. The leptin receptor belongs to the cytokine receptor family with high homology to the interleukin-6 receptor. The receptor exists in several alternatively spliced isoforms with a common extracellular domain and a variable intracellular domain. The db mutation is due to an abnormally spliced leptin receptor in the hypothalamus [42]. The mutant protein lacks the cytoplasmic region, and it has been suggested that the defect involves impaired leptin signaling in the hypothalamus. Although the leptin signaling pathway has not yet been described in detail, it has been suggested that the leptin signal leads to inhibition of neuropeptide Y, which otherwise stimulates food intake and decreases thermogenesis [43]. Early-onset obesity and hypogonadism segregated with mutations in the leptin receptor gene in one known family [44]. Contribution of more common variants in *LEPR* to obesity and obesity-related phenotypes including leptin levels has remained elusive [45,46]. A lysine to arginine *LEPR* variant (Lys109Arg) has been associated with higher leptin levels in postmenopausal overweight women and a polymorphism resulting in a glutamine to arginine substitution (Gln223Arg) with elevated glucose and insulin levels in response to overfeeding [47,48]. Male monozygotic twins with the Gln223 allele exhibited higher leptin levels after overfeeding than male carriers of the Arg223 allele [48]. A pentanucleotide insertion/deletion (I/D) polymorphism in the 3'-untranslated region (3'UTR) of *LEPR* has been associated with lower glucose levels after a glucose load and reduced fasting insulin levels in obese subjects [46,49,50]. It has been suggested that leptin might inhibit insulin release from the pancreatic β-cells and that the I/D polymorphism could modify this effect by affecting the amount of *LEPR* mRNA in β-cells [51-54].

Pro-Opiomelanocortin, Agouti, FAT and Melanocortin Receptors

In contrast to the forms of murine obesity above, *agouti* is a dominantly inherited late-onset form of obesity resulting from ectopic expression of the agouti protein in the hypothalamus. Normally the α-melanocyte-stimulating hormone (α-MSH) binds to the melanocortin 1 receptor (MCR1) in the skin to control pigmentation and to MCR4 in the hypothalamus to suppress appetite [55]. The agouti protein is normally expressed in the hair follicles where it by antagonizing the effect of α-MSH on MCR1 and causes a characteristic yellow color of the fur. When the mutated protein is ectopically expressed in the hypothalamus it also antagonizes the effect of α-MSH on MCR4 resulting in uncontrolled appetite. In humans the counterpart of the agouti protein is the agouti-related peptide (56). Mutations in the MCR4 gene have also been associated with morbid obesity in some families [57,58].

Together with β-MSH, γ-MSH and adrenocorticotropic hormone (ACTH), α-MSH is processed from the pro-opiomelanocortin gene (*POMC*) by different peptidases. There are several pieces of evidence supporting a role for *POMC* in the pathogenesis of obesity. Neuropeptide Y (NPY), which normally stimulates appetite, down-regulates the expression of *POMC* mRNA in the brain, whereas leptin, which suppresses appetite up-regulates *POMC* expression. Linkage to the *POMC* region on chromosome 2p21 has been reported to leptin levels and resting metabolic rate [59,60]. In one family, mutations in the *POMC* gene segregated with progressing obesity, ACTH deficiency and red hair, analogous to the yellow fur of the agouti mouse [61]. We have recently shown that monogenic forms of obesity due to mutations in the POMC and MC4R genes are rare but that lean carriers of the C-allele in a *POMC* polymorphism (C8246T) exhibit increased leptin levels. This was especially pronounced in combination with another *POMC* polymorphism (RsaI--/+- genotype) [62].

The *FAT* mouse represents another form of slowly evolving murine obesity associated with hyperinsulinemia. The mutation has been mapped to mouse chromosome 8 (syngenic with human chromosome 4) very close to the gene for carboxypeptidase E (*CpE*) [63]. *CpE* encodes a protein that processes pro-hormones like pro-insulin and POMC. Mutations in this gene could therefore result in altered processing of pro-hormones. This was also supported by findings in a female with obesity and hypogonadotropic hypogonadism associated with elevated serum levels of pro-insulin, cortisol and pro-opiomelanocortin. She was found to be composite heterozygous for a glycine to arginine mutation in position 483 resulting in skipping of exon 5 of the endopeptidase prohormone convertase 1 [64].

Beta-Adrenergic Receptors

Catecholamines stimulate lipolysis through the β-adrenergic receptors and inhibit lipolysis through α-adrenergic receptors. The β1- and β2-adrenergic receptors (β1AR and β2AR) are expressed in several tissues and they are the predominant β-receptor subclasses in cardiac myocytes and adipocytes, respectively. The b3-adrenergic receptor (β3AR) is expressed in brown adipose tissue of rodents and considered responsible for stimulation of thermogenesis [65]. Lack of brown adipose tissue in transgenic animals result in decreased thermogenesis and obesity [66]. It was long disputed whether the β3AR exists in humans since they have very little brown fat. The demonstration of β3AR mRNA in visceral fat changed this view [67]. Subsequently it was demonstrated that catecholamine-induced lipolysis was increased in visceral fat from subjects with abdominal obesity due to increased

β_3AR function [68]. The β3AR thereby became a prime candidate gene for abdominal obesity.

A few years ago we and others reported a mutation in the first intracellular loop of the receptor changing a tryptophane in position 64 to arginine [69-71]. Mutation carriers showed more abdominal obesity, higher insulin concentrations, more insulin resistance and higher blood pressure than individuals homozygous for the wild type (Trp64Trp), i.e. features of the dysmetabolic syndrome [70]. Furthermore, they had a lower metabolic rate [72] and lower resting sympathetic nervous system activity [73], features one would expect of a thrifty gene. This finding was later replicated in Mexican American sibling pairs discordant for the Trp64Arg variant but concordant for the chromosome 2p21-p23 locus linked to leptin levels close to *POMC* [74]. The region of the β3AR gene on chromosome 8p12-11.1 has also been linked the quantitative trait of a high BMI in Mexican American families [75]. A number of negative population association studies have also been reported but given the inherent problems in selecting an appropriate control group such association studies must be interpreted with caution [76,77]. The prevalence of this variant differs between populations with an allele frequency of about 10% in Finns and 30% in Japanese [78]. *In vitro*, the β3AR Trp64Arg mutation seems to be associated with impairment of catecholamine-stimulated lipolysis [79,80].

A glutamic acid to glutamine variant at codon 27 (Glu27Gln) in the β2AR gene has been associated with obesity and hypertension [81]. Carriers of this variant are resistant to catecholamine-induced downregulation of the gene [82]. A polymorphism in the 5'-leader cistron of the β2AR gene is in linkage disequilibrium with the codon 27 variant and associated with obesity and type 2 diabetes in the Japanese [83]. Using a case-control design, we have recently found that the homozygous carriers of another β2AR gene polymorphisms, the Arg16 allele, had a significantly increased risk for hypertension, particularly among individuals with both hypertension and type 2 diabetes [84]. In addition, our results suggest the haplotype Cys19-Arg16-Gln27 as a risk haplotype for hypertension and obesity, the Gln27 as a risk-allele for elevated FFA levels, and the combination of *β2AR* and *β3AR* genotypes with an increased risk for type 2 diabetes.

The third β-adrenergic receptor is encoded by the β1AR gene on chromosome 10q24-q26. β-blocking agents are commonly used to treat elevated blood pressure and the antihypertensive effect is mediated by the β1AR, leading to decreased cardiac output. Recently, an arginine to glycine polymorphism (Arg389Gly) in the intracellular cytoplasmic tail near the seventh transmembrane domain of the receptor was described and the 389Arg allele was associated with higher basal and isoproterenol-stimulated adenylyl cyclase activity compared to the 389Gly allele. [85]. Individuals homozygous for the 389Arg allele had an increased risk for hypertension as well as higher heart rate and diastolic blood pressure compared to those without this genotype but no clear association with type 2 diabetes was shown [86]. Taken together, genetic variation in all three beta-adrenergic receptor genes may form an important part of the thrifty genotype.

Lipases

Several lipases are involved in the regulation of fat metabolism such as the hepatic lipase, the endothelial lipoprotein lipase (LPL) and the hormone sensitive lipase (HSL) in adipose tissue. These are all potential candidate genes, particularly for obesity and dyslipidemia. A polymorphism at position -514 in the promoter of the hepatic lipase gene has been shown to determine variations in hepatic lipase activity and serum lipoprotein concentrations [87]. An asparagine to serine variant (Asn291Ser) in exon 6 of the LPL gene has been associated with high triglycerides, low HDL cholesterol and increased risk of cardiovascular disease [88,89]. We have found increased frequency of DMS in insulin-resistant normoglycemic carriers of the Asn291Ser variant [90].

Beta-adrenergic agonists stimulate lipolysis by activating the hormone sensitive lipase (HSL) by covalent modification (serine phosphorylation). A decrease in the lipolytic effect of catecholamines, possibly through a lesser degree of activation of HSL, has repeatedly been demonstrated in obesity and it has been suggested that impaired expression of the HSL gene (LIPE) may at least in part explain this enzymatic defect [91]. Interestingly, a C-60G LIPE promoter variant exhibits a 40 % reduction in promoter activity in vitro [92] and variation in the HSL gene has been linked to both features of DMS and type 2 diabetes [93]. Importantly, variations in the gene were shown to be overtransmitted to abdominally obese offspring from heterozygous parents in a transmission disequilibrium test.

Uncoupling Proteins

Thermogenesis in brown adipose tissue of rodents is largely determined by the activity of the mitochondrial uncoupling proteins (UCPs). The UCPs are proton channel proteins situated in the inner mitochondrial membrane and uncouple oxidative phosphorylation by converting the electrochemical potential of the mitochondria into heat instead of ATP. Somewhat surprisingly, targeted disruption of the gene encoding the first UCP, the UCP1 gene, did not result in an obese but a more cold sensitive phenotype [94]. This lead to the identification of other UCPs. The genes encoding UCP2 and UCP3 are adjacent to each other on chromosome 11. While UCP1 is expressed almost exclusively in brown adipose tissue, UCP2 is expressed in most tissues including white adipose tissue. The UCP3 gene is a particularly attractive candidate gene for insulin resistance since it is strongly expressed in skeletal muscle.

A polymorphism in the promoter region of the UCP1 gene on chromosome 4 is associated with weight gain in humans, and this is further accentuated if the patient has the Trp64Arg mutation in the β3AR gene [95]. So far no mutations in the coding sequences or promoter regions of the genes encoding UCP2 and UCP3 have been associated with human obesity [96,97]. In fact, there is a debate as to whether these proteins really are uncoupling proteins. However, a common polymorphism in the promotor of the *UCP2* gene (G-866A) has recently been shown to be associated with obesity [98]. Despite a relatively modest effect in an association study, because of its high frequency (approximately 63%), the more-common risk allele (-866A) conferred a relatively large population-attributable risk accounting for 15% of the obesity in the population studied. On the other hand, while conducive for obesity the same allele has been associated with a reduced risk for type 2 diabetes [99]. Interestingly, UCP2-deficient mice have higher islet ATP levels and increased glucose-stimulated insulin secretion, establishing that UCP2 negatively regulates insulin secretion [100].

Tumor Necrosis Factor-α

TNF-α is a cytokine which is overexpressed in adipose tissue of obese animals and humans [24,101]. TNF-α can induce insulin resistance by inhibition of tyrosine phosphorylation of the insulin receptor β chain and insulin receptor substrate-1 (IRS-1). In the ob/ob mouse, neutralizing TNF-α leads to improved insulin sensitivity although this could not be confirmed in humans [102]. A positive correlation has been demonstrated between the level of TNF-α mRNA in fat tissue and the level of hyperinsulinemia, suggesting a role for this cytokine in the pathogenesis of insulin resistance [24]. Although we have recently demonstrated a negative correlation between the plasma concentrations of TNF-α and insulin-stimulated glucose metabolism in humans [103], it is more likely that this only represents a spillover and that TNF-α exerts a paracrine rather than an endocrine effect in man. It has also been suggested that interleukin 6, another cytokine, may be more important than TNF-α in humans [104]. Two polymorphisms have been identified in the 5'-untranslated region of the human TNF-α gene (chromosome 6p21.3), one G to A polymorphism at position 238 and another at position 308. Although these polymorphisms seem to influence the host response to infections, discrepant results have been obtained regarding a possible association with human obesity and insulin resistance [105,106]. We were not able to replicate the findings of an association between the 238 polymorphism and type 2 diabetes using a family-based approach in which we studied transmission of the "disease" allele to affected offspring [107]. Taken together it may be premature to ascribe the TNF-α gene a role in the pathogenesis of human obesity and the metabolic syndrome.

Peroxisome Proliferator-Activated Receptor γ

There are three isoforms of peroxisome proliferator-activated receptors (PPARs); α, β and γ, which heterodimerize with the retinoid X receptor (RXR) to induce transcription of a number of target genes in adipose tissue [108]. Fatty acids or their derivatives are naturally occurring ligands of PPARs, in addition to drugs like thiazolidinediones (TZDs for PPARγ) and fibrates (for PPARα). The human PPARγ gene maps to chromosome 3p24, a region implicated in several genome-wide scans for type 2 diabetes. A rare proline to glutamine mutation (Pro115Gln) in the N-terminal domain of PPARγ has been described in four morbidly obese subjects [109]. This mutation leads to inhibition of phosphorylation of a serine residue at position 114 and thereby to a constitutively active PPARγ, resulting in increased adipocyte differentiation and greater cellular accumulation of triglycerides. A more common proline to alanine variant (Pro12Ala) has been associated with low BMI, increased insulin sensitivity, and lower risk for type 2 diabetes [110]. *In vitro*, this mutation leads to decreased PPARγ activity. Recently, 16 gene variants that had previously been reported to be associated with type 2 diabetes were studied within the Botnia study using a family-based association design [107]. Only one of the earlier findings was confirmed, the association of the PPARγ Pro12Ala with type 2 diabetes. A meta-analysis including 3.000 individuals from earlier studies reporting evidence both for and against association, indicated a 15% risk reduction for diabetes associated with the Ala-allele (allele frequency ~15%). Although the individual risk reduction associated with the Ala-allele is moderate, the high frequency of the Pro-allele in the population translates into a rather large population attributable risk of about 25% [107]. Whether individuals with different *PPARγ* genotypes respond differently to TZD treatment still needs to be demonstrated.

Peroxisome Proliferator-Activated Receptor γ Cofactor 1α

In addition to PPARγ its cofactor PGC1α is major metabolic determinants for differentiation of adipocytes and regulation of genes involved in glucose and lipid metabolism and as such strong a candidate gene for DSM and type 2 diabetes. A common polymorphisms in PGC-1α causing a glycine to serine substitution in the protein (Gly482Ser) have been associated with type 2diabetes and the expression of the PGC-1α gene has been shown to be reduced in the adipose tissue of insulin resistant subjects [111,112].

DNA microarrays offer the potential to identify pathways that are dysregulated in human disease. The relevant changes may be subtle at the level of individual genes, however, and difficult to recognize. We have described an analytical framework (Gene Set Enrichment Analysis, GSEA) designed to detect subtle but coordinate expression differences in *a priori* defined sets of functionally related genes. We applied GSEA to RNA expression profiles of muscle from patients with type 2 diabetes, IGT and NGT. Although no single gene differed significantly between disease states, GSEA detected that 87 of 112 genes involved in oxidative phosphorylation (OXPHOS) were downregulated in type 2 diabetes. The reduction was largely due to a subset of OXPHOS genes that were co-regulated (OXPHOS-CR), highly expressed at major sites of glucose disposal and strongly induced following forced expression of PGC-1α [113]. Thus, a more detailed investigation of the mitochondrial genome or genes involved in the regulation of these genes may be rewarding in the search for candidate genes for DSM.

Adiponectin

The adipose tissue has been ascribed a more central role in the pathogenesis of insulin resistance than previously thought. One of the main reasons for this is the identification of several hormones/cytokines secreted from adipose tissue that exert effects on insulin action in other tissues. It has recently been shown that the adipocyte-derived hormone *adiponectin* [114] reduces glucose levels through activation of AMP-activated protein kinase [115], an enzyme that also is central to the actions of leptin [116] and antidiabetic drugs such as metformin [117] and TZDs [118]. The plasma levels of adiponectin are decreased in both obesity and type 2 diabetes [119] and low levels of adiponectin predict type 2 diabetes [120,121]. This may be important as adiponectin can counteract insulin resistance (122) and enhance insulin action [123]. Genetic variants in the adiponectin gene (*APM1*; chromosome 3q27) seem to predispose to both obesity and type 2 diabetes [124-127]. This chromosomal region has also been linked to type 2 diabetes in a genome wide scan [128].

Forkhead Box C2

Another interesting adipocyte molecule is FOXC2, a winged helix transcription factor that protects from diet-induced obesity and insulin resistance when transgenically overexpressed in the adipose tissue of mice [129]. A polymorphism in the 5'-untranslated region of the FOXC2 gene seems to be associated with decreased expression of the gene in adipose tissue as well as insulin resistance in humans [130]. Several studies have failed to identify an association between *FOXC2* and type 2 diabetes but found association between –512C and dyslipidemia and BMI, suggesting that FOXC2 is a candidate gene for DMS. Interestingly, the *FOXC2 C-512T* polymorphism was recently implicated in familial combined hyperlipidemia (FCHL), a trait characterized by increased levels of triglycerides and decreased levels of HDL-cholesterol, where the common allele was associated with increased triglyceride levels and a haplotype combination consisting of the common alleles of the C-512T polymorphism and another downstream polymorphism (hCV2649496) was more often transmitted to affected subjects in families with FCHL [131]. Whether *FOXC2* is associated specifically with FCHL or dyslipidemia in general needs further investigation.

Resistin

Contrary to adiponectin and FOXC2, data obtained in mice for another adipocyte derived hormone, *resistin*, that impairs insulin action and the plasma levels of which are increased in models of obesity [132], have not been readily confirmed in humans [133-135]. So far there has only been marginal evidence for association between genetic variation in the human resistin gene (*RSTN*; chromosome 19p13) and insulin resistance, obesity or type 2 diabetes [136-140].

Calpain-10

The gene encoding calpain-10 (CAPN10; chromosome 2) illustrates the first successful positional cloning of a gene for a complex inherited polygenic disease like type 2 diabetes [141,142]. The diabetes-associated CAPN10 single nucleotide polymorphism 43 G/G genotype has further been associated with reduced muscle CAPN10 mRNA expression in skeletal muscle and impaired insulin-stimulated glucose metabolism, mainly impaired glucose oxidation [143], as well as elevated FFA levels [144]. The precise function of this cysteine protease in glucose metabolism or type 2 diabetes remains to be defined. It has been shown that calpain inhibitors decrease the insulin secretory response to glucose in mouse pancreatic islets and reduce insulin-mediated glucose transport in muscle strips and adipocytes as well as incorporation of glucose into glycogen in muscle from rat [415-147]. From a mechanistic point of view it is not surprising that a protein involved in vesicular transport has both these effect. From a genetic point of view CAPN10 represents the "perfect" candidate gene for type 2 diabetes since this would imply that it increases the susceptibility both to insulin resistance and impaired insulin secretion, a prerequisite for a diabetes-causing gene. Whether the effect on insulin sensitivity or insulin secretion dominates remains to be determined, as does the role for CAPN10 in DMS.

Glycoprotein PC-1

The membrane glycoprotein PC-1 (prohormone convertase 1) was isolated from a patient with extreme insulin resistance and found to inhibit insulin receptor tyrosine kinase activity [148]. A lysine to glutamine variant (Lys121Gln) in exon 4 of the PC-1 gene (*ENPP1*; chromosome 6q22-23) has been associated with insulin resistance and features of DMS [149,150]. *In vitro*, this variant is associated with impaired autophosphorylation of the insulin receptor tyrosine kinase. This is in line with our findings in genotype discordant sibling pairs; siblings with the Gln-allele had higher fasting glucose and impaired insulin action during an oral glucose tolerance test [150]. Similarly, carriers of the Gln-allele had impaired insulin-stimulated glucose uptake during clamp compared with carriers of the Lys-allele [151].

Insulin Receptor Substrates

The docking protein IRS-1 is an important link between the tyrosine phosphorylated insulin receptor to downstream components of the insulin signaling pathway [152]. IRS-1 is phosphorylated on multiple tyrosine residues in response to insulin and could be a candidate gene for insulin resistance. Two amino acid polymorphisms, a glycine to arginine variant (Gly972Arg) and an alanine to proline variant (Ala513Pro), have been described in the IRS-1 gene [153]. Both these amino acid substitutions, located close to tyrosine phosphorylation motifs, were slightly more frequent in type 2 diabetic patients than in control subjects. Furthermore, the presence of the codon 972 polymorphism was associated with insulin resistance and clustering of several other features of DMS in obese non-diabetic Danish subjects [154]. Subsequently, several other insulin receptor substrates (*IRS2* [chromosome 13q34], *IRS3* and *IRS4* [chromosome Xq22]) have been discovered but no consistent variations in these genes have been found. It seems that the different IRS proteins play very different overlapping rather than redundant roles in the insulin signaling pathway. Whereas *IRS1* knockout mice suffer from embryonic and postnatal growth retardation and muscle insulin resistance, *IRS2* knockout animals are normal in size but develop diabetes due to liver insulin resistance and lack of pancreatic β-cell compensation [155,156]. In fact, the *IRS1* knock-out mice maintained normoglycaemia by compensatory β-cell hyperplasia, while the amount of β-cells was reduced in the *IRS2* knock-out mouse underlining the importance of *IRS2* as a regulator of β-cell mass [156]. Moreover, the IRS-2 gene (but not *IRS1*) was recently reported as a target for TZDs. In differentiated 3T3-L1 adipocytes as well as in human adipose tissue cultures, TZDs had a rapid and marked stimulatory effect on *IRS2* expression [157].

Glycogen Synthase

Impaired insulin stimulation of glycogen synthesis is a hallmark feature of insulin resistance in type 2 diabetes and impaired glucose tolerance [13,158]. The key enzyme of this pathway, skeletal muscle glycogen synthase (GS) could therefore be an important candidate for a genetic defect causing insulin resistance. We have described the genomic structure of the human GS gene (*GYS1*) and assigned it to chromosome 19q13.3 [159,160]. An XbaI polymorphism of the *GYS1* gene has been associated with type 2 diabetes and insulin resistance, particularly impaired insulin-stimulated glycogen synthesis in skeletal muscle [161,162]. We applied the genotype discordant sibling pair approach to explore this association further. The sibling with the rare A2 allele had more features of DMS (obesity, hypertension and microalbuminuria) and an increased risk of myocardial infarction compared to siblings with the A1 allele [163]. In addition, diabetic A2 carriers were more severely dyslipidemic and insulin resistant compared to those without A2 allele. Recently, similar results were reported in a Danish twin study. Twins with the A2 allele were significantly more insulin resistant, and had higher diastolic blood pressure compared to their genotype discordant dizygotic twin [164]. Another recent study provides some evidence for how this variant may lead to insulin resistance. Neuromuscular electrical stimulation of muscle (and most likely exercise) increases the amount of GS protein in carriers of the A1 variant whereas this increase is impaired in carriers of the A2 allele [165]. In a meta-analysis, the *GYS1* gene showed evidence of ethnic heterogeneity [166]. A plausible explanation is that multiple alleles are contributing to the *GYS1* association.

Further support for a role of the *GYS1* gene in the pathogenesis of insulin resistance comes from studies in the diabetes-prone C57BL/6J mouse [167]. This mouse strain becomes obese, insulin-resistant, and develops diabetes when fed a diabetogenic diet. The phenotype of developing hyperglycemia when fed such a diet was linked to a locus on chromosome 7. This putative susceptibility locus is consistent with that of the *GYS1* gene. The diabetes-prone mouse had decreased GS activity in muscle even when fed a control diet. However, insulin resistance as demonstrated by elevated plasma insulin levels was seen only when the mouse was fed a diabetogenic diet, suggesting that for insulin resistance to become manifest, an interaction between genetic and environmental factors is necessary.

Insulin Gene Variable Number of Tandem Repeats

The insulin gene is located on human chromosome 11. A variable number of tandem repeats (INS-VNTR) 0.5 kb upstream of the gene has received a lot of attention in the past years not only as a potential susceptibility gene for type 1 and type 2 diabetes but also for obesity and low birth weight [168-172]. Depending on the number of repeats, INS-VNTR can be divided into class I (26-63 repeats), II (64-104 repeats) and III (141-209 repeats). The number of repeats is considered to influence expression of the insulin gene in both the thymus and in the pancreas [173-177]. Whereas the class I allele has been associated with an increased risk of type 1 diabetes the class III allele has been suggested to increase the risk for type 2 diabetes. Several studies have shown that the class I allele is associated with elevated insulin concentrations in children, particularly in juvenile obesity [171,177]. A parent of origin effect has also been proposed in that this is particularly due to paternal expression of the class I allele [170,178]. The association with type 2 diabetes is, however, less consistent and might be secondary to hyperinsulinemia and obesity.

Kir 6.2 and SUR1

As per definition genes affecting insulin secretion should perhaps not be considered as candidate genes for DMS but for diabetes only. However, given the high prevalence of DMS in type 2 diabetes we feel that it may be worthwhile keeping them in mind. In pancreatic β-cells ATP-sensitive potassium (K_{ATP}) channels control insulin secretion by coupling metabolism to changes in electrical activity. The K_{ATP} channels are composed of two subunits; the sulfonylurea receptor (*SUR1 or ABCC8*) and the inwardly rectifying potassium channel Kir 6.2 [179]. These two genes are located 5 kb from each other on the short arm of chromosome 11. Sulfonylureas stimulate insulin secretion by closing the K_{ATP} channels, which in turn results in opening of voltage-gated calcium channels. A glutamic acid to lysine variant (E23K) variant in the *Kir 6.2* gene has been associated with type 2 diabetes in several studies and been suggested to explain about 12% of the population attributable risk of type 2 diabetes [180-183]. This variant seems to induce spontaneous over-activity in the pancreatic β-cells thereby decreasing the sensitivity of the β-cells to ATP [184].

Mutations in the *SUR1* gene cause decreased K_{ATP} channel activity and congenital hyperinsulinemia [185,186]. Recently it was shown that a dominant mutation in the *SUR1* gene causing a glutamic acid to lysine substitution (E1506K), resulting in neonatal hypoglycemia, in its heterozygous form increases susceptibility to type 2 diabetes later in life [187]. It can thus be assumed that continuous over-stimulation of insulin secretion might lead to subsequent insulin deficiency and diabetes. Several other variants have been identified in the *SUR1* gene but none of these have been consistently associated with type 2 diabetes [182,188].

Genome Wide Scans

The advantage of the genome wide scan approach is that it does not assume any knowledge about the pathophysiological mechanisms leading to DMS. The disadvantages are that it requires large family resources and that it encompasses a high risk of false positive results. Several genome wide scans have been carried out with either obesity or type 2 diabetes as phenotype. Alternatively, BMI, leptin concentrations or metabolic rates have been used as quantitative traits. In obese Mexican Americans, linkage was observed between fat mass or leptin concentrations and a region on chromosome 2 [59]. *POMC* is the most interesting candidate gene in this chromosomal region. In the Quebec family study linkage was found between percent body fat and a region on the long arm of chromosome 20. This region is syngenic to a region on mouse chromosome 2, to which linkage first was observed [189]. More recently, linkage between basal metabolic rate and a region on chromosome 11 was reported in the Quebec study. This region contains both the UCP2 and UCP3 genes. Linkage between percent body fat and a region on chromosome 11 has also been found in Pima Indians, but it does not seem to be identical to the UCP2/UCP3 region [190]. In type 2 diabetic subjects, linkage has been reported to several regions including 2q [191-194]. To date, no genome wide scan has been performed using DMS as the phenotype under study.

Concluding Remarks

The genetics of the dysmetabolic syndrome is still a puzzle although no longer a nightmare. It has become evident that concerning the underlying genetics, this complex cluster of risk factors may not be as heterogeneous as the risk factors themselves since some genes contribute to the risk for developing several of the components of the syndrome. Among genes contributing to DMS those regulating lipolysis and thermogenesis remain prime candidates. So far, mutations in candidate genes can only explain a few rare cases of monogenic forms of obesity. Abdominal obesity most likely results from the interplay between several genes and an affluent environment and these interactions need further study. In fact, the interplay between common variants in candidate genes and an affluent environment may explain most of the genetic component of the disease. Despite substantial progress in our understanding of the physiology of DMS, the pathophysiology of the condition remains obscure. The limited knowledge about the pathophysiological events emphasizes the continued use for random approaches. A prerequisite is that the search is focused on families with a clearly defined inherited genetic risk of developing abdominal obesity and/or insulin resistance.

References

[1] Groop, L., Orho-Melander, M. (2001) The dysmetabolic syndrome. *J. Intern. Med.* 250:105-120

[2] Alberti KG, Zimmet PZ (1998) Definition, diagnosis and classification of diabetes mellitus and its complications. Part 1: diagnosis and classification of diabetes mellitus provisional report of a WHO consultation. *Diabet. Med.* 15:539-553

[3] World Health Organisation, 1999. *Report of a WHO consultation:definition of metabolic syndrome in definition, diagnosis, and classification of diabetes mellitus and its complications. I. Diagnosis and classification of diabetes mellitus.* World Health Organisation, Department of Noncommunicable Disease Surveillance, Geneva

[4] Balkau, B., Charles, M.A. (1999) Comment of the provisional report from the WHO consultation: European Group for the Study of Insulin Resistance (EGIR). *Diabet. Med.*. 16:442-443

[5] Third report of the National Cholesterol Education Program (NCEP) Expert Panel on detection, evaluation and treatment of high blood cholesterol in adults (Adult Treatment Panel III). *JAMA* 285:2486-2497

[6] Isomaa, B. (2003) A major health hazard: The metabolic syndrome. *Life Sci.* 73:2395-2411

[7] Eschwège, E. (2003) The dysmetabolic syndrome, insulin resistance and increased cardiovascular (CV) morbidity and mortality in type 2 diabetes: aetiological factors in the development of CV complications. *Diabetes Metab.* 29:S19-S27

[8] Groop, L., Forsblom , C., Lehtovirta, M., Tuomi, T., Karanko, S., Nissén, M., Ehrnström, B.-O., Forsén, B., Isomaa, B., Snickars, B., Taskinen, M.-R. (1996) Metabolic consequences of a family history of NIDDM (The Botnia Study). *Diabetes* 45:1585-1593

[9] Isomaa, B., Almgren, P., Tuomi, T., Forsen, B., Lahti, K., Nissen, M., Taskinen, M.R., Groop, L. (2001) Cardiovascular morbidity and mortality associated with the metabolic syndrome. *Diabetes Care* 24:683-689

[10] Eriksson, K.F., Lindgärde, F. (1998) No excess 12-year mortality in men with impaired glucose tolerance who participated in the Malmö Preventive Trial with diet and exercise. *Diabetologia* 41:1010-1016

[11] Tuomilehto, J., Lindstrom, J., Eriksson, J.G., Valle, T.T., Hamalainen, H., Ilanne-Parikka, P., Keinanen-Kiukaanniemi, S., Laakso, M., Louheranta, A., Rastas, M., Salminen, V., Uusitupa, M.; Finnish Diabetes Prevention Study Group. (2001) Prevention of type 2 diabetes mellitus by changes in lifestyle among subjects with impaired glucose tolerance. *N. Engl. J. Med.* 344:1343-1350

[12] Knowler, W.C., Barrett-Connor, E., Fowler, S.E., Hamman, R.F., Lachin, J.M., Walker, E.A., Nathan, D.M.; Diabetes Prevention Program Research Group. (2002) Reduction in the incidence of type 2 diabetes with lifestyle intervention or metformin. *N. Engl. J. Med.* 346:393-403

[13] Beck-Nielsen, H., Groop, L. (1994) Metabolic and genetic characterization of prediabetic states. Sequence of events leading to non-insulin-dependent diabetes mellitus. *J. Clin. Invest.* 94:1714-1721

[14] Groop, L., Tuomi, T. (1997) Non-insulin-dependent diabetes mellitus - a collision between thrifty genes and an affluent society. *Ann. Med.* 29:37-53

[15] Bouchard, C., Perusse, L., Leblanc, C., Tremblay, A., Theriault, G. (1988) Inheritance of the amount and distribution of human body fat. *Int. J. Obesity.* 12:205-215

[16] Bouchard, C. (1996) Genetics of body fat content. In *Progress in Obesity Research 7*, Angel, H., Anderson, H., Bouchard, C., Lau, D., Leiter, L., Mendelson, R. (eds), Vol. 7. pp. 33-41. John Libbey: London

[17] Carey, D., Nguyen, T., Campbell, L., Chisholm, D., Kelly, P. (1996) Genetic influences on central abdominal fat: a twin study. *Int. J. Obesity* 20:722-726

[18] Samaras, K., Spector, T., Nguyen, T., Baan, K., Campbell, L., Kelly, P. (1997) Independent genetic factors determine the amount and distribution of fat in women after the menopause. *J. Clin. Endocrinol. Metab.* 82:781-785

[19] Lönnqvist, F., Thörne, A., Nilsell, K., Hoffstedt, J., Arner, P. (1995) A pathogenetic role of visceral fat beta-3-adrenoreceptors in obesity. *J. Clin. Invest.* 95:1109-1116

[20] Krief, S., Lönnqvist, F., Raimbault, S., Baude, B., Van Spronsen, A., Arner, P., Strosberg, A., Ricquier, D., Emorine, L. (1993) Tissue distribution of beta-3-adrenergic receptor mRNA in man. *J. Clin. Invest.* 91:344-349

[21] Reynisdotter, S., Wahrenberg, H., Carlström, K., Rössner, S., Arner, P. (1994) Catecholamine resistance in fat cells of women with upper-body obesity due to decreased expression of beta-2-adrenoceptors. *Diabetologia* 37:428-435

[22] Banerji, M., Chaiken, R., Gordon, D., Kral, J., Lebovitz, H. (1995) Does intraabdominal adipose tissue in black men determine whether NIDDM is insulin-resistant or insulin-sensitive? *Diabetes* 44:141-146

[23] Zhang, Y., Proenca, R., Maffei, M., Baron, M., Leopold, L., Friedman, J. (1994) Positional cloning of the mouse obese gene and its human homologue. *Nature* 372:425-432

[24] Hotamisligil, G., Shargill, N., Spiegelman, B. (1993) Adipose expression of tumor necrosis factor-a: Direct role in obesity-linked insulin resistance. *Science* 259:87-91

[25] Storlien, L., Jenkins, A., Chisholm, D., Pasqoe, W., Kohouri, S., Kraegen, E. (1991) Influence of dietary fat composition on development of insulin resistance in rats. Relationship to muscle triglyceride and omega-3 fatty acids in muscle phospholipid. *Diabetes* 40:280-289

[26] Groop, L., Ferrannini, E. (1993) Insulin action and substrate competition. *Baillière's Clinical Endocrinology and Metabolism* 7:1007-1032

[27] Neel, V. (1962) Diabetes mellitus: a "thrifty" genotype rendered detrimental by progress? *Am. J. Hum. Genet.* 14:352-362

[28] Coleman, D. (1979) Obesity genes: beneficial effects in heterozygous mice. *Science* 203:663-665

[29] Walder, K., Oakes, N., Fahey, R.P., Cooney, G., Zimmet, P.Z., Collier, G.R. (2002) Profile of dyslipidemia in Psammomys obesus, an animal model of the metabolic syndrome. *Endocr. Regul.* 36:1-8

[30] Hales, C., Barker, D. (1992) Type 2 diabetes mellitus: the thrifty phenotype hypothesis. *Diabetologia* 35:595-601

[31] Melander, O., Mattiasson, I., K, M., Groop, L., Hulthén, L. (1999) Heredity for hypertension influences intrauterine growth and the relation between foetal growth and adult blood pressure. *J. Hypertension* 17:1557-1561

[32] Hattersley, A., Beards, F., Ballantyne, E., Appleton, M., Harvey, R., Ellard, S. (1998) Mutations in the glucokinase gene of the fetus result in reduced birth weight. *Nature Genetics* 19:268-270

[33] Hästbacka, J., De la Chapelle, A., Mahtani, M., Clines, G., Reeve-Daly, M., Daly, M., Hamilton, B., Kusumi, K., Trivedi, B., Weawer, A., Coloma, A., Lovett, M., Buckler, A., Kaitila, I., Lander, E. (1994) The diastrophic dysplasia gene encodes a novel sulfate

transporter: positional cloning by fine-structure linkage disequilibrium mapping. *Cell* 78:1073-1087

[34] Bouchard, C., Rice, T., Lemieux, S., Despres, J., Perusse, L., Rao, D. (1996) Major gene for abdominal visceral fat area in the Quebec Family Study. *Int. J. Obesity.* 20:420-427

[35] Coleman, D. (1973) Effects of parabiosis of obese with diabetes and normal mice. *Diabetologia* 9:294-298

[36] Pelleymounter, M., Cullen, M., Baker, M., Hecht, R., Winters, D., Boone, T., Collins, F. (1995). Effects of the obese gene product on body weight regulation in ob/ob mice. *Science* 269:540-542

[37] Consindine, R., Consindine, E., William, C., Nyce, M., Magosin, S., Bauer, T., Rosato, E., Colberg, J., Caro, J. (1995) Evidence against either a premature stop codon or the abscence of obese gene mRNA in human obesity. *J. Clin. Invest.* 95:2986-2988

[38] Maffei, M., Halaas, J., Ravussin, E., Pratley, R., Lee, G., Zhang, Y., Fei, H., Kim, S., Lallone, R., Ranganathan, S., Kern, P., Friedman, J. (1995) Leptin levels in human and rodent: measurement of plasma leptin and ob RNA in obese and weight-reduced subjects. *Nature Medicine* 1:1155-1161

[39] Ogawa, Y., Masuzaki, H., Isse, N., Okazaki, T., Mori, K., Shigemoto, M., Satoh, N., Tamura, N., Hosohoda, K., Yoshimasa, Y., Jingami, H., Kawada, T., Nakao, K. (1995) Molecular cloning of rat obese cDNA and augmented gene expression in genetically obese Zucker fatty (fa/fa) rats. *J. Clin. Invest.* 96:1647-1652

[40] Montague, C., Farroqi, S., Whitehead, J., Soos, M., Rau, H., Wareham, N., Sewter, C., Digby, J., Mohammed, S., Hurst, J., Cheetham, C., Earley, A., Barnett, A., Prins, J., O'Rahilly, S. (1997) Congenital leptin deficiency is associated with severe early-onset obesity in humans. *Nature* 387:903-908

[41] Tartaglia, L., Dembski, M., Weng, X., Deng , N., Culpepper, J., Devos, R., Richards, G., Campfield, L., Clark, F., Dees, J., Muir, C., Sanker, S., Moriarty, A., Moore, K., Smutko, J., Mays, G., Woolf, E., Monroe, C., Tepper, R. (1996) Identification and expression cloning of a leptin receptor, ob-R. *Cell* 83:1263-1271

[42] Lee, G-H., Proenca, R., Montez, J., Carroll, K., Darvishzadeh, J., Lee, J., Friedman, J. (1996) Abnormal splicing of the leptin receptor in diabetic mice. *Nature* 379:632-635

[43] Stephens, T., Basinski, M., Bristow, P., Bue-Valleskey, J., Burgett, S., Craft, L., Hale, J., Hoffmann, J., Hsiung, H., Kriauciunas, A., MacKellar, W., Rosteck Jr, P., Schoner, B., Smith, D., Tinsley, F., Zhang, X.-Y., Heiman, M. (1995) The role of neuropeptide Y in the antiobesity action of the obese gene product. *Nature* 377:530-532

[44] Clement, K., Vaisse, C., Lahlou, N., Cabrol, S., Pelloux, V., Cassuto, D., Gourmelen, M., Dina, C., Chambaz, J., Lacorte, J., Basdevant, A., Bougneres, P., Lebouc, Y., Froguel, P., Guy-Grand, B. (1998). A mutation in the leptin receptor gene causes obesity and pituitary dysfunction. *Nature* 392:398-401

[45] Silver, K., Walston, J., Chung, W.K., Yao, F., Parikh, V.V., Andersen, R., Cheskin, L.J., Elahi, D., Muller, D., Leibel, R.L., Shuldiner, A.R. (1997) The Gln223Arg and Lys656Asn polymorphisms in the human leptin receptor do not associate with traits related to obesity. *Diabetes* 46:1898-1900

[46] Francke, S., Clement, K., Dina, C., Inoue, H., Behn, P., Vatin, V., Basdevant, A., Guy-Grand, B., Permutt, M.A., Froguel, P., Hager, J. (1997) Genetic studies of the leptin receptor gene in morbidly obese French Caucasian families. *Hum. Genet.* 100:491-496

[47] Wauters, M., Mertens, I., Chagnon, M., Rankinen, T., Considine, R.V., Chagnon, Y.C., Van Gaal, L.F., Bouchard, C. (2001) Polymorphisms in the leptin receptor gene, body composition and fat distribution in overweight and obese women. *Int. J. Obes. Relat. Metab. Disord.* 25:714-720

[48] Ukkola, O., Tremblay, A., Despres, J.P., Chagnon, Y.C., Campfield, L.A., Bouchard, C. (2000) Leptin receptor Gln223Arg variant is associated with a cluster of metabolic abnormalities in response to long-term overfeeding. *J. Intern. Med.* 248:435-439

[49] Oksanen, L., Kaprio, J., Mustajoki, P., Kontula, K. (1998) A common pentanucleotide polymorphism of the 3'-untranslated part of the leptin receptor gene generates a putative stem-loop motif in the mRNA and is associated with serum insulin levels in obese individuals. *Int. J. Obese.* 22:634-640

[50] Lakka, H.M., Oksanen, L., Tuomainen, T.P., Kontula, K., Salonen, J.T. (2000) The common pentanucleotide polymorphism of the 3'-untranslated region of the leptin receptor gene is associated with serum insulin levels and the risk of type 2 diabetes in non-diabetic men: a prospective case-control study. *J Intern Med* 248:77-83

[51] Kieffer, T.J., Heller, R.S., Habener, J.F. (1996) Leptin receptors expressed on pancreatic beta-cells. *Biochem. Biophys. Res. Commun.* 224:522-527

[52] Vickers, M.H., Reddy, S., Ikenasio, B.A., Breier, B.H. (2001) Dysregulation of the adipoinsular axis - a mechanism for the pathogenesis of hyperleptinemia and adipogenic diabetes induced by fetal programming. *J. Endocrinol.* 170:323-332

[53] Kieffer, T.J., Heller, R.S., Leech, C.A., Holz, G.G., Habener, J.F. (1997) Leptin suppression of insulin secretion by the activation of ATP-sensitive K+ channels in pancreatic beta-cells. *Diabetes* 46:1087-1093

[54] Seufert, J., Kieffer, T.J., Leech, C.A., Holz, G.G., Moritz, W., Ricordi, C., Habener, J.F. (1999) Leptin suppression of insulin secretion and gene expression in human pancreatic islets: implications for the development of adipogenic diabetes mellitus. *J Clin. Endocrinol. Metab.* 84:670-676

[55] Fan, W., Boston, B., Kesterson, R., Hurby, V., Cone, R. (1997) Role of melanocrotinergic neurons in feeding and the agouti obesity syndrome. *Nature* 385:165-168

[56] Ollman, M., Wilson, B., Yang, Y., Kerns, J., Chen, Y., Gantz, I., Barsch, G. (1997) Antagonism of central melanocortin receptors in-vitro and in-vivo by agouti-related protein. *Science* 278:135-138

[57] Vaisse, C., Clement, K., Guy-Grand, B., Froguel, P. (1998) A frameshift mutation in human MCR4 is associated with a dominant form of obesity. *Nature Genetics* 20:113-114

[58] Yeo, G., Farooqi, I., Aminian, S., Halsell, D., Stanhope, R., O'Rahilly, S. (1998) A frameshift mutation in MCR4R associated with dominantly inherited human obesity. *Nature Genetics* 20:111-112

[59] Comuzzie, A., Hixson, J., Almasy, L., Mitchell, B., Mahaney, M., Dyer, T., Stern, M., MacCluer, J., Blangero, J. (1997) A major quantitative trait locus determining serum

leptin levels and fat mass is located on human chromosome 2. *Nature Genetics* 15:273-276

[60] Chagnon, Y., Chen, W., Perusse, L., Chagnon, M., Nadeau, A., Wilkinson, B, Bouchard, C. (1997) Linkage and association studies between the melanocortin receptor-4 and receptor-5 genes and obesity-related phenotypes in the Quebec family study. *Molecular Medicine* 3:663-673

[61] Krude, H., Biebermann, H., Luck, W., Horn, R., Brabant, G., Grueters, A. (1998) Severe early-onset obesity, adrenal insufficiency and red hair pigmentation caused by POMC mutations in humans. *Nat. Genet.* 19:155-157

[62] Suviolahti, E., Ridderstråle, M., Klannemark, M., Melander, O., Carlsson, E., Carlsson, M., Hedenbro, J., Orho-Melander, M. (2003) The pro-opiomelanocortin gene is associated with serum leptin levels in lean but not in obese individuals *Int. J. Obesity.* 27:1204-1211

[63] Naggert, J., Fricker, L., Varlamov, O., Nishina, P., Roille, Y., Steiner, D., Carroll, R., Paigen, B., Leiter, E. (1995) Hyperproinsulinemia in obese fat/fat mice associated with a carboxypeptidase E mutation which reduces enzyme activity. *Nature Genetics* 10:135-142

[64] Jackson, R., Creemers, J., Ohagi, S., Raffin-Sanson, M.-L., Sanders, L., Montague, C., Hutton, J., O'Rahilly, S. (1997) Obesity and impaired prohormone processing associated with mutations in the human prohormone convertase 1 gene. *Nature Genetics* 16:303-306

[65] Emorine, L., Marullo, S., Briend-Sutren, M., Patey, G., Tate, K., Delavier-Klutchko, C., Strosberg, A. (1989) Molecular characterization of the human beta-3-adrenergic receptor. *Science* 245:1118-1121

[66] Lowell, B., Susulic, V., Hamman, A., Lawitts, J., Himms-Hagen, J., Boyer, B., Kozak, L., Flier, J. (1993) Development of obesity in transgenic mice after genetic ablation of brown adipose tissue. *Nature* 366:740-742

[67] Krief, S., Lönnqvist, F., Raimbault, S., Baude, B., Van Spronsen, A., Arner, P., Strosberg, A., Ricquier, D., Emorine, L. (1993) Tissue distribution of beta-3-adrenergic receptor mRNA in man. *J. Clin. Invest.* 91:344-349

[68] Lönnqvist, F., Thörne, A., Nilsell, K., Hoffstedt, J., Arner, P. (1995) A pathogenetic role of visceral fat beta-3-adrenoreceptors in obesity. *J. Clin. Invest.* 95:1109-1116

[69] Walston, J., Silver, K., Bogardus, C., Knowler, W., Celi, F., Austin, S., Manning, B., Strosberg, D., Stern, M., Raben, N., Sorkin, J., Roth, J., Shuldiner, A. (1995) Time of onset of non-insulin-dependent diabetes mellitus and genetic variation in the beta3-adrenergic-receptor gene. *New Engl. J. Med.* 333:343-347

[70] Widén, E., Lehto, M., Kanninen, T., Walston, J., Shuldiner, A., Groop, L. (1995) Association of a polymorphism in the beta-3-adrenergic-receptor gene with features of the insulin resistance syndrome in Finns. *New Engl. J. Med.* 333:348-351

[71] Clement, K., Vaisse, C., Manning, B., Basdevant, A., Guy-Grand, B., Ruiz, J., Silver, K., Shuldiner, A., Froguel, P., Strosberg, A. (1995) Genetic variation in the beta3-adrenergic receptor and an increased capacity to gain weight in patients with morbid obesity. *New Engl. J. Med.* 333:352-354

[72] Sipiläinen, R., Uusitupa, M., Heikkinen, S., Rissanen, A., Laakso, M. (1997) Polymorphism of the beta-3-adrenergic receptor gene affects basal metabolic rate in obese Finns. *Diabetes* 46:77-80

[73] Shihara, N., Yasuda, K., Moritani, T., Ue, H., Adachi, T., Tanaka, H., Tsuda, K., Seino, Y. (1999) The association between Trp 64Arg polymorphism of the beta-3-adrenergic receptor and autonomic nervous system activity. *J. Clin. Endocrinol. Metab.* 84:1623-1627

[74] Mitchell, B., Blangero, J., Comuzzie, A., Almasy, L., Shuldiner, A., Silver, K., Stern, M., MacCluer, J., Hixson, J. (1998) A paired sibling analysis of the beta-3 adrenergic receptor and obesity in Mexican americans. *J. Clin. Invest.* 101:584-587

[75] Mitchell, B., Cole, S., Comuzzie, A., Almasy, L., Blangero, J., MacCluer, J., Hixson, J. (1999) A quantitative trait locus influencing BMI maps to the region of beta-3-adrenergic receptor. *Diabetes* 48:1863-1867

[76] Gagnon, J., Mauriege, P., Roy, S., Sjöström, D., Chagnon, Y., Dionne, F., Oppert, J.-M., Perussé, L., Sjöström, L., Bouchard, C. (1996) The Trp64Arg mutation of the beta-3-adrenergic receptor gene has no effect on obesity phenotypes in the Quebec family study and Swedish Obese subjects cohort. *J. Clin. Invest.* 98:2086-2093

[77] Fujisawa, T., Ikegami, H., Kawaguchi, Y., Ogihara, T. (1998) Meta-analysis of the association of the Trp64Arg polyomorphism of the beta-3-adrenergic receptor gene with body mass index. *J. Clin. Endocrinol. Metab.* 83:2441-2444

[78] Sakane, N., Yoshida, T., Umekawa, T., Kondo, M., Sakai, Y., Takahashi, T. (1997) Beta-3-adrenergic receptor polymorphism: a genetic marker for visceral fat obesity and the insulin resistance syndrome. *Diabetologia* 40:200-204

[79] Pietro-Rouxel, F., Manning, B., Gros, J., Strosberg, D. (1997) The biological effect of the naturally occurring Trp64-Arg mutation on human beta-3-adrenoceptor activity. *Eur. J. Biochemistry.* 247:1174-1179

[80] Hoffstedt, J., Poirier, O., Thörne, A., Lönnqvist, F., Herrrmann, S., Cambien, F., Arner, P. (1999) Polymorphism of the human beta-3-adrenoceptir gene forms a well-conserved haplotype that is associated with moderate obesity and altered receptor function. *Diabetes* 48:203-205

[81] Large, V., Hellström, I., Reynisdottir, S., Lönnqvist, F., Eriksson, P., Lannfelt, L., Arner, P. (1997) Human beta-2-adrenoceptor gene polymorphisms are highly frequent in obesity and associate with altered adiipocyte beta-2-adrenoceptor function. *J. Clin. Invest.* 100:3005-3013

[82] Green, S., Turki, J., Innis, M., Liggett, S. (1994) Aminoterminal polymorphisms of the human beta-2-adrenergic receptor impart distinct agonist-promoted regulatory properties. *Biochemistry* 33:9414-9419

[83] Yamada, K., Ishiyama-Shigemoto, S., Ichikawa, F., Yuan, X., Koyanagi, A., Koyama, W., Nonaka, K. (1999) Polymorphism in the 5'-leader cistron of the beta-2-adrenergic receptor gene associated with obesity and type 2 diabetes. *J. Edocrinol. Metab.* 84:1754-1757

[84] Bengtsson, K., Orho-Melander, M., Melander, O., Lindblad, U., Ranstam, J., Rastam, L., Groop, L. (2001) Beta(2)-adrenergic receptor gene variation and hypertension in subjects with type 2 diabetes. *Hypertension* 37:1303-1308

[85] Mason, D. A., Moore, J. D., Green, S. A., Liggett, S. B. (1999) A gain-of-function polymorphism in a G-protein coupling domain of the human beta-1-adrenergic receptor. *J. Biol. Chem.* 274:12670-12674

[86] Bengtsson, K., Melander, O., Orho-Melander, M., Lindblad, U., Ranstam, J., Rastam, L., Groop, L. (2001) Polymorphism in the beta(1)-adrenergic receptor gene and hypertension. *Circulation* 104:187-190

[87] Tahvanainen, E., Syvänne, M., Frick, M., Murtomäki-Repo, S., Antikainen, M., Kesäniemi, A., Kauma, H., Pasternak, A., Taskinen, M.-R., Ehnholm, C., Study, L. (1998) Association of variation in hepatic lipase activity with promoter variation in the hepatic lipase gene. *J. Clin. Invest.* 101:956-960

[88] Reymer, P., Gagné, E., Groenemeyer, B. (1995) A lipoprotein lipase mutation (Asn291Ser) is associated with reduced HDL cholesterol levels in premature atherosclerosis. *Nature Genetics* 10:28-34

[89] Knudsen, P., Murtomäki, S., Antikainen, M., Ehnholm, S., Lahdenperä, S., Ehnholm, C., Taskinen, M.-R. (1997) The Asn291-Ser and Ser-477-stop mutations of the lipoprotein lipase gene and their significance for lipid metabolism in patients with hypertriglyceridemia. *Eur. J. Clin. Invest.* 27:928-935

[90] Klannemark, M., Suurinkeroinen, L., Orho-Melander, M., Groop, L., Taskinen, M.R. (2000) Interaction between the Asn291Ser variant of the LPL gene and insulin resistance on dyslipidaemia in high risk individuals for Type 2 diabetes mellitus. *Diabet. Med.* 17:599-605

[91] Large, V., Reynisdottir, S., Langin, D., Fredby, D., Klannemark, M., Holm, C., Arner, P. (1999) Decreased expression and function of adipocyte hormone-sensitive lipase in subcutaneous fat cells of obese subjects. *J. Lipid Res.* 40:2059-2065

[92] Talmud, P.J., Palmen, J., Walker, M. (1998) Identification of genetic variation in the human hormone-sensitive lipase gene and 5''sequences: homology of 5''sequences with mouse promoter and identification of potential regulatory elements. *Biochem. Biophys. Res. Commun.* 252:661-668

[93] Klannemark, M., Orho, M., Langin, D., Laurell, H., Holm, C., Reynisdottir, S., Arner, P., Groop, L. (1998) The putative role of the hormone sensitive lipase gene in the pathogenesis of the metabolic syndrome. *Diabetologia* 41:1515-1522

[94] Enerbäck, S., Jacobsson, A., Simpson, E., Guerra, C., Yamashita, H., Harper, M.-E., Kozak, L. (1997) Mice lacking mitochondrial uncoupling protein are cold -sensitive but not obese. *Nature* 387:90-93

[95] Clement, K., Ruiz, J., Cassard-Doulcier, A. (1996) Additve effect of A-G(-3826) variant of the uncoupling protein gene and the Trp64Arg mutation of the beta-3-adrenergic receptor gene on weight gain in morbid obesity. *Int J obesity* 20:1062-1066

[96] Klannemark, M., Orho, M., Groop, L. (1998) No relationship between variants in the uncoupling protein 2 gene and energy expenditure. *Eur. J. Endocrinol.* 139:217-221

[97] Chung, W., Luke, A., Cooper, R., Royni, C., Vidal-Puig, A., Rosenbaum, M., Chua, M., Solanes, G., Zheng, M., Zhao, L., LeDuc, C., Eisberg, A., Chu, F., Murphy, E., Schreier, M., Aronne, L., Caprio, S., Kahle, B., Gordon, D., Leal, S., Goldsmith, R., Andreau, A., Bruno, C., DiMauro, S., Heo, M., LoweJr, W., Lowell, B., allison, D.,

Leibel, R. (1999) Genetic and physiologic analysis of the role of uncoupling protein 3 in human energy homeostasis. *Diabetes* 48:1890-1895

[98] Esterbauer, H., Schneitler, C., Oberkofler, H., Ebenbichler, C., Paulweber, B., Sandhofer, F., Ladurner, G., Hell, E., Strosberg, A.D., Patsch, J.R., Krempler, F., Patsch, W. (2001) A common polymorphism in the promoter of UCP2 is associated with decreased risk of obesity in middle-aged humans. *Nat. Genet.* 28:178-183

[99] Krempler, F., Esterbauer, H., Weitgasser, R., Ebenbichler, C., Patsch, J.R., Miller, K., Xie, M., Linnemayr, V., Oberkofler, H., Patsch, W. (2001) A functional polymorphism in the promoter of UCP2 enhances obesity risk but reduces type 2 diabetes risk in obese middle-aged humans. *Diabetes* 51:3331-3335

[100] Zhang, C.Y., Baffy, G., Perret, P., Krauss, S., Peroni, O., Grujic, D., Hagen, T., Vidal-Puig, A.J., Boss, O., Kim, Y.B., Zheng, X.X., Wheeler, M.B., Shulman, G.I., Chan, C.B., Lowell, B.B. (2001) Uncoupling protein-2 negatively regulates insulin secretion and is a major link between obesity, beta cell dysfunction, and type 2 diabetes. *Cell* 105:745-755

[101] Hotamisigil, G., Arner, P., Caro, J., Atkinson, R., Spiegelman, B. (1995) Increased adipose tissue expression of tumor necrosis factor-□ in human obesity and insulin resistance. *J. Clin. Invest.* 95:2409-2415

[102] Saghizadeh, M., Ong, J., Garvey, W., Henry, R., Kern, P. (1996) The expression of TNF alfa by human muscle. Relationship to insulin resistance. *J. Clin. Invest.* 97:1111-1116

[103] Kellerer, M., Rett, K., Renn, W., Groop, L., Häring, H. (1996) Circulating TNF-alpha and leptin levels in offspring of NIDDM patients do not correlate to individual insulin sensitivityand insulin sensitivity in man. *Horm. Metab. Res.* 28:737-743

[104] Mohamed-Ali, A., Goodrick, S., Rawesh, A., Katz, D.R., Miles, J.M., Yudkin, J.S., Klein, S., Coppack, S.W. (1997) Subcutaneous adipose tissue secretes interleukin-6 but not tumor necrosis factor-□ in vivo. *J. Clin. Endocrinol. Metab.* 82:4196-4200

[105] Fernandéz-Real, J., Gutierrez, C., Ricart, W., Casamitjana, R., Fernandéz-Castanér, M., Vendrell, J., Richart, C., Soler, J. (1997) The TNF-alpha gene Nco I polymorphism influences the relationship among insulin resistance, percent body fat, and increased serum leptin levels. *Diabetes* 46:1468-1472

[106] Walston, J., Seibert, M., Jen-Yen, C., Cheskin, L., Andersen, R. (1999) Tumor necrosis factor-alpha-238 and-308 polymorhisms do not associate with traits related to obesity and insulin resistance. *Diabetes* 48:2096-2098

[107] Altshuler, D., Hirschorn, J.N., Klannemark, M., Lindgren, C.M., Vohl, M.-C., Nemesh, J., Lane, C.R., Schaffner, S.F., Bolk, S., Brewer, C., Tuomi, T., Gaudet, D., Hudson, T.J., Daly, M, Groop, L., Lander, E.S. (2000) The common PPARγ Pro12Ala polymorphism is associated with decreased risk of type 2 diabetes. *Nat Genet* 26:76-80

[108] Auwerx, J. (1999) PPARgamma, the ultimate thriphty gene. *Diabetologia* 42:1033-1049

[109] Ristow, M., Muller-Wieland, D., Pfeiffer, A., Krone, W., Kahn, C. (1998) Obesity associated with a mutation in a genetic regulator of adipocyte differentiation. *New Engl. J. Med.* 339:953-959

[110] Deeb, S., Fajas, L., Nemoto, M., Laakso, M., Fujimoto, W., Auwerx, J. (1998) A Pro 12Ala substitution in the human peroxisome proliferator-activated receptor gamma2 is associated with decreased receptor activity, improved insulin sensitivity and lowered body mass index. *Nature Genetics* 20:284-287

[111] Ek, J., Andersen, G., Urhammer, S.A, Gaede, P.H., Drivsholm, T., Borch-Johnsen, K., Hansen, T, Pedersen, O. (2001) Mutation analysis of peroxisome proliferator-activated receptor-gamma coactivator-1 (PGC-1) and relationships of identified amino acid polymorphisms to Type II diabetes mellitus. *Diabetologia* 44: 2220-2226.

[112] Hammarstedt, A., Jansson, P.A., Wesslau, C., Yang, X., Smith, U. (2003) Reduced expression of PGC-1 and insulin-signaling molecules in adipose tissue is associated with insulin resistance. *Biochem. Biophys. Res. Commun.* 301:578-582

[113] Mootha, V.K., Lindgren, C.M, Eriksson, K-F., Subramanian, A., Sihag, S., Lehar, J., Hirsschorn, J., Puigserver, P., Carlsson, E., Ridderstråle, M., Laurila, E., Daly, M.J., Patterson, N., Mesirov, J.P., Golub, T.R., Tamayo, P., Spiegelman, B., Lander, E.S., Hirschhorn, J.N., Altshuler, D., Groop, L.C. (2003) PGC-1□ responsive genes involved in oxidative phosphorylation are coordinately downregulated in human diabetes. *Nature Genet* 34:267-273

[114] Scherer, P.E., Williams, S., Fogliano, M., Baldini, G., Lodish, H.F. (1995) A novel serum protein similar to C1q, produced exclusively in adipocytes. *J. Biol. Chem.* 270:26746-26749

[115] Yamauchi, T., Kamon, J., Minokoshi, Y., Ito, Y., Waki, H., Uchida, S., Yamashita, S., Noda, M., Kita, S., Ueki, K., Eto, K., Akanuma, Y., Froguel, P., Foufelle, F., Ferre, P., Carling, D., Kimura, S., Nagai, R., Kahn, B.B., Kadowaki, T. (2002) Adiponectin stimulates glucose utilization and fatty-acid oxidation by activating AMP-activated protein kinase. *Nature Medicine* 8, 1288-1295

[116] Minokoshi, Y., Kim, Y.B., Peroni, O.D., Fryer, L.G., Muller, C., Carling, D., Kahn, B.B. (2002) Leptin stimulates fatty-acid oxidation by activating AMP-activated protein kinase. *Nature* 415:339-343

[117] Zhou, G., Myers, R., Li, Y., Chen, Y., Shen, X., Fenyk-Melody, J., Wu, M., Ventre, J., Doebber, T., Fujii, N., Musi, N., Hirshman, M.F., Goodyear, L.J., Moller, D.E. (2001) Role of AMP-activated protein kinase in mechanism of metformin action. *J. Clin. Invest.* 108:1167-1174

[118] Fryer, L.G., Parbu-Patel, A., Carling, D. (2002) The anti-diabetic drugs rosiglitazone and metformin stimulate AMP-activated protein kinase through distinct signaling pathways. *J. Biol. Chem.* 277:25226-25232

[119] Arita, Y., Kihara, S., Ouchi, N., Takahaschi, M., Maeda, K., Miyagawa, J., Hotta, K., Shimomura, I., Nakamura, T., Miyaoka, K., Kuriyama, H., Nishida, M., Yamashita, S., Okubo, K., Matsubara, K., Muraguchi, M., Ohmoto, Y., Funahashi, T., Matsuzawa, Y. (1999) Paradoxical decrease of an adipose-specific protein, adiponectin, in obesity. *Biochem. Biophys. Res. Commun.* 275:79-83

[120] Lindsay, R.S., Funahashi, T., Hanson, R.L., Matsuzawa, Y., Tanaka, S., Tataranni, P.A., Knowler, W.C., Krakoff, J. (2002) Adiponectin and development of type 2 diabetes in Pima Indian population. *Lancet* 360:57-58

[121] Spranger, J., Kroke, A., Möhlig, M., Bergmann, M.M., Ristow, M., Boening, H., Pfeiffer, A.F.H. (2003) Adiponectin and protection against type 2 diabetes mellitus. *Lancet* 361:226-228

[122] Yamauchi, T., Kamon, J., Waki, H., Terauchi, Y., Kubota, N., Hara, K., Mori, Y., Ide, T., Murakami, K., Tsuboyama-Kasaoka, N., Ezaki, O., Akanuma, Y., Gavrilova, O., Vinson, C., Reitman, M.L., Kagechika, H., Shudo, K., Yoda, M., Nakano, Y., Tobe, K., Nagai, R., Kimura, S., Tmoita, M., Froguel, P., Kadowaki, T. (2001) The fat-derived hormone adiponectin reverses insulin resistance associated with both lipoatrophy and obesity. *Nat. Medicine.* 7:941-946

[123] Berg, A.H., Combs, T.P., Du, X., Brownlee, M., Scherer, P.E. (2001) The adipocyte-ecreted protein Arp30 enhances hepatic insulin action. *Nat. Medicine.* 7:947-953

[124] Stumvoll, M., Tschritter, O., Fritsche, A., Staiger, H., Renn, H., Weisser, M., Machicao, F., Häring, H. (2002) Association of the T-G polymorphism in adiponectin (exon 2) with obesity and insulin sensitivity. *Diabetes* 51:37-41

[125] Hara, K., Boutin, P., Mori, Y., Tobe, K., Dina, C., Yasada, K., Yamauchi, T., Otabe, S., Okada, T., Eto, K., Kadowaki, H., Hagura, R., Akanuma, Y., Yazaki, Y., Nagai, R., Taniyama, M., Matsubara, K., Yoda, M., Nakano, Y., Kimura, S., Tomita, M., Kimura, S., Ito, C., Froguel, P., Kadowaki, T. (2002) Genetic variation in the gene encoding adiponectin is associated with an increased risk of type 2 diabetes in the Japanese population. *Diabetes* 51:536-540

[126] Menzaghi, C., Ercolino, T., Di Paola, R., Berg, A.H., Warram, J.H., Scherer, P.E., Trischitta, V., Doria, A. (2002) A haplotype at the adiponectin locus is associated with obesity and other features of the insulin resistance syndrome. *Diabetes* 51:2306-2312

[127] Vasseur, F., Helbecque, N., Dina, C., Lobbens, S., Delannoy, V., Gaget, S., Boutin, P., Vaxillaire, M., Leprêtre, F., Dupont, S., Hara, K., Clément, K., Bilhain, B., Kadowaki, T., Froguel, P. (2002) Single-nucleotide polymorphism haplotypes in both the proximal promoter and exon 3 of the *APM1* gene modulate adipocyte-secreted adiponectin hormone levels and contribute to the genetic risk for type 2 diabetes in French Caucasians. *Hum. Mol. Gen.* 11:2607-2624

[128] Vionnet, N., Hani, El-H., Dupont, S., Gallina, S., Francke, S., Dotte, S., De Matos, F., Durand, E., Leprêtre, F., Lecoeur, C., Gallina, P., Zekiri, L., Dina., Froguel, P. (2000) Genome wide search for type 2 diabetes-susceptibility genes in French whites: evidence for a novel susceptibility locus for early-onset diabetes on chromosome 3q27-qter and independent replication of a type 2-diabetes locus on chromosome 1q21-q24. *Am. J. Hum. Genet.* 67:1470-1480

[129] Cederberg, A., Grönning, L.M., Ahrén, B., Taskén, K., Carlsson, P., Enerbäck, S. (2001) FOXC2 is a winged helix gene that counteracts obesity, hypertriglyceridemia, and diet-induced insulin resistance. *Cell* 106:563-573

[130] Ridderstråle, M., Carlsson, E., Klannemark, M., Cederberg, M., Kösters, C., Tornqvist, H., Storgaard, H., Vaag, A., Enerbäck, S., Groop, L. (2002) *FOXC2* mRNA and a 5'UTR polymorphism of the gene are associated with insulin resistance. *Diabetes* 51:3554-3560

[131] Pajukanta, P., Allayee, H., Krass, K.L., Kuraishy, A., Soro, A., Lilja, H.E., Mar, R., Taskinen, M.-R., Nuotio, I., Laakso, M., Rotter, J.I., de Bruin, T.W.A., Cantor, R.M.,

Lusis, A.J., Peltonen, L. (2003) Combined analysis of genome scans of Dutch and Finnish families reveals a susceptibility locus for high-density lipoprotein cholesterol on chromosome 16q. *Am. J. Hum. Genet.* 72: 903-917

[132] Steppan, C.M., Bailey, S.T., Bhat, S., Brown, E.J., Banerjee, R.R., Wright, C.M., Patel, H.R., Ahima, R.S., Lazar, M.A. (2001) The hormone resistin links obesity to diabetes. *Nature* 409:307-312

[133] Nagaev, I., Smith, U. (2001) Insulin resistance and type 2 diabetes are not related to resistin expression in human fat cells or skelatel muscle. *Biochem. Biophys. Res. Commun.* 285:561-564

[134] Savage, D.B., Sewter, C.P., Klenk, E.S., Segal, D.G., Vidal-Puig, A., Considine, R.V., O'Rahilly, S. (2001) Resistin/Fizz3 expression in relation to obesity and peroxisome proliferator-activated receptor-□ action in humans. *Diabetes* 50:2199-2202

[135] Janke, J., Engeli, S., Gorzelniak, K., Luft, F.C., Sharma, A.M. (2002) Resistin gene expression in human adipocytes is not related to insulin resistance. *Obesity Research* 10:1-5

[136] Sentinelli, F., Romeo, S., Arca, M., Filippi, E., Leonetti, F., Banchieri, M., Di Mario, U., Baroni, M.G. (2002) Human resistin gene, obesity, and type 2 diabetes. *Diabetes* 51:860-862

[137] Osawa, H., Onuma, H., Murakami, A., Ochi, M., Nishimiya, T., Kato, K., Shimizu, I., Fujii, Y., Ohashi, J., Makino, H. (2002) Systematic search for single nucleotide polymorphisms in the resistin gene: the absence of evidence for the association of three identified single nucleotide polymorphisms with Japanese type 2 diabetes. *Diabetes* 51:863-866

[138] Engert, J.C., Vohl, M-C., Williams, S.M., Lepage, P., Loredo-Osti, J.C., Faith, J., Doré, C., Renaud, Y., Burtt, N.P., Villeneuve, A., Hirschhorn, J.N., Altshuler, D., Groop, L.C., Després, J-P., Gaudet, D., Hudson, T.J. (2002) 5' flanking variants of resistin are associated with obesity. *Diabetes* 51:1629-1634

[139] Wang, H., Chu, W.S., Hemphill, C., Elbein, S.C. (2002) Human resistin gene: molecular scanning and evaluation of association with insulin sensitivity and type 2 diabetes in caucasians. *J. Clin. Endocrinol. Metab.* 87:2520-2524

[140] Pizzuti, A., Frititta, L., Argiolas, A., Baratta, R., Goldfine, I., Bozzali, M., Ercolino, T., Scarlato, G., Iacovello, L., Vigneri, R., Tassi, V., Trischitta, V. (1999) A polymorphism (K121Q) of the human glycoprotein PC-1 gene coding region is strongly associated with insulin resistance. *Diabetes* 48:1881-1884

[141] Hanis, C., Boerwinkle, E., Chakraborty, R., Ellsworth, D., Concannon, P., Stirling, B., Morrison, V., Wapelhorst, B., Spielman, R., Goglin-Ewens, K., Shephard, J., Williams, S., Risch, N., Hinds, D., Iwasaki, N., Ogata, M., Omori, Y., Petzold, C., Rietsch, H., Schröder, H.-E., Schulze, J., Cox, N., Menzel, S., Boriraj, V., Chen, X., Lim, L., Lindner, T., Mereu, L., Wang, Y.-Q., Xiang, K., Yamagata, K., Yang, Y., Bell, G. (1996) A genome-wide search for human non-insulin-dependent (type 2) diabetes genes reveals a major susceptibility locus on chromosome 2. *Nat. Genet.* 13:161-166

[142] Horikawa Y., Oda, N., Cox, N.J., Li, X., Orho-Melander, M., Hara, M., Hinokio, Y., Lindner, T.H., Mashima, H., Schwarz, P.E., del Bosque-Plata, L., Horikawa, Y., Oda, Y., Yoshiuchi, I., Colilla, S., Polonsky, K.S., Wei, S., Concannon, P., Iwasaki, N.,

Schulze, J., Baier, L.J., Bogardus, C., Groop, L., Boerwinkle, E., Hanis, C.L., Bell, G.I. (2000) Genetic variation in the gene encoding calpain-10 is associated with type 2 diabetes mellitus. *Nat. Genet.* 26:163-175

[143] Baier, L.J., Permana, P.A., Yang, X., Pratley, R.E., Hanson, R.L., Shen, G.-Q., Mott, D., Knowler, W.C., Cox, N.J., Horikawa, Y., Oda, N., Bell, G.I., Bogardus, C. (2000) A calpain-10 gene polymorphism is associated with reduced muscle mRNA levels and insulin resistance. *J. Clin. Invest.* 106:R69-R73

[144] Orho-Melander, M., Klannemark, M., Svensson, M., Ridderstråle, M., Lindgren, C., Groop, L. (2002) Variants in the calpain-10 gene predispose to insulin resistance and elevated free fatty acid levels. *Diabetes* 51:2658-2664

[145] Sreenan, S.K., Zhou, Y.-P., Otani, K., Hansen, P.A., Currie, K.P.M., Pan, C.-Y., Lee, J.-P., Ostrega, D.M., Pugh, W., Horikawa, Y., Cox, N.J., Hanis, C.L., Burant, C.F., Fox, A.P., Bell, G.I., Polonsky, K.S. (2001) Calpains play a role in insulin secretion and action. *Diabetes* 50:2013-2020

[146] Zhou, Y.P, Sreenan, S., Pan, C.Y., Currie, K.B., Bindokas, V.P., Horikawa, Y., Lee, J.P., Ostrega, D., Ahmed, N., Baldwin, A.C., Cox, N.J., Fox, A.P., Miller, R.J., Bell, G.I., Polonsky, K.S. (2003) A 48-hour exposure of pancreatic islets to calpain inhibitors impairs mitochondrial fuel metabolism and exocytosis of insulin. *Metabolism* 52:528-534

[147] Paul, D.S., Harmon, A.W., Winston, C.P, Patel, Y.M. (2003) Calpain facilitates GLUT4 vesicle translocation during insulin-stimulated glucose uptake in adipocytes. *Biochem. J.* (Epub ahead of print)

[148] Maddux, B., Sbraccia, P., Kumakura, S., Sasson, S., Youngren, J., Fisher, A., Spemcer, S., Grupe, A., Henzel, W., Stewart, T., Reaven, G., Goldfine, I. (1995) Membrane glycoprotein PC-1 and insulin resistance in non-insulin dependent diabetes mellitus. *Nature* 373:448-451

[149] Pizzuti, A., Frititta, L., Argiolas, A., Baratta, R., Goldfine, I., Bozzali, M., Ercolino, T., Scarlato, G., Iacovello, L., Vigneri, R., Tassi, V., Trischitta, V. (1999) A polymorphism (K12Q) of the human glycoprotein PC-1 gene coding region is strongly associated with insulin resistance. *Diabetes* 48:1881-1884

[150] Gu, H.F., Almgren, P., Lindholm, E., Frittitta, L., Pizzuti, A., Trischitta, V., Groop, L.C. (2000) Association between the human glycoprotein PC-1 gene and elevated glucose and insulin levels in a paired -sibling analysis. *Diabetes* 49:1601-1603

[151] Kubaszek, A., Pihlajamäki, J., Karhapää, P., Vauhkonen, I., Laakso, M. (2003) The K121Q polymorphism of the PC-1 gene is associated with insulin resistance but not with dyslipidemia. *Diabetes Care* 26:464-467

[152] Sun, X., Rothenberg, P., Kahn, R., Backer, J., Arakai, E., Wilden, P., Cahill, D., Goldhill, B., White, M. (1991) Structure of the insulin receptor substrate IRS-1 defines a unique signal transduction protein. *Nature* 352:73-77

[153] Almind, K., Bjoerbaek, C., Vestergaard, H., Hansen, T., Echwald, S., Pedersen, O. (1993) Aminoacid polymorphism of the insulin receptor substrate -1 in non-insulin-dependent diabetes mellitus. *Lancet* 342:828-832

[154] Clausen, J., Hansen, T., Bjoerbaek, C., Echwald, S., Urhammer, S., Rasmussen, S., Andersen, C., Hansen, L., Almind, K., Winther, K., Haraldsdottir, J., Borch-Johnsen,

K., Pedersen, O. (1995) Insulin resistance:interactions between obesity and a common variant of the insulin receptor substrate-1. *Lancet* 346:397-402

[155] Abe, H., Yamada, N., Kamata, K., Kuwaki, T., Shimada, M., Osuga, j., Shionoiri, F., Yahagi, N., Kadowaki, T., Tamemoto, H., Ishibashi, S., Yazaki, Y., Makuuchi, M. (1998) Hypertension, hypertriglyceridemia, and impaired endothelium-dependent vascular relaxation in mice lacking insulin receptor substrate-1. *J. Clin. Invest.* 101:1784-1788

[156] Kubota, N., Tobe, K., Terauchi, Y., Eto, K., Yamauchi, T., Suzuki, R., Tsubamoto, Y., Komeda, K., Nakano, R., Miki, H., Satoh, S., Sekihara, H., Sciacchitano, S., Lesniak, M., Aizawa, S., Nagai, R., Kimura, S., Akanuma, Y., Taylor, S.I., Kadowaki, T. (2000) Disruption of insulin receptor substrate 2 causes type 2 diabetes because of liver insulin resistance and lack of compensatory beta-cell hyperplasia. *Diabetes* 50:1880-1889

[157] Smith, U., Gogg, S., Johansson, A., Olausson, T., Rotter, V., Svalstedt, B. (2001) Thiazolidinediones (PPARgamma agonists) but not PPARalpha agonists increase IRS-2 gene expression in 3T3-L1 and human adipocytes. *FASEB* 15:215-220

[158] Eriksson, J., Franssila-Kallunki, A., Ekstrand, A., Saloranta, C., Widen, E., Schalin, C., Groop, L. (1989) Early metabolic defects in persons at increased risk for non-insulin-dependent diabetes mellitus. *New Engl J Med* 321:337-343

[159] Lehto, M., Stoffel, M., Groop, L., Espinosa III, R., LeBeau, M., Bell, G. (1993) Assignment of the gene encoding gycogen synthase to human chromosome 19, band q13.3. *Genomics* 15:460-461

[160] Orho, M., Nikula-Ijäs, P., Schalin-Jäntti, C., Permutt, M., Groop, L. (1995) Isolation and characterization of the human muscle glycogen synthase gene. *Diabetes* 44:1099-1105

[161] Groop, L., Kankuri, M., Schalin-Jäntti , C., Ekstrand, A., Nikula-Ijäs, P., Widèn, E., Kuismanen, E., Eriksson, J., Franssila-Kallunki, A., Saloranta, C., Koskimies, S. (1993) Association between polymorphism of the glycogen synthase gene and non-insulin-dependent diabetes mellitus. *New Engl. J. Med.* 328:10-14

[162] Majer, M., Mott, D., Mochizuki, H., Rowles, J., Pedersen, O., Knowler, W., Bogardus, C., Prochazka, M. (1996) Association of the glycogen synthase locus 19q13 with NIDDM in Pima Indians. *Diabetologia* 39:314-321

[163] Orho-Melander, M., Almgren, P., Kanninen, T., Forsblom, C., Groop, L. (1999) A paired sibling analysis of the XbaI polymorphism in the muscle glycogen synthase gene. *Diabetologia* 42:1138-1145

[164] Fenger, M., Poulsen, P., Beck-Nielsen, H., Vaag, A. (2000) Impact of the Xba1-polymorphism of the human muscle glycogen synthase gene on parameters of the insulin resistance syndrome in a Danish twin population. *Diabet Med.* 17:735-740

[165] St-Onge, J., Joanisse, D.R., Simoneau, J.A. (2001) The stimulation-induced increase in skeletal muscle glycogen synthase content is impaired in carriers of the glycogen synthase XbaI gene polymorphism. *Diabetes* 50:195-198

[166] Lohmueller, K.E., Pearce, C.L., Pike, M., Lander, E.S., Hieschhorn, J.N. (2003) Meta-analysis of genetic association studies supports a contribution of common variants to susceptibility to common disease. *Nat. Genet.* 33:177-182

[167] Seldin, M., Mott, D., Bhat, D., Petro, A., Kuhn, C., Kingsmore, S., Bogardus, C., Opara, E., Feinglos, M., Surwit, R. (1994) Glycogen synthase: a putative locus for diet-induced hyperglycemia. *J. Clin. Invest.* 94:1-8.

[168] Bell, G.I., Selby, M.J., Rutter, W.J. (1982) The highly polymorphic region near the human insulin gene is composed of simple tandemly repeating sequences. *Nature* 295:31-35

[169] Lucassen, A.M., Juloer, C., Beressi, J.-P., Boitard, C., Froguel, P., Lathrop, M., Bell, J.I. (1993) Susceptibility to insulin dependent diabetes mellitus maps to a 4.1 kb segment of DNA spanning the insulin gene and associated VNTR. *Nat. Genet.* 4:305-310

[170] Bennett, S.T., Wilson, A.J., Esposito, L., Bouzekri, N., Undlien, D.E., Cucca, F., Nistico, L., Buzzetti, R., the IMDIAB Group, Bosi, E., Pociot, F., Nerup, J., Cambon-Thomsen, A., Pugliese, A., Shield. J.P.H., Kinney, P.A., Bain, S.C., Polychronakos, C., Todd. J.A. (1997) insulin VNTR allele-specific effect in type 1 diabetes depends on identity of untransmitted paternal allele. *Nat. Genet.* 17:350-352

[171] Le Stunff, C., Fallin, D., Bougnères, P. (2001) paternal transmission of the very common class I INS VNTR alleles predisposes to childhood obesity. *Nat. Genet.* 29:96-99

[172] Lindsay, R.S., Hanson, R.L., Wiedrich, C., Knowler, W.C., Bennett, P.H., Baier, L.J. (2003) The insulin gene variable number tandem repeat class I/III polymorphism is in linkage disequilibrium with birth weight but not type 2 diabetes in the Pima population. *Diabetes* 52:187-193

[173] Kennedy, G.C., German, M.S., Rutter, W.J. (1995) The minisatellite in the diabetes susceptibility locus IDDM2 regulates insulin transcription. *Nat. Genet.* 9:293-298

[174] Lucassen, A.M., Screaton, G.R., Julier, C., Elliott, T.J., Lathrop, M., Bell, J.I. (1995) Regulation of insulin gene expression by the IDDM associated, insulin locus haplotype. *Hum. Mol. Genet.* 4:501-506

[175] Vafiadis, P., Bennett, S.T., Colle, E., Grabs, R., Goodyer, C.G., Polychronakos, C. (1996) Imprinted and genotype-specific expression of genes at the IDDM2 locus in pancreas and leucocytes. *J. Autoimmun.*. 9:397-403

[176] Pugliese, A., Zeller, M., Fernandez, A., Jr., Zalcberg, L.J., Bartlett, R.J., Ricordi, C., Pietropaolo, M., Eisenbarth, G.S., Bennett, S.T., Patel, D.D. (1997) The insulin gene is transcribed in the human thymus and transcription levels correlated with allelic variation at the INS VNTR-IDDM2 susceptibility locus for type 1 diabetes. *Nat. Genet.* 15:293-297

[177] Undlien, D.E., Berg, J.P. (2001) Common variants in the regulatory region of the insulin gene are associated with fasting plasma insulin levels in juvenile obesity. *Eur. J. Endocrinol.* 5:457-459

[178] Huxtable, S.J., Saker, P.J., Haddad, L., Walker, M., Frayling, T.M., Levy, J.C., Hitman, G.A., O'Rahilly, S., Hattersley, A.T., McCarthy, M.I. (2000) Analysis of parent-offspring trios provides evidence for linkage and association between the insulin gene and type 2 diabetes mediated exclusively through paternally transmitted class III variable number tandem repeat alleles. *Diabetes* 49:126-130

[179] Aguilar-Bryan, L., Bryan, J. (1999) Molecular biology of triphosphate-sensitive potassium channels. *Endocrine Rev.* 20:101-135

[180] Hani, E.H, Boutin, P., Durand, E., Inoue, H., Permutt, M.A., Velho, G., Froguel, P. (1998) Missense mutations in the pancreatic islet beta cell inwardly rectifying K+ channel gene (KIR6.2/BIR): a meta-analysis suggests a role in the polygenic basis of Type II diabetes mellitus in Caucasians. *Diabetologia* 41:1511-1515

[181] Love-Gregory, L., Wasson, J., Lin, J., Skolnick, G., Suarez, B., Permutt, M.A. (2002) An E23K single nucleotide polymorphism in the islet ATP-sensitive potassium channel gene (Kir6.2) contributes as much to the risk of type II diabetes in Caucasians as the PPARγPro12Ala variant. *Diabetologia* 43:136-137

[182] Gloyn, A.L., Weedon, M.N., Owen, K.R., Turner, M.J., Knight, B.A., Hitman, G., Walker, M., Levy, J.C., Sampson, M., Halford, S., McCarthy, M., Hattersley, A.T., Frayling, T.M. (2003) Large scale association studies of variants in genes encoding the pancreatic β-cell KATP channel subunits Kir 6.2 (KCNJ11) and <SUR1 (ABCC8) confirm that the KCNJ11 E23K variant is<associated with type 2 diabetes. *Diabetes* 52:568-572

[183] Nielsen, E.M., Hansen, L., Carstensen, B., Echwald, S.M., Drivsholm, T., Glumer, C., Thorsteinsson, B., Borch-Johnsen, K., Hansen, T., Pedersen, O. (2003) The E23K variant of Kir6.2 associates with impaired post-OGTT serum insulin response and increased risk of type 2 diabetes. *Diabetes* 52:573-577

[184] Schwanstecher, C., Neugebauer, B., Schulz, M., Schwanstecher, M. (2002) The common single nucleotide polymorphism E23K in K(IR)6.2 sensitizes pancreatic beta-cell ATP-sensitive potassium channels toward activation through nucleoside diphosphates. *Diabetes* 51(Suppl 3):S363-S367

[185] Thomas, P.M., Cote, G.J., Wohllk, N., Haddad, B., Mathew, P.M., Rabl, W., Aguilar-Bryan, L., Gagel, R.F., Bryan, J. (1995) Mutations in the sulfonylurea receptor gene in familial persistent hyperinsulinemic hypoglycemia of infancy. *Science* 268:426-429

[186] Huopio, H., Reimann, F., Ashfield, R., Komulainen, J., Lenko, H-L., Rahier, J., Vauhkonen, I., Kere, J., Laakso, M., Aschcroft, F., Otonkoski, T. (2000) Dominantly inherited hyperinsulinism caused by a mutation in the sulfonylrea receptor type 1. *J. Clin. Invest* 106:897-906

[187] Huopio, H., Otonkoski, T., Vauhkonen, I., Reimann, F., Aschcroft, F.M., Laakso, M. (2003) A new subtype of autosomal dominant diabetes attributable to a mutation in the gene for sulfonylurea receptor 1. *Lancet* 361:301-307

[188] Hansen, T., Ambye, L., Grarup, N., Hansen, L., Echwald, S.M., Ferrer, J., Pedersen, O. (2001) Genetic variability of the SUR1 promoter in relation to beta-cell function and Type II diabetes mellitus. *Diabetologia* 44:1330-1334

[189] Lembertas, A., Perusse, L., Chagnon, Y., Fisler, J., Warden, C., Purcell-Huynh, D., Dionne, F., Gagnon, J., Nadeau, A., Lusis, A., Bouchard, C. (1997) Identification of an obesity quantitative trait locus on mouse chromosome 2 and evidence of linkage to body fat and insulin on human homologous region 20q. *J. Clin. Invest.* 100:1240-1247

[190] Norman, R., Thompson, D., Foroud, T., Garvey, W., Bennett, P., Bogardus, C., Ravussin, E. (1996) Genomewide search for genes influencing percent body fat in Pima Indians: suggestive linkage at chromosome 11q21-q22. *Am. J. Hum. Genet.* 60:166-173

[191] Hanis, C., Boerwinkle, E., Chakraborty, R., Ellsworth, D., Concannon, P., Stirling, B., Morrison, V., Wapelhorst, B., Spielman, R., Goglin-Ewens, K., Shephard, J., Williams, S., Risch, N., Hinds, D., Iwasaki, N., Ogata, M., Omori, Y., Petzold, C., Rietsch, H., Schröder, H.-E., Schulze, J., Cox, N., Menzel, S., Boriraj, V., Chen, X., Lim, L., Lindner, T., Mereu, L., Wang, Y.-Q., Xiang, K., Yamagata, K., Yang, Y., Bell, G. (1996) A genome-wide search for human non-insulin-dependent (type 2) diabetes genes reveals a major susceptibility locus on chromosome 2. *Nat. Genet.* 13:161-166

[192] Mahtani, M.M., Widen, E., Lehto, M., Thomas, J., McCarthy, M., Brayer, J., Bryant, B., Chan, G., Daly, M., Forsblom, C., Kanninen, T., Kirby, A., Kruglyak, L., Munnelly, K., Parkkonen, M., Reeve Daly, M.P., Weaver, A., Brettin, T., Duyk, G., Lander, E.S., Groop, L.C. (1996) Mapping of a gene for type 2 diabetes associated with an insulin secretion defect by a genome scan in Finnish families. *Nat. Genet.* 14:90-94

[193] Zouali, H., Hani, E., Philippi, A., Vionnet, N., Beckmann, J., Demenais, F., Froguel, P. (1997) A susceptibility locus for early-onset non-insulin dependent (type 2) diabetes mellitus maps to chromosome 20q, proximal to the phosphoenolpyruvate carboxykinase gene. *Hum. Mol. Gen.* 6:1401-1408

[194] Ghosh, S., Watanabe, R., Hauser, E., Valle, T., Magnuson, V., Erdos, M., Langefeld, C., BalowJr, J., Ally, D., Kohtamäki, K., Chines, P., Birznieks, G., Kaleta, H.-S., Musick, A., Te, C., Tannenbaum, J., Eldridge, W., Shapiro, S., Martin, C., Alyson, W., So, A., Chang, J., Shurtleff, B., Porter, R., Kudelko, K., Unni, A., Segal, L., Sharaf, R., Blaschak-Harvan, J., Eriksson, J., Tenkula, T., Vidgren, G., Ehnholm, C., Tuomilehto-Wolf, E., Hagopian, W., Buchanan, T., Tuomilehto, J., Bergman, R., Collins, F., Boehnke, M. (1999) Type 2 diabetes: evidence for linkage on chromosome 20 in 716 Finnish affected sib pairs. *Proc. Natl. Acad. Sci. USA* 96:2198-2203

In: Trends in Diabetes Research
Editor: Ashley M. Ford, pp. 71-106
ISBN: 1-59454-796-3

Chapter IV

Reactive Oxygen Species and K^+ Channel Function in Diabetes and Insulin Resistance

Yanping Liu[1*], *Jefferson C. Frisbee*[2] *and David D. Gutterman*[1]
[1] Cardiovascular Center, VA Medical Center, Medical College of Wisconsin, 8701 Watertown Plank Road, Milwaukee, WI 53226
[2] Center for Interdisciplinary Research in Cardiovascular Sciences Department of Physiology and Pharmacology, West Virginia University Morgantown, West Virginia 26506

Abstract

Diabetes mellitus is associated with an increased prevalence of cardiovascular disease. Enhanced oxidative stress has been implicated in impaired vasomotor responsiveness in diabetes. Recent evidence suggests that reactive oxygen species (ROS) induced by hyperglycemia play an essential role in altered activity of potassium (K^+) channels, a target of endothelium-dependent hyperpolarizing factors (EDHFs). The enhanced oxidative stress may occur prior to the development of frank diabetes, such as insulin resistance. This review focuses on the mechanism of ROS production in hyperglycemia and insulin resistance and describes the consequences on hyperpolarization-mediated vasodilation.

Several pathways have been proposed as mechanisms for hyperglycemia-induced-superoxide overproduction, including activation of polyol pathway, activation of the diacylglycerol-protein kinase C pathway, upregulation of NADPH oxidase and mitochondrial generation of ROS. The resulting excess production of superoxide has been implicated in the impaired dilator responses to K_{ATP} channel openers in aorta,

* Correspondence to: Yanping Liu, M.D., Ph.D.Cardiovascular Center, Medical College of Wisconsin 8701 Watertown Plank Road, Milwaukee, WI 53226 (414) 456-5633 Phone (414) 456-6572 Fax E-mail: ypliu@mcw.edu

mesenteric and cerebral arteries of streptozotosin-induced diabetic rats and in coronary arterioles from patients with diabetes. This may have important implications in ischemia-mediated vasodilation. The effect of ROS on K_v channel function has been examined in xenopus oocytes where shaker and shaw channel were expressed. Reduced K^+ currents were observed in most shaker channels. Incubation of small rat coronary arteries in high glucose for 24 hours increases both superoxide and peroxynitrite generation, which greatly reduces K_v channel activity and functional responses, both of which can be partially restored by antioxidant treatment. In contrast to K_{ATP} and K_v channels, Ca^{2+}-activated K^+ channels are refractory to superoxide providing a compensatory mechanism for reduced dilator response to activation of other K^+ channels. However, in conditions where peroxynitrite is increased, K_{Ca} channel function is inhibited. In this circumstance, compensatory dilator mechanism acting through hyperpolarization may fail.
Insulin resistance, a condition where insulin-induced glucose uptake is reduced, is considered to be a precursor to the development of type II diabetes mellitus. In hyperinsulinemia, impaired vasodilator responses are observed in variety of vascular beds of obesity animals even in normoglycemia or mild hyperglycemia. Reduced K^+ channel function, such as K_{Ca} and K_{ATP} channels, may be a mechanism responsible for the impaired vascular reactivity in insulin resistance. Treatment with antioxidants such as superoxide dismutase restores the dilator response in obese animals supporting an inhibitory role of ROS in vasomotor function in the insulin resistant state.
In summary, determining the effect of ROS on K^+ channel mediated dilation is important for understanding the pathophysiology of vascular dysfunction in diabetes and insulin resistance and may suggest new therapies to improve tissue perfusion.

Introduction

Diabetes mellitus is a major source of morbidity in the United States, almost exclusively due to concomitant vascular disease. Substantial evidence suggests that endothelial dependent dilation is reduced in diabetes largely due to reduced bioavailability of nitric oxide (NO) [1,13,39,51]. Enhanced oxidative stress has been postulated as one of the mechanisms for the impaired NO-mediated dilation, since treatment with free radical scavengers provides protection against impaired dilation [35,56,73]. It is widely recognized that in certain vascular beds especially in microcirculation, a major class of compounds distinct from NO, endothelial derived hyperpolarization factors (EDHF's), are released from the endothelium and are responsible for vasodilation by opening K^+ channels. Although it has been suggested that EDHF may compensate for loss of NO in certain disease situations, such as hypercholesterolemia[141,142], reactive oxygen species (ROS) may globally affect endothelium-dependent dilator mechanisms including EDHF.

ROS interactions with EDHF may take place at the vascular smooth muscle cell (VSMC) K^+ channels, the target site of EDHF. However knowledge about redox modulation of K^+-channel activity is limited. Understanding these mechanisms is important for developing therapeutic strategies to reverse vascular dysfunction. This review will focus on the interaction of oxidative stress with K^+ channel activity in the vasculature.

Physiological Importance and Basic Structure of K^+ Channels

There are many types of K^+ channels have been identified in vasculature. Among them, there are three major types of potassium (K^+) channels, including ATP-sensitive K^+ (K_{ATP}) channels, voltage-gated K^+ (K_v) channels and calcium-activated K^+ (K_{Ca}) channels have been proposed playing critical role in regulating vasomotor function. Their physiological importance and basic structures are summarized below.

K_{ATP} Channels

K_{ATP} channels exist in pancreatic β cells, neurons, skeletal muscle, vascular and non-vascular smooth muscle [75]. The physiologic role of K_{ATP} channels is to couple the electrical activity of the cells to their metabolic rate by sensing changes in the concentrations of adenine nucleotides (ATP and ADP). In pancreatic β cells, ATP increases when the plasma glucose level rises. The closure of K_{ATP} channels by ATP induces depolarization of cell membrane, which triggers calcium entry and insulin release [75]. In cardiac myocytes, ATP falls as a result of hypoxia, opening of K_{ATP} channels shortens the cardiac action potential and reduces cardiac work [18,48]. K_{ATP} channel in vascular smooth muscle senses changes in oxygen [54,118,133], pH [67] and metabolic products, such as adenosine [143], and opening of these channels produces vasodilation. Growing evidence also suggests that K_{ATP} channels in the inner membrane of the mitochondria play an important role in cardiac ischemic preconditioning [86,120].

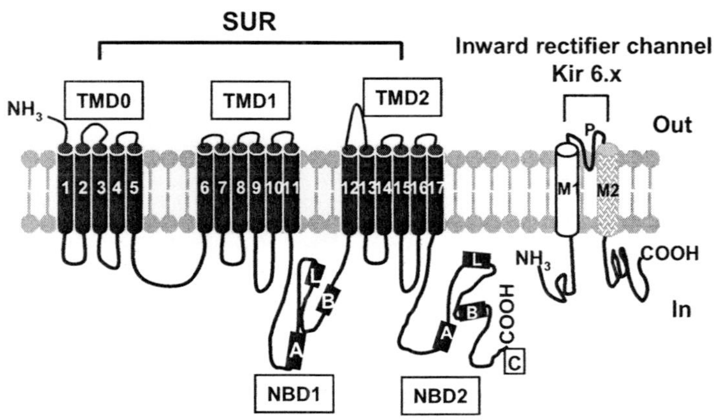

Figure 1. K_{ATP} channels are composed of an ATP-binding cassette protein (the sulfonylurea receptor, SUR) and Kir 6.X subunits. SUR is consisted of three transmembrane domains (TMD0, TMD1 and TMD2) and two nucleotide-binding domains (NBD1 and NBD2). The NBDs are characterized by conserved sequence motifs involved in the binding and hydrolysis of ATP at sites labeled A and B and in the transmission of the signal to transmembrane domain through linker (L). The TM 16 and 17, the intracellular loop between TM13 and TM14, and the region termed C are the binging areas for K^+ channel openers. In Kir 6.0, M1 and M2 represent the transmembrane domains, with a pore region (P). Adapted from reference [177]

At the molecular level the channel is a complex of two subunits (Fig. 1), namely the sulphonylurea receptor (SUR), a member of the ATP binding cassette family of proteins, and a channel pore forming subunit (K_{ir} 6.x), a member of the inwardly rectifying family of K^+ channels.

SUR is composed of two intracellular nucleotide binding domains (NBD1 and NBD2) and three transmembrane domains (TMD0, TMD1 and TMD2) that contain five, six and six transmembrane helix (TMs), respectively [75]. The TM 16 and 17, the intracellular loop between TM13 and TM14, and at the $COOH^-$ terminal are the binding areas for potassium channel openers. Two genes for SUR receptors have been identified, encoding the proteins SUR1 and SUR2 which are expressed in different tissues [3,93]. SUR1 is predominantly found in pancreatic β-cells and neurons. Alternative splicing of SUR2 produces a cardiac/skeletal muscle isoform (SUR2A) [101] and smooth muscle isoform (SUR2B) [101]. In addition to tissue specificity of SUR isoforms, the sensitivity to K_{ATP} channel openers between SUR1 and SUR2 type K_{ATP} channel are also different. For example, pinacidil, P1075, cromakalim and nicorandil, activate SUR2-type K_{ATP} channels, but have little effect on SUR1-type channels [162,163]. These properties are of therapeutic importance for selecting K_{ATP} channel opener therapy. For instance, nicroandil is used as a vasodilator for the treatment of angina, and does not impair insulin secretion from the pancreatic β-cells [17,162]. In contrast, diazoxide, has both vasodilatory and insulin inhibitory effects [17].

Two clones of the inwardly rectifying component, K_{ir} 6.1 and K_{ir} 6.2, have been isolated. Studies examining the distribution of K_{ir} 6.x in variety of tissues indicate that K_{ir} 6.2 is expressed in heart [92], brain[91], skeletal muscle[92], smooth muscl[101] and pancreatic tissue[91], but not in visceral smooth muscle or lung[16], whereas K_{ir} 6.1 is more widely expressed in these tissues as well as in visceral smooth muscle [191].

Voltage-Gated K⁺ Channels

Numerous studies have demonstrated that K_v channels contribute to the resting membrane potential in coronary [49,114,122], cerebral [4], and pulmonary [87,108,174] circulations, and that pharmacological inhibition of these channels depolarizes and constricts arteries and arterioles. Several studies have shown that K_v channels mediate pharmacological dilator responses. The β-adrenoceptor agonist isoproterenol, or the adenylate cyclase activator forskolin, increases 4-AP sensitive K^+ currents in rabbit portal veins and coronary arteries [5,6]. Studies from our laboratory indicate that 4-aminopyridine (4-AP), a K_v channel blocker, reduces dilation of rat small coronary arteries to isoproterenol and to forskolin [114] suggesting an important role of K_v channels in the coronary microcirculation. K_v channels are also involved in a variety of other vasomotor responses. Inhibition of K_v channels is a mechanism for hypoxic pulmonary vasoconstriction[87,159]. In the coronary circulation, activation of histamine H_1-receptors inhibits 4-AP sensitive K^+ channels consistent with a role for K_v channels in coronary vasospasm[100]. The vasoconstrictor effect of angiotensin II is, in part, mediated by a reduction in K_v current[47]. K_v channels also have been shown to regulate coronary vascular tone in response to changes in pH of rat coronary arterial myocytes[22].

K_v channels have been described in most types of vascular smooth muscle cells [12]. They emanate from at least 11 gene families (*i.e.*, K_v1 – K_v11). *Drosophila* channels including *Shaker* (K_v1), *Shab* (K_v2), *Shaw* (K_v3) and *Shal* (K_v4) have been well characterized. Recent reports have document the expression of three *Shaker* K^+ channel subtypes (K_v 1.2, 1.4 1.5) in vascular smooth muscle cells from several critical regulatory beds, including the coronary, pulmonary and renal circulations [66,87,122,131,149,186]. As shown in Figure 2, K_v channels have four transmembrane domains. Each domain is composed of two subunits, α and β.

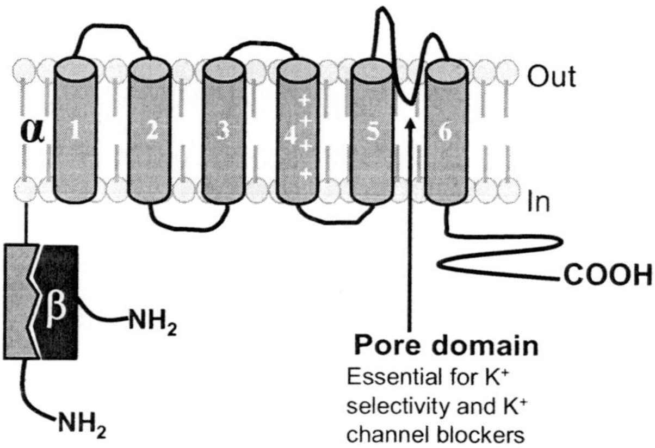

Figure 2. The putative membrane-spanning segments of the α-subunit of K_v channel are designated as S1-S6. S4 segment is considered as a voltage sensor. P loop of α-subunit is a critical portion for K^+ ion selectivity and conductivity. The extracellular portion of P loop contains the binding sites for toxins. The intracellular side of P loop has the binding sites for compounds such as 4-AP, tetraethylammonium, and quinidine. The N-terminal domain of the α-subunit contains the binding site for β-subunit (black area). Adapted from reference [193]

There are six transmembrane segments (S1-S6) and a pore-forming region between S5 and S6 in the α subunit[44,158]. Three amino acid residues containing an aromatic ring located in the S5-S6 linker, namely, two tryptophans and one tyrosine, are common to the pore or P loop and are considered as a critical site for K^+ ion selectivity and conductivity. The extracellular portion of the P loop contains the binding sites for toxins, such as iberiotoxin and charybdotoxin. The intracellular side of P loop has the binding sites for compounds such as 4-AP, tetraethylammonium, and quinidine [172]. S4 segment is considered a voltage sensor. This segment contains positively charged residues (lysine, arginine and histidine) at approximately every third position. Membrane depolarization causes S4 conformational changes, which interact with S5 and S6 leading to channel opening. $K_v\beta$ subunits that are attached to NH_3 terminals of α-subunits alter channel kinetics and modify cell surface expression. [32,61,140,161,164,170]. Recent studies suggest that K_v β may have NADPH oxidoreductase activity. Therefore the N-terminal domain of K_v channel may redox-sensitive [2].

Ca^{2+}-Activated K^+ Channels

An important physiological role of K_{Ca} channels in vascular smooth muscle stems from the fact that these channels serve a negative feedback role, opposing depolarization, VSMC Ca^{2+} entry, and vasoconstriction. In the vasculature, K_{Ca} and K_v channels open at different stages of depolarization. In response to initial depolarizing stimuli, the opening of K_v channels provides the initial negative feedback to attenuate vasoconstriction. The subsequent increase in cytosolic free Ca^{2+}, however, closes the K_v channels resulting in further depolarization. Both membrane depolarization and the rise in cytosolic Ca^{2+} act synergistically to enhance the opening of K_{Ca} channels and limit arterial constriction. K_{Ca} channels have also been postulated to respond directly to several endogenous vasodilators. For instance, nitric oxide induced relaxation are inhibited by K_{Ca} channel blockers such as tetraethylammonium [11,12,23] and iberiotoxin [23,58,146] in variety of vascular beds. Li et al demonstrated that K_{Ca} channels are involved in response to cytochrome P450 metabolites, such as epoxyeicosatrienoic acid [116,117]. In pathological conditions such as hypertension, overexpression of K_{Ca} channels is observed in cerebral [119], coronary[76], renal[127] and mesenteric microcirculation [14,52] and activation of these channels permits small arteries to maintain an optimal diameter for the perfusion of distal tissues.

Most of molecular studies of K_{Ca} channel structure have focused on large conductance Ca^{2+}-activated K^+ channels. Unlike K_v channels that originate from multiple gene familes, K_{Ca} channel α-subunits appear to arise from a single gene family [132]. K_{Ca} channel shares partial homology with the shaker K_v channels, containing six transmembrane segments (S1-S6) and a highly conserved pore region between S5 and S6 [132]. Similar to K_v channels, the voltage sensor is located at S4. Ca^{2+} sensitivity of the K_{Ca} channels is conferred by an extra four transmembrane segments (S7-S10) at the C-terminal region of the α-subunit, and by close association with a single regulatory β-subunit [187]. A Ca^{2+} binding motif composed of a string of aspartate residues may provide a site for Ca^{2+} binding on the C-terminal region. Additionally, interaction between the α-subunit and β-subunit greatly enhances Ca^{2+} sensitivity to the K_{Ca} channels. Studies by Hanner et al [78] suggest that co-expression of β-subunits also increases the binding of high-affinity peptidyl toxin blockers, such as iberiotoxin, to the mouth of the α-subunit of the K_{Ca} channels, thereby occluding the passage of ions through the pore.

Impaired Vasomotor Function in Diabetes and Insulin Resistance

Vascular endothelial cells play an important role in maintaining cardiovascular homeostasis. In addition to providing a physical barrier between the vessel wall and circulating blood, the endothelium secretes mediators that regulate platelet aggregation [53,85,111], coagulation [151,180], fibrinolysis [41,168,175] and vessel tone [79,126]. Endothelial dysfunction results from an imbalance in the production of these mediators, which may reduce dilation, and promote vasoconstriction and thrombosis.

The role of the endothelium in regulating vasomotor tone is one of the most widely studied aspects of vascular function. Endothelial cells release vasodilator substances including nitric oxide (NO), prostacyclin (PGI_2) and endothelium-derived hyperpolarizing factor (EDHF). NO is the major contributor to endothelium-dependent relaxation in large arteries with PGI_2 and EDHF playing a less prominent role. In addition to regulating vessel tone, NO protects the blood vessel from atherosclerosis by stimulating molecular signals that prevent platelet and leukocyte interaction with the vascular wall and inhibit vascular smooth muscle proliferation. In small resistance arteries, EDHF predominates as a mediator of endothelium-dependent dilation by opening K^+ channels in vascular smooth muscle membranes.

In diabetes, including both type 1 and type 2, numerous studies have shown the impairment of endothelium-dependent relaxation to various receptor-mediated agonists, including acetylcholine [1,13,55], bradykinin [74,155], and flow-mediated dilation [13,71] in different vascular beds from human [45,153] or animal tissue [71,102,150]. Endothelial dysfunction in diabetes appears to be associated specifically with hyperglycemia rather than other metabolic disturbances. As gleaned from vitro studies, exposure of arteries to high glucose mimics impaired endothelium-dependent dilation, that occurs in diabetes. However altered vasomotor function in diabetes is not only due to endothelial dysfunction. Previous studies [114,122] from our laboratory suggest that vascular smooth muscle cell are also involved, particularly, K^+ channel mechanisms as is discussed in detail below.

Insulin resistance states typified by obesity, type 2 diabetes and polycystic ovarian syndrome are associated with impaired glucose uptake into skeletal muscle and fat cells, and inhibition of lipolysis in adipose tissue resulting in increase systemic free fatty acid release.. Insulin resistance has been extensively studied with respect to its role in the pathogenesis of type 2 diabetes. However, recent studies in animals and humans demonstrate that in addition to the impaired classic actions of insulin, dilations to endothelium-dependent pharmacological stimuli are also decreased in insulin resistance. The impaired vasomotor function involving both endothelium and smooth muscle cells is independent of hyperglycemia as discussed below.

Hyperglycemia, Oxidative Stress and Sources for Generating Reactive Oxygen Species

The Enhanced oxidative stress of hyperglycemia has been linked to the vascular complications of diabetes[88]. Several lines of evidence suggest that the production of superoxide is increased when levels of glucose are elevated. Tesfamarian and Cohen showed that incubation of rabbit aorta in 44 mM glucose impaired NO-mediated dilation by an SOD-inhibitable mechanism [178]. Similarly, studies performed in our laboratory demonstrated increased superoxide production by fluorescence microscopy with hydroethidine as a probe, in rat coronary resistance arteries exposed to 23 mM glucose for 24 hours [122]. The enhanced fluorescence intensity can be reversed by superoxide dismutase indicating the contribution of superoxide.

As a consequence of the quenching of superoxide by NO, a potent antioxidant byproduct is formed, peroxynitrite. Peroxynitrite ($ONOO^-$) is a strong and relatively stable oxidant species capable of causing lipid peroxidation and nitration of tyrosine residues on key cellular proteins[125,165,194,195). An elevated level of peroxynitrite has been reported in diabetic patients [34,36,37] and in rat small coronary arteries [115] incubated in vitro in high glucose , and in aortic endothelial cells [195].

Since glucose and its metabolites can affect multiple pathways, there are several biochemical mechanisms that appear to explain the sources for generating reactive oxygen species in hyperglycemia. For instance, glucose is transported into the vascular cells mostly by GLUT-1 transporters, which can be regulated by extracellular glucose concentration. Once glucose is transported, it is metabolized to alter signal transduction pathways, such as activation of diacylglycerol and protein kinase C, or to increase flux through the mitochondria to change the redox states. The common pathways of sources for generating reactive oxygen species are described below.

Activation of Polyol Pathway

The polyol pathway consists of two enzymes, aldose reductase which reduces glucose to sorbitol in the presence of NADPH, and sorbitol dehydrogenase which converts sorbitol to fructose with its co-factor NAD. Under conditions of euglycemia, the intracellular concentration of sorbitol is very low due to high enzyme kinetics of aldose reductase. However, when glucose level is elevated, more glucose is channeled into polyol pathway. The conversion of glucose to sorbitol in cells by aldose reductase has been associated with microvascular complications and enhanced oxidative stress in diabetes [31,43,60]. In animal models, treatment with aldose reductase inhibitors effectively prevents the development of various diabetic complications, including cataract [68], neuropathy [40,60,192], and nephropathy [20].

There are three potential mechanisms by which the polyol pathway can contribute to oxidative stress. First, activation of the polyol pathway depletes the co-factor NADPH, which is required for generating glutathione, a key intracellular antioxidant. Second, the production of NADH is increased in the process of oxidation of sorbitol to fructose. NADH is a substrate for NADPH oxidase for generating reactive oxygen species (ROS). Finally, fructose, the product of polyol pathway and its metabolites, fructose 3-phosphate and 3-deoxyglucosone are glycation agents, which increase in the formation of advanced glycation end products (AGE) and cause oxidative stress.

However, enhanced oxidative stress in diabetes can not be fully explained by activation of the polyol pathway. For example, aldose reductase inhibitor, sobinil or tolrestat, caused only a modest improvement in the impaired endothelium-dependent dilation by glucose exposed platelets in rabbit carotid arteries [148]. In sciatic nerve, the level of sorbitol does not correspond to the severity of neural dysfunction [145]. These observations suggest that other mechanisms may also be involved in the generation of ROS in diabetes.

Activation of Diacylglycerol-Protein Kinase C Pathway

In animals with chemically or genetically induced diabetes, enhanced protein kinase C (PKC) activity has been observed in many vascular tissues such as the aorta, heart, retina, and renal glomeruli [27,72,82,95,97,97,99,112]. The diacylglycerol (DAG) level has also been shown to be increased parallel with PKC. Increasing glucose levels from 5 to 22 mmol/L in the culture media elevated cellular DAG levels in aortic endothelial and smooth muscle cells [94], retinal endothelial cells [171] and renal mesangial cells [15,176] suggesting the important contribution of DAG in elevated level of PKC in diabetes. DAG can be generated from multiple pathways. Several studies examining the source of generation of DAG associated with high glucose indicate that increased level of DAG by high glucose are derived partly from the *de novo* pathway. For example, in labeling studies using [6-3H]- or [U-14C]-glucose, elevated glucose increased the incorporation of glucose into the glycerol backbone of DAG in aortic endothelial cells, aortic smooth muscle cells and renal glomeruli. Another pathway for excess DAG production in high glucose is the result of glycol-oxidation induced activation of the DAG pathway, since oxidants such as H_2O_2 are known to activate the DAG-PKC pathway. One of the actions of PKC is to activate NAD(P)H oxidase, an enzyme for generation of superoxide. Exposure of cultured bovine aortic endothelial and smooth muscle cells in glucose (400 mg/dl for 72 hours) significantly increased free radical generation measured by electron spin resonance, compared to the cells incubated in 100 mg/dl glucose. A similar increment in free radical formation was also observed in cells treated with phorbol myristic acid (PMA), a PKC activator. The enhanced free radical production by high glucose or by PMC can be restored by diphenylene iodonium (DPI), a NADPH oxidase inhibitor and PKC inhibitor, calphosin C or GF109203X indicating that high glucose stimulates ROS generation via a PKC-dependent activation of NADPH oxidases in vascular cells.

The activation of PKC by hyperglycemia appears to be tissue specific, since it has been noted in the retina, aorta, heart and glomeruli but not in the brain and peripheral nerves in diabetic animals. Therefore other pathways may also be involved in the production of ROS in diabetes.

Upregulation of NADPH Oxidase

NADPH oxidases of the cardiovascular system are membrane-associated enzymes that catalyze the production of superoxide from molecular oxygen and NADPH. This enzymatic activity has been shown to be the major oxidase in vascular tissue [139,160,189] and in cardiac cells [138] as compared with production of ROS from xanthine oxidase, arachidonic acid, and mitochondrial oxidases.

The vascular form of the NADPH oxidase consists of two membrane-bound elements, gp91phox and p22phox, two cytosolic components, p67phox and p47phox, and a low molecular weight G protein, either rac 2 or rac 1. The essential subunit of the NADPH oxidase is gp91phox, to which are bound the electron carrying components of the oxidase. p22phox has a tail in the cytosol. When p47phox is phosphorylated, it binds to p67phox and brings the entire cytosolic oxidase complex to the membrane to assemble the active oxidase. p67phox is generally thought of as an accessory protein whose exact function is unclear, although it is required for the activity of the oxidase. p47phox is the protein that carries the cytosolic proteins to the membrane proteins as described above.

Several reports have recently shown that the expression of NADPH oxidase subunit proteins, including p22phox, p47phox, or p67phox, is upregulated in aorta from animal models of diabetes [42,82,96,106]and in saphenous vein and internal mammary arteries from patients with diabetes and coronary artery disease [77]. Studies by Hink et al [82] demonstrated a 7-fold increase in gp91phox mRNA accompanied by an increase in superoxide in aorta from chemically-induced diabetic rats. Studies from our laboratory showed an elevated level of superoxide production in rat small coronary arteries exposed to 23 mmol/l glucose for 24 hours [122]. The enhanced superoxide production was reduced by co-incubation of arteries with DPI, an NADPH oxidase inhibitor. DPI also restored the whole cell K^+ current density in cells from arteries incubated with high glucose (unpublished data). These results support the idea that vascular NADPH oxidase may play a role in generation of superoxide in hyperglycemia.

Mitochondrial Generation of ROS

The mitochondrial respiratory chain consists of four inner membrane associated enzyme complexes, with cytochrome c and the mobile carrier ubiquinone,[38,113,183,185] by which electrons donated by NADH derived from both cytosol and mitochondrial TCA cycle are transported to NADH:ubiquinone oxidoreductase (complex I). Complex I ultimately transfers its electrons to succinate:ubiquinone oxidoreductase (complex II). Electrons from reduced ubiquinone are then transferred to ubiquinol:cytochrome c oxidoreductase (complex III) by the ubisemiquinone radical-generating Q cycle[184]. Electron transport proceeds through cytochrome c, cytochrome c oxidase (complex IV) and, finally, molecular oxygen. The mitochondrial respiratory chain is the major site of ROS production within the cell. Superoxide is produced continually as byproduct of normal respiration. The main source of superoxide in mitochondria is from ubisemiquinone formed during the Q cycle of complex III. Complex I is also a source for ROS. Evidence that supports mitochondrial ROS production during hyperglycemia is based on experiments using bovine aortic endothelial cells exposed to 5 mmol/l or 30 mmol/l glucose. Increased ROS generation was observed in cells incubated with 30 mmol/l glucose. The enhanced ROS by high glucose can be normalized by co-incubation of cells with thenoyltrifluoroacetone (TTFA), an inhibitor of complex II or carbonyl cyanide *m*-chlorophenylhydrazone (CCCP), an uncoupler of oxidative phosphorylation that abolishes the mitochondrial membrane proton gradient. The data suggest that mitochondria play an important role in generating superoxide during hyperglycemia.

In summary, multiple pathways have been proposed as responsible for generating superoxide during hyperglycemia, including increased polyol pathway flux, activation of DAG-PKC pathway, upregulation of NADPH oxidase and mitochondrial electron transport chain. The contribution of each pathway to the generation of ROS in hyperglycemia varies between tissue type, animal species and experimental conditions. A unifying linking mechanism of these pathways in hyperglycemia remains to be further investigated.

Hyperglycemia, Reactive Oxygen Species and K^+ Channel Function

Potassium efflux through K^+ channels regulates membrane potential and vascular tone in response to a variety of pharmacological dilator agents including EDHF, and in response to hypoxia and ischemia. Alterations in the activity of these K^+ channels by ROS during the enhanced oxidative stress of diabetes are likely to modulate vascular resistance. Understanding the mechanisms by which ROS affects K^+ channels may suggest new therapeutic approaches for the treatment of the vascular dysfunction associated with this disease. The effect of hyperglycemia on three major types of K^+ channels, including K_{ATP}, K_v and K_{Ca}, should be considered.

K_{ATP} Channels

In diabetes, the role of the K_{ATP} channel in vasodilation has been studied by several laboratories [103,129,129,166,166]. Impaired dilation to the K_{ATP} channel openers aprikalim, levcromakalim and cromakalim has been observed in aorta [103], mesenteric [25] and cerebral arteries [129,130,130] of streptozotocin-induced diabetic rats. In human coronary arteriolar dilation to aprikalim, a selective K_{ATP} opener, is reduced in subjects with type 1 or type 2 diabetes and coronary artery disease (CAD) compared to those with CAD but without diabetes. K_{ATP} channels contribute substantially to the dilation to hypoxia in these patients. Consistent with this finding, hypoxic dilation is reduced in subjects with diabetes.

Surprisingly, enhanced vasodilator responses to aprikalim have been observed in coronary microvessels of diabetic and hyperglycemic dogs, and these enhanced dilator responses persist during coronary occlusion [169]. It remains unclear whether the expression or properties of the K_{ATP} channel are altered in diabetes, and how this would affect K_{ATP} channel-mediated vasodilator properties when diabetes co-exists with ischemic heart disease.

In contrast to the vascular response, the effect of ROS on K_{ATP} channel activity in cardiac myocytes is different. Studies by Tokube et al [181] reported that $O_2^{\bullet-}$ increases the open state probability of K_{ATP} channels in ventricular cells from guinea pigs in cell-attached and inside out patches. This effect is enhanced by ADP, and abolished by either radical scavengers or glibenclamide suggesting the contribution of $O_2^{\bullet-}$ in mediating K_{ATP} channel function. It has been also reported that hydroxyl radicals and hydrogen peroxide activate cardiac K_{ATP} channels [182], which could be one of the mechanisms contributing to the phenomenon of ischemic preconditioning [89]. The increased K_{ATP} channel activity by $O_2^{\bullet-}$ may involves modulation of the ATP binding site of the SUR subunit of the channel [188]. Data showing $O_2^{\bullet-}$ -induced activation of cardiac K_{ATP} channels contrast with the inhibitory effect of ROS on K_{ATP} channels in the vasculature, suggesting that major differences in the regulation or subunit composition of K_{ATP} channels exist between cardiac and vascular channels.

Since vascular K_{ATP} channels, in contrast to cardiac K_{ATP} channels, demonstrate reduced activity when exposed to $O_2^{\bullet-}$, it may be expected that the interaction between ROS and K_{ATP} channels during diabetes will be a complex relationship with qualitatively different effects on vascular *vs* myocardial K_{ATP} channels. Additional studies involving electrophysiological, molecular and functional approaches will be needed to determine the mechanisms by which hyperglycemia influences K_{ATP} channel -induced vasodilation.

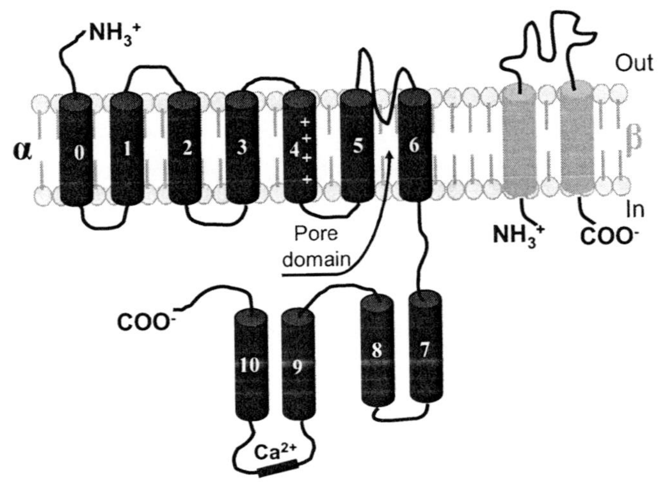

Figure 3. α-subunit of K_{Ca} channel consists of ten transmembrane segments (S1-S10). Voltage sensor is located at S4. The region between S5 and S6 is the pore forming region. The Ca^{2+} sensitivity of the K_{Ca} channels is conferred by transmembrane segments, S7-S10 at the C-terminal region of the α-subunit, and by close association with a single regulatory β-subunit. Adapted from reference [107]

K_v Channels

The effect of oxidative stress on K_v channel activity has been examined in Xenopus oocytes where *shaker* channel (K_v1.3, K_v1.4 and K_v1.5) and *shaw* channel (K_v4.3) were expressed [59]. Exogenous generation of ROS markedly inhibited K_v1.3, K_v1.4, and K_v1.5, but not K_v1.2, K_v2.1, and K_v4.1. It is likely that ROS other than superoxide were responsible for these effects since exposure to xanthine plus xanthine oxidase had no effect on any of the channels studied[59].

We have examined the effect of redox stress on K_v channels in rat coronary small arteries. 4-aminopyridine, a broad spectrum inhibitor of the Kv channels, produces a dose-dependent constriction [21,24,122]. When vessels are incubated in elevated levels of glucose, an SOD-inhibitable reduction in constriction to 4-AP is observed [122].

This effect of oxidative stress on K_v channel function was confirmed in separate studies. Dilation to the beta-adrenergic agonist, isoproterenol which increases production of cAMP, is mediated in part by K_v channels since the dilation is blocked by 4-AP[114]. Exposure to elevated levels of glucose inhibits coronary dilation to both isoproterenol and forskolin, a selective activator of adenylate cyclase. Interestingly the production of cAMP was not affected by high glucose[114] suggesting that the inhibitory effect occurs distal in the signaling pathway. The 4-AP inhibitable component of the dilation was reduced by incubation in high glucose, supporting the idea that ROS inhibit dilation through an effect on K_v channels.

We examined more directly the effect of superoxide generated by the reaction of xanthine and xanthine oxidase on K_v channel activity in freshly isolated rat coronary smooth muscle cells using patch clamping whole-cell configuration [122]. Superoxide reduced 4-AP sensitive K$^+$ current density. A similar reduction in 4-AP sensitive current was also observed in cells from arteries exposed to high glucose (figure 4). The reduced whole cell current is not due to changes in osmolarity since increasing osmolarity with L-glucose (not metabolized) had no effect on either the dilator response or current density. The role of ROS in this response to high glucose is evident by the fact that SOD and catalase partially restored the voltage-dependent potassium channel current density (figure 5). Catalase alone had little effect on K_v channel currents. Thus ROS, probably superoxide, impair K_v channel function in the coronary vasculature either directly or through the effects of elevations in glucose.

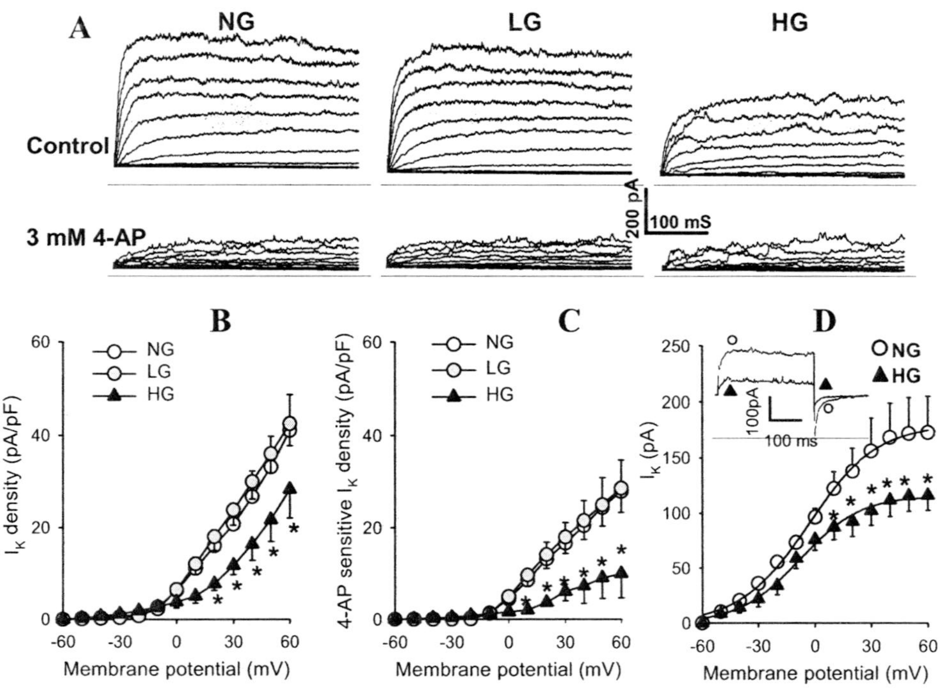

Figure 4. Whole cell K$^+$ currents in coronary VSMCs from arteries incubated with normal glucose (NG), L-glucose (LG) and high glucose (HG). Outward currents in cells from arteries exposed to HG were reduced compared to cells from arteries incubated in NG or LG. 4-aminopyridine (4-AP, 3 mmol/L) blocked a large component of the outward current in cells from NG and LG arteries, but caused less inhibition in cells from HG arteries. B: I-V relationships of K$^+$ current (I_k) densities in cells from arteries exposed to NG, LG or HG. Density was significantly reduced in cells from HG arteries compared to cells from NG and LG arteries (*$P<0.05$ vs NG and LG). C: I-V relationships showing the effect of 4-AP on macroscopic K$^+$ current in NG, LG and HG cells. VSMCs from arteries incubated with HG show less 4-AP sensitive K_v current compared to

cells from arteries exposed to NG and LG (* P< 0.05 vs NG and LG). D: Comparison of voltage dependence of K^+ current between cells from NG and HG arteries. Inset shows sample traces of tail currents recorded at –60 mV after a prepulse step to +60 mV to maximally activated K^+ current. The plot of peak tail current amplitudes versus prepulse potentials indicates that tail currents were reduced in cells from HG arteries, whereas voltage dependence of K^+ current was not altered. Data is adopted from reference [122] with permission.

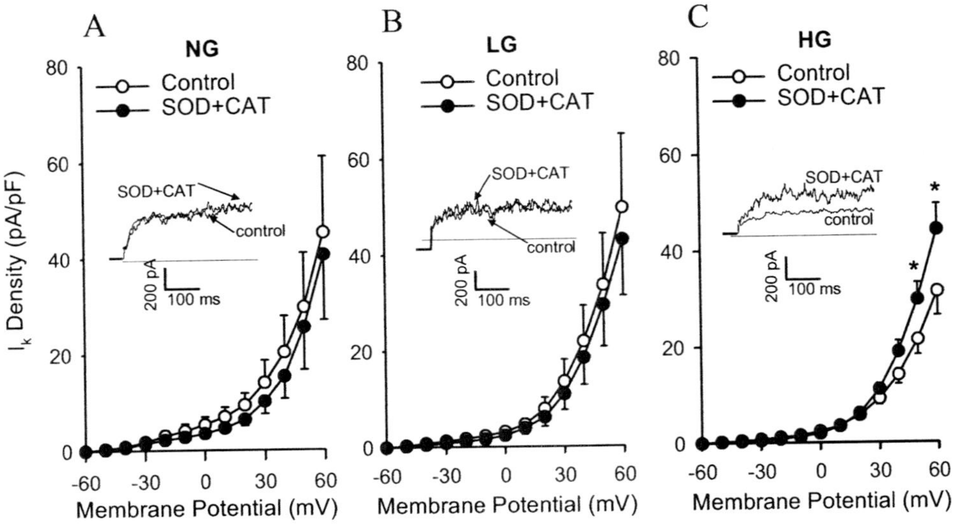

Figure 5. A, B and C: Current-voltage relationships comparing K^+ current densities of patch-clamped NG, LG or HG cells in response to SOD (150 U/ml) and CAT (500 U/ml). A, B: SOD and CAT did not alter K^+ current (I_k) density in cells from arteries incubated in NG or LG. C: However, SOD and CAT partially restored K^+ current in cells from arteries incubated in HG (*p<0.05 vs control). Insets show original currents recorded at +60 mV before and after cells were superfused with SOD and CAT. Data is adopted from reference [122] with permission.

Several studies have shown an increased level of peroxynitrite ($ONOO^-$), a product formed by reaction of $O_2^{\bullet-}$ and NO in diabetes and in hyperglycemia [194,195]. One of the detrimental effects of $ONOO^-$ is nitration of tyrosine residues that alters the function of proteins, as occurs with superoxide dismutase [125], cytochrome P450 [165] and prostacyclin synthase[194,195]. Based on these findings, we have performed studies to examine the effect of $ONOO^-$ on K_v channel function, particularly the K_v1 family. The contractile response to 4-AP was greatly attenuated by authentic $ONOO^-$, but not decomposed $ONOO^-$ (DC-$ONOO^-$). Further study identifying the involvement of K_v channel subtype family was performed in freshly isolated rat coronary smooth muscle cells using patch clamp whole-cell recording. Correolide, a specific blocker of K_v1 family[7,115], reduced whole-cell K^+ current when cells were exposed to DC-$ONOO^-$. Authentic $ONOO^-$ decreased K^+ currents. Correolide had no further effect on K^+ current in the presence of $ONOO^-$ suggesting the reduced currents by $ONOO^-$ were K_v1 channel currents. Generation $ONOO^-$ by high glucose was confirmed by immunohistochemistry using antibodies to nitrotyrosine in rat small coronary arteries exposed to normal or high glucose for 24 hours. Augmentation of nitrotyrosine staining was observed in high glucose vessels and prevented by co-incubation of urate, a scavenger of $ONOO^-$. In addition, video microscopic study revealed a partial restoration of the impaired constriction to 4-AP in vessels exposed to high glucose by urate or ebselen, two chemically distinct $ONOO^-$ scavengers. The impairment of K_v1 channels by high glucose may be due to tyrosine nitration of K_v channels[115]. However, the relative contribution of $O_2^{\bullet-}$ and $ONOO^-$ to the reduction of K_v channel function in hyperglycemia remains to be determined.

K_{ca} Channels

Our laboratory examined the direct effects of ROS on K_{Ca} activity. $O_2^{\bullet-}$ was formed by xanthine and xanthine oxidase. Freshly isolated human coronary arteriolar smooth muscle cells were examined with the cell-attached patch clamp technique. Open state probability of K_{Ca} channels was not altered by incubation in superoxide[121]. We also examined responses to bradykinin, an endothelium-dependent dilator of human coronary arterioles that operates through an EDHF mechanism activating K_{Ca} channels in the underlying smooth muscle[137]. Bradykinin dilation of isolated arterioles was not affected by treatment with xanthine+xanthine oxidase. In contrast, Ross et al observed an impaired dilation to NS1619, a K_{Ca} channel opener, in piglet cerebral arterioles exposed to hypoxanthine and xanthine oxidase to generate superoxide [167]. However, the limitation of this study is that direct effect of superoxide on K_{Ca} channel activity was not determined, and the role of hydrogen peroxide, hydroxyl radical, or peroxynitrite were not examined. In addition, NS1619 is not a specific blocker for K_{Ca}. It also opens Ca^{2+} channel. Therefore, pharmacological study would not be sufficient to evaluate K_{Ca} channel function.

Hydrogen peroxide, formed by the spontaneous or catalyzed dismutation of superoxide, is a strong vasodilator[29,136] and activator of K_{Ca} channel activity in several vascular beds[90,157,179] including the coronary circulation[19], although other mechanisms exist for H_2O_2 –induced dilation[29,109]. Vasodilation in response to exogenously generated superoxide is generally mediated by the hydrogen peroxide[157]. Oxidizing agents directly open K_{Ca} channels in isolated inside-out patches[152], and H_2O_2 specifically hyperpolarizes vascular smooth muscle[136] as well as endothelial cell membranes[30] by opening K_{Ca} channels.

Although, the K_{Ca} channel is not altered by $O_2^{\bullet-}$, the product formed from reaction of $O_2^{\bullet-}$ with NO, peroxynitrite ($ONOO^-$), does inhibit K_{Ca} channels in smooth muscle cell membranes of rat cerebral arteries [28]. Reduced small conductance K_{Ca} channel activity in response to high concentration of NO donors has also been observed in renal cortical collecting duct [124]. The inhibitory effect of NO can be abolished by treatment with Tiron indicating involvement of ROS, probably $ONOO^-$. Our laboratory has examined the effect of $ONOO^-$ in human coronary arterioles on K_{Ca} function. Impaired dilation to bradykinin was observed when vessels exposed to authentic $ONOO^-$ (figure 6A). In a separate study $ONOO^-$ was generated by combination of xanthine, xanthine oxidase and an NO donor, either sodium nitroprusside (figure 6B) or spermine nonoate (figure 6C). Dilation to bradykinin was reduced when vessels were incubated with any three ONOO-generating chemicals together. The reduced K_{Ca} channel function is localized in smooth muscle cells since decreased dilation to NS1619, a K_{Ca} channel opener, was found following denudation of endothelium of human coronary arterioles.

The mechanisms of impaired K_{Ca} channel activity by $ONOO^-$ was further investigated using patch clamp techniques. Open state probability was greatly reduced in inside-out patches in response to $ONOO^-$ but not DC-$ONOO^-$ suggesting that $ONOO^-$ inhibits K_{Ca} channel activity possibly by a direct effect.

In summary, oxidative stress clearly affects the activity of several vascular K^+ channels, and therefore plays an important role in mediating vasomotor tone and tissue perfusion during ischemia, changes in metabolism, and in response to agonists. ROS generated within the vascular wall or from underlying tissue reduce bioactivity of NO, thereby impairing an important mechanism of vasodilation and promoting atherogenesis. Especially in the microvasculature hyperpolarization mechanisms of dilation compensate for loss of NO-dilator responses. However these responses are affected by the oxidative milieu and in the presence of redox species such as peroxynitrite, even compensatory dilator mechanisms acting through hyperpolarization may fail.

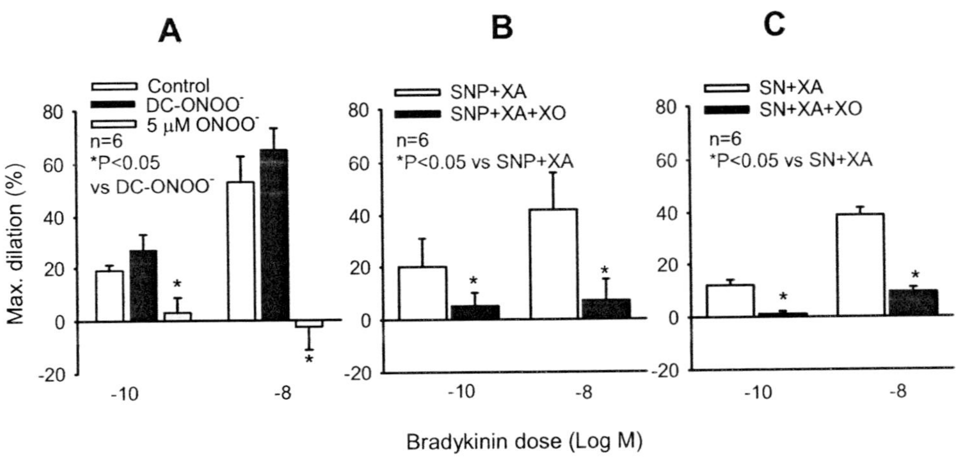

Figure 6. Effect of authentic $ONOO^-$ (A) or exogenous formation of $ONOO^-$ (B, C) on BK-induced dilation in human coronary arterioles. Dilations to BK were significantly reduced in arterioles exposed to authentic $ONOO^-$, or $ONOO^-$ generated by sodium nitroprusside (SNP) or spermine nonoate (SN) plus XA+XO (n=6, each group, *$P<0.05$). Data is adopted from reference [80] with permission.

Insulin Resistance and Vascular Disease

The pathological condition of insulin resistance has generally been defined as the progressive decay in the body's ability to respond to insulin secreted by the pancreas and is characterized by the presence of normoglycemia or mild hyperglycemia and significant hyperinsulinemia in the fasting state [8,9]. Specifically, the condition of insulin resistance refers to an inability of secreted insulin to lower plasma glucose levels via effective suppression of hepatic glucose production and/or the stimulation of glucose utilization in skeletal muscle and adipose tissue. Additionally, the insulin-resistant state can be characterized by the failure of normal insulin levels to suppress lipolysis by adipocytes, ultimately causing an elevated plasma free fatty acid concentration, which can stimulate both triglyceride and glucose production within the liver.

The genesis of the insulin resistant state can be extremely heterogeneous between afflicted individuals, with its origins within both genetic and environmental inputs. While a partial genetic contribution to insulin resistance cannot be denied, there appears to be little evidence for a single gene which is responsible for the full manifestation of the disease. Rather, insulin resistance, especially under conditions of obesity, appears to be transmitted as a polygenic familial trait, although the specific genes responsible remain undetermined [154]. Clearly, genetic mutations compromising the efficacy of the insulin receptor can underlie insulin resistance, however, these appear to be relatively rare in the human population. While other impairments have been identified that exist downstream of insulin binding with its receptor, including a reduced tyrosine kinase activity within the receptor, the reduced activities of both the insulin-sensitive GLUT-4 glucose transporter and glycogen synthase, the extent to which these impairments represent a cause of insulin resistance rather than an effect of the pathology remains unclear [154]. Additionally, polymorphisms for genes encoding insulin receptor substrate 1 [46], glycogen synthase [196] and the regulatory subunits of protein tyrosine phosphatase 1 [147] have all been associated with resistance to insulin, but their importance as a cause of insulin resistance remains undetermined.

The insulin resistant condition is considered to be a core precursor for the development of type II diabetes mellitus and has itself become an increasingly strong challenge to public health issues confronting not only Western society, but also much of the world. Currently, greater than 60 million Americans are afflicted with some degree of insulin resistance, and it has been estimated that approximately 25% of these individuals will ultimately develop type II diabetes mellitus [8,9]. Further, while the presence of insulin resistance represents a key risk factor for the incidence of heart disease and stroke, the progressive inability of the body to utilize insulin and tolerate glucose efficiently leads to imbalances in the lipid profile of the blood; including an increased ratio of low-density to high density lipoproteins and an increased level of circulating triglycerides; also risk factors for the accelerated evolution of atherosclerosis [9]. Clearly, investigation into the effects of insulin resistance on vascular function, and in particular the behavior of K^+ channels underlying vascular reactivity, represents a vital avenue for further study.

From an environmental perspective, the consumption of an energy-rich diet, coupled with a sedentary lifestyle predisposes an individual to the development of central obesity, one of the key predictors of the development of insulin resistance, particularly for skeletal muscle [9]. The increased metabolic activity of intra-abdominal adipose tissue, increased sympathetic activity and an elevated β-adrenoreceptor mediated lipolysis, leads to an elevated triglyceride and free fatty acid turnover which is associated with skeletal muscle insulin resistance [123]

Within biomedical research, numerous animal models of insulin resistance have been used to study the development of this pathological condition on basic vascular function, including a myriad of mouse knockout models for elements of both insulin receptors and sites within the insulin signaling cascade [144], and a series of rat models, including the JCR:LC-cp and other corpulent rats strains [26]. With specific regard to the alterations in vascular dilator reactivity and the role of the relevant K^+ channels and oxidant stress, two rat models of insulin resistance have recently undergone intensive study; the obese Zucker rat (*fa/fa*) and the high fructose-diet fed rat. The obese Zucker rat (OZR) possesses a dysfunctional leptin receptor gene, and as such is severely resistant to the effects of leptin. Due to this genetic alteration, the OZR fed *ad libitum*, experiences chronic hyperphagia [128], with the ensuing development of obesity, insulin resistance, dyslipidemia and moderate hypertension versus its control strain, the lean Zucker rat. The OZR represents an excellent candidate model for the study of the effects of insulin resistance, as this condition develops naturally, as a result of a chronically elevated caloric intake, an evolution of the condition that can closely mimic that identified in the human population [8,9]. In contrast, the fructose-fed rat (FFR) model of insulin resistance employs a normal rat ingesting an artificial diet consisting of approximately 66% fructose [104]. After several weeks on this fructose rich diet, rats develop severe insulin resistance, without the confounding influences of obesity, which is consistently present in the OZR model, or fasting hyperglycemia, which can be variably present in the OZR. Severe hypertriglyceridemia and a moderate, clinically relevant, hypertension are present to a comparable extent in both the OZR and the fructose-fed rat (FFR) models of insulin resistance. When taken as a whole, however, the combination of the OZR model and the FFR model of insulin resistance comprise two major platforms for the investigation of altered vascular function in the insulin resistant state, as both of these models provide physiological information regarding alterations in vascular reactivity which mirror those found in clinical studies using insulin-resistant human subjects [83,98,173].

Insulin Resistance and Vascular Reactivity

Almost without exception, the existing literature clearly indicates that the evolution of insulin resistance in both the OZR and in the FFR models results in a dramatic impairment in the dilator reactivity of small arteries and arterioles throughout the body.

Using the OZR, endothelial dependent dilator responses of intestinal [102], skeletal muscle [69,110], cerebral [65], renal [81], epineurial [50] and mesenteric [190] arteries and arterioles have routinely been found to be strongly impaired versus responses in control rats. As representative examples, the ability of renal arterioles to dilate in response to challenge with acetylcholine in the insulin resistant OZR was significantly impaired versus responses determined in control strains [81]. Similarly, dilator responses of intestinal arterioles to both application of acetylcholine or elevated intraluminal flow were significantly lower than in control animals [102]. Further, the ability of norepinephrine-preconstricted mesenteric arteries to dilate in response to challenge with acetylcholine or sodium nitroprusside was reduced in OZR versus lean Zucker rat controls [190]. More recently, Frisbee and colleagues demonstrated that the ability of skeletal muscle arterioles to dilate in response to the physiologically relevant stimuli of reduced oxygen tension in isolated vessels; and elevated wall shear rate in *in situ* microvessels, is strongly impaired in OZR as compared to lean Zucker rat control animals.

Microvessels from the multiple tissues and organs within the FFR demonstrate a similar pattern of impaired dilator reactivity to endothelium-dependent stimuli as demonstrated in the Zucker rat model of insulin resistance. Initial studies by Miller and colleagues have clearly demonstrated that the dilator responses of isolated coronary arteries [135] and mesenteric arteries [105] in response to acetylcholine was impaired in FFR as compared to responses determined in vessels from rats fed a normal diet. Specifically, the authors demonstrated that the acetylcholine-induced dilation of phenylephrine-preconstricted mesenteric arteries was significantly impaired in vessels from FFR, and that this was not due to any contribution from cyclooxygenase metabolites [105], while a supplemental study by this same group found that this similar pattern of impaired vasodilator responses was also present in coronary arteries of FFR, as vasodilation in response to application of acetylcholine was impaired in these vessels as well [135], and that this was independent of cyclooxygenase metabolites. However, Miller *et al.* suggested that this impaired reactivity might be due to a decrease in an endothelial-derived hyperpolarizing factor, as a broad band pharmacological blockade of Ca^{2+}-actrivated K^+ channels with a combination of charybdotoxin and apamin, while severely attenuating acetylcholine-induced dilation of coronary arteries of control rats, had a negligible effect in insulin resistant animals. Further, Katakam *et al.* determined that this pattern of impaired vasomotor responses in mesenteric arteries of FFR was most likely due to the progression of insulin resistance, *per se*, as the impaired dilator responses of these vessels in response to application of acetylcholine significantly preceded the evolution of any elevation in mean arterial pressure [104]. These observations were recently extended to the cerebral circulation, as Erdos *et al.* [63] demonstrated an impaired dilator response of isolated middle cerebral arteries of fructose-fed, insulin resistant rats to bradykinin versus responses in control animals.

Insulin Resistance and Potassium Channel Function

A recent study, using primarily the FFR model of insulin resistance, has specifically addressed alterations to the behavior of K^+ channels in vascular smooth muscle which could contribute to the demonstrated impairments in dilator reactivity. In insulin-resistant FFR, mesenteric arterial dilation in response to application of 11, 12-epoxyeicosatrienoic acids (11,12 EETs) and 14,15-EETs [dependent primarily on an increased open probability of K_{Ca} in vascular smooth muscle] was significantly reduced compared to responses determined in arteries from control rats [134]. Further, arterial dilation in response to EET application was attenuated in vessels from control animals following application of either iberiotoxin and apamin or charybdotoxin and apamin, although treatment of vessels from FFR with these agents had no effect on vascular responses to exposure to EETs. Additional investigation of K^+ channel function in mesenteric arterial myocytes from FFR indicated that, in the cell-attached configuration, the ability of exogenously applied EETs to increase the activity of K_{Ca} channels was substantially reduced in cells from FFR versus those in cells from control animals (Figure 7). In contrast, in the inside-out (I/O) patch clamp configuration, K_{Ca} channel activity was elevated following application of EETs to a comparable extent between insulin resistant rats and control animals. The results from this study clearly suggested that the impaired dilator reactivity to EET application in vessels from insulin-resistant rats may be due to an alteration in the signal transduction pathways regulating the open state probability of K_{Ca} channels rather than a specific alteration in their function of these channels *per se*.

In a follow-up study, Dimitropoulou *et al.* [57] demonstrated that the macroscopic current density via K_{Ca} channels was reduced in mesenteric microvessels from insulin-resistant FFR versus control animals. Further, the authors demonstrated that pharmacological inhibition of K_{Ca} channels from FFR (with tetraethylammonium or iberiotoxin) caused a significantly greater reduction in the K^+ current in arterial myocytes from control animals than from insulin resistant ones, while pharmacological activation of K_{Ca} channels with NS-1619 was substantially more effective at increasing outward current in control versus insulin-resistant rats.

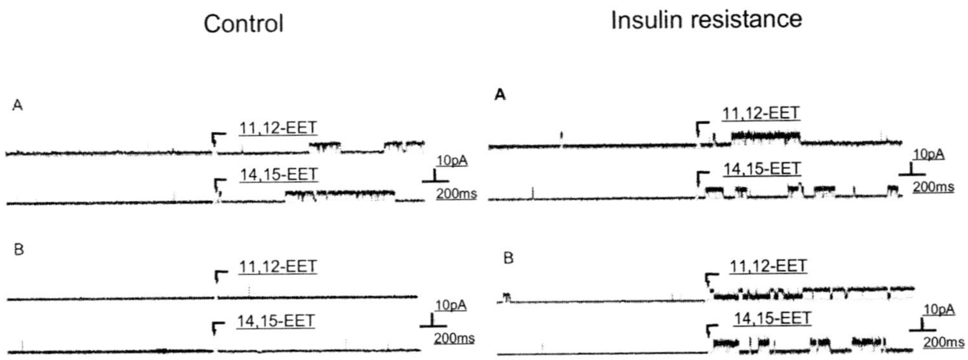

Figure 7. Continuous recordings of K_{Ca} channel openings in the cell-attached (A) and inside-out (B) configuration (+50 mV) before and after addition of 1 μM 11,12- or 14,15-EET. Channel openings are upward deflections from baseline (dashed line) or closed state. K_{Ca} channel openings are from mesenteric arterial myocytes from control (Left) or insulin-resistant (Right) rats. Data is adopted from reference [134] with permission.

More detailed analyses employing patch clamp techniques and Western blotting analyses demonstrated that K_{Ca} channels had comparable mean single channel slope conductances, sensitivity to both voltage and to increased intracellular Ca^{2+} levels and patterns of protein expression between the two groups. These results strongly suggested that a decreased K^+ current in vessels from insulin-resistant rats was not due to alterations in either channel expression or the inherent physical properties of individual channels themselves, rather that a distinct external mechanism might contribute to impaired K_{Ca} channel function.

Additional study by Erdos *et al.* [62] and Katakam *et al.* [105] has supported these observations, demonstrating that a qualitatively similar impairment in the function of both K_{ATP} (using cromakalim and pinacidil, respectively) and K_{Ca} channel activity was also occurring in the middle cerebral arteries [62] and mesenteric arteries [105] of FFR and may contribute to the compromised dilator reactivity of those vessels as well. Interestingly, a somewhat divergent set of results was identified by Frisbee and colleagues using the OZR model of insulin resistance, as dilator responses of skeletal muscle microvessels was not significantly impaired in response to application of the K_{ATP} channel activator aprikalim [69, although the effects of application of iberiotoxin on vascular tone [70] were similar to that determined in mesenteric and cerebral arteries in the FFR, discussed above.

Reactive Oxygen Species and Potassium Channel Function in Insulin Resistance

Recently, Brzezinska *et al.* [28] demonstrated that the production of peroxynitrite, via the interaction of superoxide anion with nitric oxide, had the potential to impact the regulation of vascular tone by inhibiting the open state probability of vascular K_{Ca} channels. Building on this novel observation, Frisbee *et al.* [70] determined that this oxidant stress-based inhibition of K_{Ca} channels may contribute to altered skeletal muscle microvessel reactivity in the OZR model of insulin resistance, as an enhanced myogenic activation of skeletal muscle resistance arterioles following elevations in intralumenal pressure was nearly normalized to levels found in vessels from control lean Zucker rats by either treatment of vessels with a free radical scavenger polyethyleneglycol-superoxide dismutase (PEG-SOD), or incubation of vessels with the K_{Ca} channel blocker, iberiotoxin. Further, the direct application of peroxynitrite to skeletal muscle arterioles of OZR caused a pronounced pressure-dependent vasoconstriction, which was completely blocked by prior incubation of vessels with iberiotoxin (Figure 8). Taken together, these initial results strongly suggested that oxidant stress-based inhibition of K_{Ca} channel function could contribute to the altered peripheral vascular reactivity that had been demonstrated in OZR.

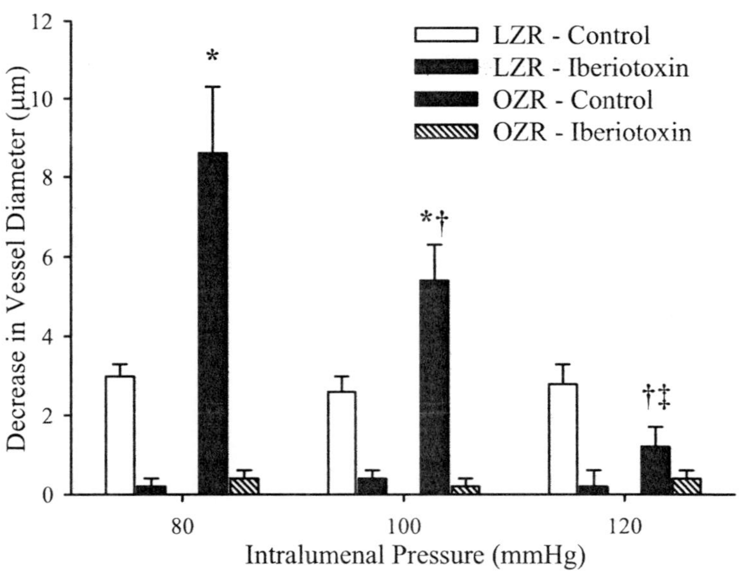

Figure 8. Change in diameter of skeletal muscle arteries from lean and obese Zucker rats in response to application of 100 nM peroxynitrite under control conditions and following treatment of vessels with the K_{Ca} channel antagonist iberiotoxin. * $p<0.05$ versus LZR at that pressure. † $p<0.05$ versus OZR-control at 80 mmHg pressure. ‡ $p<0.05$ versus OZR-control at 100 mmHg pressure. Data is adopted from reference (70) with permission.

More recently, Erdos and colleagues examined the role of elevated oxidant tone in contributing to the altered vascular reactivity determined in small resistance arteries of the cerebral circulation within both the FFR [64] and OZR [65] models of insulin resistance.

Using isolated middle cerebral arteries, Erdos *et al.* [64] demonstrated that dilator responses to both K_{Ca} channel-dependent (iloprost) and K_{ATP} channel-dependent (pinacidil) dilator agonists were impaired in FFR versus responses in vessels from control animals. However, incubation of vessels with SOD restored the dilator reactivity of vessels from FFR rats in response to application of either iloprost and pinacidil. Interestingly, vasodilator responses mediated through the inward-rectifier K^+ channels (K_{IR}, elevated extracellular K^+), were unaltered between vessels of the two animal groups, and pharmacological blockade of both K_{IR} (barium) and K_v channels (4-aminopyridine) resulted in a comparable constriction of middle cerebral arteries between the two groups.

Subsequently, using the OZR model of insulin resistance, Erdos *et al.* [65] demonstrated that the dilator responses of *in situ* basilar arteries its side branches was significantly impaired in insulin-resistant rats in response to stimuli dependent on an intact endothelium (acetylcholine), K_{Ca} channels (iloprost), K_{ATP} channels (cromakalim) and K_{IR} channels (elevated extracellular K^+) versus dilator responses in lean Zucker rats. Further, the authors demonstrated that the incubation of vessels with the SOD (added topically) restored dilator reactivity in OZR to levels determined in lean control animals (Figure 9). In contrast, treatment of vessels with either of the protein kinase C inhibitors Ro31-8220 or chelerythrine improved only the dilator responses to acetylcholine, while responses to stimuli which directly effect K^+ channels remained impaired in basilar arteries/arterioles of obese animals versus lean.

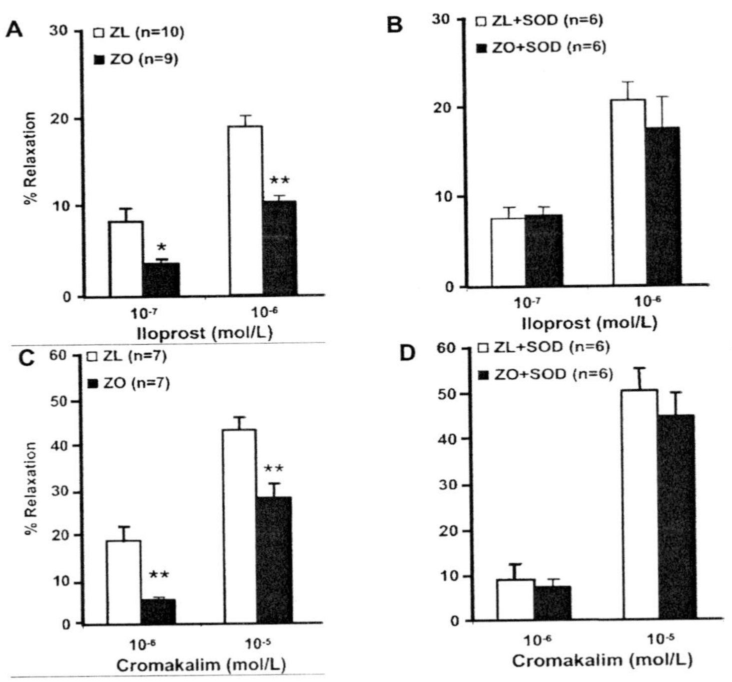

Figure 9. Responses to iloprost (Panel A,B) or cromakalim (C,D) in basilar arteries of control and SOD-treated rats. Relaxation was impaired in obese Zucker rats compared with lean Zucker rats, and SOD treatment restored relaxation to normal. * $p<0.05$; ** $p<0.01$ vs. responses in lean Zucker rats. Data is adopted from reference [65] with permission.

Summary and Conclusions

As summarized in figure 10, in diabetes or hyperglycemia, enhance oxidative stress occurs. $O_2^{\bullet-}$, one of the prominent ROS generated from multiple pathways, impairs vascular K_v and K_{ATP} channel function, but had little effect on K_{Ca} channels. $ONOO^-$, a product formed by reaction of $O_2^{\bullet-}$ and NO, inhibits both K_v and K_{Ca} channels, possibly by direct effect. The development of the insulin resistant condition, prior to the manifestation of type II diabetes mellitus, is associated with a significant impairment in the vascular dilator reactivity across a wide array of organs and tissues. In large measure, this impaired reactivity has a foundation in a compromised function of multiple subtypes of K^+ channels within vascular smooth muscle, and that an elevated oxidative stress underlies much of this altered channel behavior. While there is some evidence that treatment of insulin-resistance people with anti-oxidants may improve vascular reactivity [10,84,156], the underlying nature of the causes of the elevated oxidant tone, from reduced anti-oxidant defense mechanisms [33] to increased free radical production [173] [95], and their effects on the ion channels which underlie the regulation of vascular tone are unclear. While the study of insulin resistance on the behavior of K^+ channels in vascular smooth muscle and the role of oxidative radicals in this process may still be in the early stages, given the ongoing trends in the epidemiological status of insulin resistance and the metabolic syndrome, this clearly represents a vital avenue for future investigation.

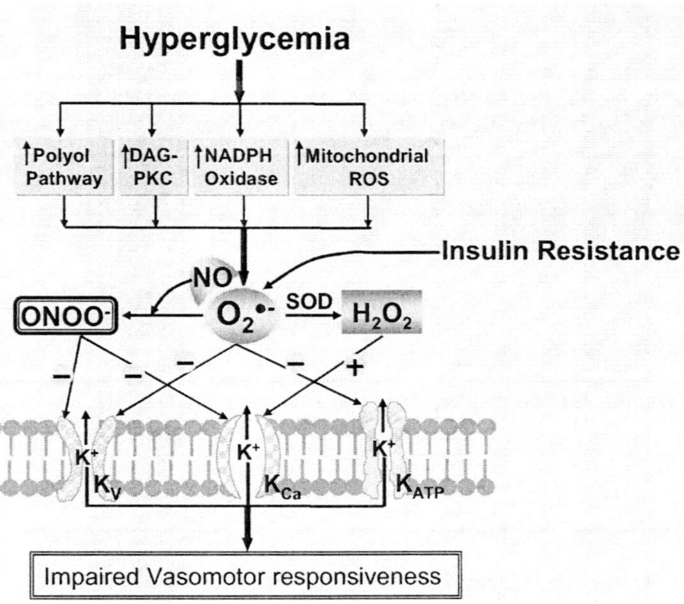

Figure 10. Schematic summary of several pathways for generation of ROS in hyperglycemia and interactions between ROS and vascular K^+channels.

References

[1] Abiru T, Watanabe Y, Kamata K, Miyata N, and Kasuya Y. Decrease in endothelium-dependent relaxation and levels of cyclic nucleotides in aorta from rabbits with alloxan-induced diabetes. *Research Communications in Chemical Pathology and Pharmacology* 68:13-25, 1990

[2] Acker H: Reactive oxygen intermediates as mediators for regulaing ion channel activity. In Oxygen Regulation of Ion Channels and Gene Expression. Lopez-Barneo J, Weir EK, Eds. N.Y., *Futura,* 1998, p. 9-18

[3] Aguilar-Bryan L, Nichols CG, Wechsler SW, Clement JP, Boyd AE, III, Gonzalez G, Herrera-Sosa H, Nguy K, Bryan J, and Nelson DA. Cloning of the beta cell high-affinity sulfonylurea receptor: a regulator of insulin secretion. *Science* 268:423-426, 1995

[4] Ahmed A, Waters CM, Leffler CW, and Jaggar JH. Ionic mechanisms mediating the myogenic response in newborn porcine cerebral arteries. *Am.J.Physiol Heart Circ.Physiol* 2004

[5] Aiello EA, Malcolm AT, Walsh MP, and Cole WC. Beta-adrenoceptor activation and PKA regulate delayed rectifier K^+ channels of vascular smooth muscle cells. *Am. J. Physiol.* 275:H448-H459, 1998

[6] Aiello EA, Walsh MP, and Cole WC. Phosphorylation by protein kinase A enhances delayed rectifier K+ current in rabbit vascular smooth muscle cells. *Am. J. Physiol.* 268:H926-H934, 1995

[7] Albarwani S, Nemetz LT, Madden JA, Tobin AA, England SK, Pratt PF, and Rusch NJ. Voltage-gated K+ channels in rat small cerebral arteries: molecular identity of the functional channels. *J.Physiol.* 551:751-763, 2003

[8] American Diabetes Association. All About Insulin Resistance, Toolkit No. 5. *American Diabetes Association* Type II Diabetes Information: 2004

[9] American Heart Association. Insulin Resistance. *American Heart Association* Diseases and Conditions: 2004

[10] Arcaro G, Cretti A, Balzano S, Lechi A, Muggeo M, Bonora E, and Bonadonna RC. Insulin causes endothelial dysfunction in humans: sites and mechanisms. *Circ.* 105:576-582, 2002

[11] Archer SL, Huang JM, Hampl V, Nelson DP, Shultz PJ, and Weir EK. Nitric oxide and cGMP cause vasorelaxation by activation of a charybdotoxin-sensitive K channel by cGMP-dependent protein kinase. *Proc.Natl.Acad.Sci.U.S.A* 91:7583-7587, 1994

[12] Archer SL, Huang JMC, Reeve HL, Hampl V, Tolarova S, Michelakis E, and Weirnik PH. Differential distribution of electrophysiologically distinct myocytes in conduit and resistance arteries determines their response to nitric oxide and hypoxia. *Circ.Res.* 78:431-442, 1996

[13] Arnal JF, Dinh-Xuan AT, Pueyo M, Darblade B, and Rami J. Endothelium-derived nitric oxide and vascular physiology and pathology. *Cell Mol.Life Sci.* 55:1078-1087, 1999

[14] Asano M, Masuzawa-Ito K, and Matsuda T. Charybdotoxin-sensitive K+ channels regulate the myogenic tone in the resting state of arteries from spontaneously hypertensive rats. *Br.J.Pharmacol.* 108:214-222, 1993

[15] Ayo SH, Radnik R, Garoni JA, Troyer DA, and Kreisberg JI. High glucose increases diacylglycerol mass and activates protein kinase C in mesangial cell cultures. *Am.J.Physiol* 261:F571-F577, 1991

[16] Babenko AP, Aguilar-Bryan L, and Bryan J. A view of sur/KIR6.X, KATP channels. *Annu.Rev.Physiol* 60:667-687, 1998

[17] Babenko AP, Gonzalez G, and Bryan J. Pharmaco-topology of sulfonylurea receptors. Separate domains of the regulatory subunits of K(ATP) channel isoforms are required for selective interaction with K(+) channel openers. *J.Biol.Chem.* 275:717-720, 2000

[18] Baker JE, Holman P, and Gross GJ. Preconditioning in immature rabbit hearts: role of KATP channels. *Circ.* 99:1249-1254, 1999

[19] 9. Barlow RS, White RE. Hydrogen peroxide relaxes porcine coronary arteries by stimulating BKCa channel activity. *Am.J.Physiol* 275:H1283-H1289, 1998

[20] Baynes JW, Thorpe SR. Role of oxidative stress in diabetic complications: a new perspective on an old paradigm. *Diabetes* 48:1-9, 1999

[21] Belevych AE, Beck R, Tammaro P, Poston L, and Smirnov SV. Developmental changes in the functional characteristics and expression of voltage-gated K+ channel currents in rat aortic myocytes. *Cardiovasc.Res.* 54:152-161, 2002

[22] Berger MG, Vandier C, Bonnet P, Jackson WF, and Rusch NJ. Intracellular acidosis differentially regulates KV channels in coronary and pulmonary vascular muscle. *Am J Physiol* 275:H1351-H1359, 1998

[23] Bialecki RA, Stinson-Fisher C. Kca channel antagonists reduce NO donor-mediated relaxation of vascular and tracheal smooth muscle. *Am.J.Physiol.* 268:L152-L159, 1995

[24] Bonnet P, Rusch NJ, and Harder DR. Characterization of an outward K+ current in freshly dispersed cerebral arterial muscle cells. *Pflugers Arch.* 418:292-296, 1991

[25] Bouchard JF, Dumont EC, and Lamontagne D. Modification of vasodilator response in streptozotocin-induced diabetic rat. *Can.J.Physiol Pharmacol.* 77:980-985, 1999

[26] Brindley DN, Russell JC. Animal models of insulin resistance and cardiovascular disease: some therapeutic approaches using JCR:LA-cp rat. *Diabetes Obes.Metab* 4:1-10, 2002

[27] Brownlee M. Biochemistry and molecular cell biology of diabetic complications. *Nature* 414:813-820, 2001

[28] Brzezinska AK, Gebremedhin D, Chilian WM, Kalyanaraman B, and Elliott SJ. Peroxynitrite reversibly inhibits Ca(2+)-activated K(+) channels in rat cerebral artery smooth muscle cells. *Am.J.Physiol Heart Circ.Physiol* 278:H1883-H1890, 2000

[29] Burke-Wolin T, Abate CJ, Wolin MS, and Gurtner GH. Hydrogen peroxide-induced pulmonary vasodilation: role of guanosine 3',5'-cyclic monophosphate. *Am.J.Physiol.* 261:L393-L398, 1991

[30] Bychkov R, Pieper K, Ried C, Milosheva M, Bychkov E, Luft FC, and Haller H. Hydrogen peroxide, potassium currents, and membrane potential in human endothelial cells. *Circ.* 99:1719-1725, 1999

[31] Cameron NE, Cotter MA, and Maxfield EK. Anti-oxidant treatment prevents the development of periperal nerve dysfunction in streptozotocin-diabetic rats. *Diabetologia* 36:299-304, 1993
[32] Castellino RC, Morales MJ, Strauss HC, and Rasmusson RL. Time- and voltage-dependent modulation of a Kv1.4 channel by a beta-subunit (Kv beta 3) cloned from ferret ventricle. *Am.J.Physiol* 269:H385-H391, 1995
[33] Cavarape A, Feletto F, Mercuri F, Quagliaro L, Daman G, and Ceriello A. High-fructose diet decreases catalase mRNA levels in rat tissues. *J.Endocrinol.Invest* 24:838-845, 2001
[34] Ceriello A. Nitrotyrosine: new findings as a marker of postprandial oxidative stress. *Int.J.Clin.Pract.Suppl*51-58, 2002
[35] Ceriello A. New insights on oxidative stress and diabetic complications may lead to a "causal" antioxidant therapy. *Diab.Care* 26:1589-1596, 2003
[36] Ceriello A, Mercuri F, Quagliaro L, Assaloni R, Motz E, Tonutti L, and Taboga C. Detection of nitrotyrosine in the diabetic plasma: evidence of oxidative stress. *Diabetologia* 44:834-838, 2001
[37] Ceriello A, Quagliaro L, Catone B, Pascon R, Piazzola M, Bais B, Marra G, Tonutti L, Taboga C, and Motz E. Role of hyperglycemia in nitrotyrosine postprandial generation. *Diab.Care* 25:1439-1443, 2002
[38] Chakraborti T, Das S, Mondal M, Roychoudhury S, and Chakraborti S. Oxidant, mitochondria and calcium: an overview. *Cell Signal.* 11:77-85, 1999
[39] NN, Vallance P, and Colhoun HM. Nitric oxide and vascular responses in Type I diabetes. *Diabetologia* 43:137-147, 2000
[40] Chang K, Ido Y, Lejeune W, Williamson JR, and Tilton RG. Increased sciatic nerve blood flow in diabetic rats: assessment by "molecular" vs. particulate microspheres. *Am.J.Physiol.* 273:E164-E173, 1997
[41] Chikani G, Zhu W, and Smart EJ. Lipids: potential regulators of nitric oxide generation. *Am.J.Physiol Endocrinol.Metab* 287:E386-E389, 2004
[42] Christ M, Bauersachs J, Liebetrau C, Heck M, Gunther A, and Wehling M. Glucose increases endothelial-dependent superoxide formation in coronary arteries by NAD(P)H oxidase activation: attenuation by the 3-hydroxy-3-methylglutaryl coenzyme A reductase inhibitor atorvastatin. *Diabetes* 51:2648-2652, 2002
[43] Chung SS, Ho EC, Lam KS, and Chung SK. Contribution of polyol pathway to diabetes-induced oxidative stress. *J.Amer.Soc.Nephrol.* 14:S233-S236, 2003
[44] Clapp LH, Tinker A. Potassium channels in the vasculature. *Current Opinion in Nephrology and Hypertension* 7:91-98, 1998
[45] Clarkson P, Celermajer DS, Powe AJ, Donald AE, Henry RM, and Deanfield JE. Endothelium-dependent dilatation is impaired in young healthy subjects with a family history of premature coronary disease. *Circ.* 96:3378-3383, 1997
[46] Clausen JO, Hansen T, Bjorbaek C, Echwald SM, Urhammer SA, Rasmussen S, Andersen CB, Hansen L, Almind K, Winther K, and . Insulin resistance: interactions between obesity and a common variant of insulin receptor substrate-1. *Lancet* 346:397-402, 1995

[47] Clement-Chomienne O, Walsh MP, and Cole WC. Angiotensin II activation of protein kinase C decreases delayed rectifier K+ current in rabbit vascular myocytes. *J. Physiol. (Lond)* 495 (Pt 3):689-700, 1996

[48] Cleveland JCJ, Meldrum DR, Cain BS, Banerjee A, and Harken AH. Oral sulfonylurea hypoglycemic agents prevent ischemic preconditioning in human myocardium. Two paradoxes revisited. *Circ.* 96:29-32, 1997

[49] Cole WC, Clement-Chomienne O, and Aiello EA. Regulation of 4-aminopyridine-sensitive, delayed rectifier K^+ channels in vascular smooth muscle by phosphorylation. [Review]. *Biochemistry and Cell Biology* 74:439-447, 1996

[50] Coppey LJ, Gellett JS, and Yorek MA. Mediation of vascular relaxation in epineurial arterioles of the sciatic nerve: effect of diabetes in type 1 and type 2 diabetic rat models. *Endothelium* 10:89-94, 2003

[51] Cosentino F, Luscher TF. Endothelial dysfunction in diabetes mellitus. *J.Cardiovasc.Pharmacol.* 32 Suppl 3:S54-S61, 1998

[52] Cox RH, Lozinskaya I, and Dietz NJ. Differences in K^+ current components in mesenteric artery myocytes from WKY and SHR. *Am.J Hypertens.* 14:897-907, 2001

[53] Czervionke RL, Hoak JC, Haycraft DL, Fry GL, and Mann KG. Contribution of a platelet component to endothelial prostacyclin production despite inhibition of platelet cyclooxygenase activity. *Trans.Assoc.Am.Physicians* 95:272-279, 1982

[54] Daut J, Klieber HG, Cyrys S, and Noack T. K_{ATP} channels and basal coronary vascular tone. *Cardiovasc.Res.* 28:811-817, 1994

[55] Dellsperger KC, Brooks LA, Eastham CL, Gutterman DD: Coronary microvascular vasodilator responses in diabetic dogs (Abstract). *Circ.* 84, 1992

[56] Diederich D, Skopec J, Diederich A, and Dai F-X. Endothelial dysfunction in mesenteric resistance arteries of diabetic rats: role of free radicals. *Am.J.Physiol.* 266:H1153-H1161, 1994

[57] Dimitropoulou C, Han G, Miller AW, Molero M, Fuchs LC, White RE, and Carrier GO. Potassium (BK_{Ca}) currents are reduced in microvascular smooth muscle cells from insulin-resistant rats. *Am.J.Physiol Heart Circ.Physiol* 282:H908-H917, 2002

[58] Dong H, Waldron GJ, Galipeau D, Cole WC, and Triggle CR. NO/PGI2-independent vasorelaxation and the cytochrome P450 pathway in rabbit carotid artery. *Br.J.Pharmacol.* 120:695-701, 1997

[59] Duprat F, Guillemare E, Romey G, Fink M, Lesage F, Lazdunski M, and Honore E. Susceptibility of cloned K+ channels to reactive oxygen species. *Proc.Natl.Acad.Sci.U.S.A* 92:11796-11800, 1995

[60] Dyck PJ, Zimmerman BR, Vilen TH, Minnerath SR, Karnes JL, Yao JK, and Poduslo JF. Nerve glucose, fructose, sorbitol, myo-inositol, and fiber degenertation and regeneration in diabetic neuropathy. *NEJM* 319:542-548, 1988

[61] England SK, Uebele VN, Shear H, Kodali J, Bennett PB, and Tamkun MM. Characterization of a voltage-gated K+ channel beta subunit expressed in human heart. *Proc.Natl.Acad.Sci.U.S.A* 92:6309-6313, 1995

[62] Erdos B, Miller AW, and Busija DW. Alterations in KATP and KCa channel function in cerebral arteries of insulin-resistant rats. *Am.J.Physiol Heart Circ.Physiol* 283:H2472-H2477, 2002

[63] Erdos B, Miller AW, and Busija DW. Impaired endothelium-mediated relaxation in isolated cerebral arteries from insulin-resistant rats. *Am.J.Physiol Heart Circ.Physiol* 282:H2060-H2065, 2002

[64] Erdos B, Simandle SA, Snipes JA, Miller AW, and Busija DW. Potassium channel dysfunction in cerebral arteries of insulin-resistant rats is mediated by reactive oxygen species. *Stroke* 35:964-969, 2004

[65] Erdos B, Snipes JA, Miller AW, and Busija DW. Cerebrovascular dysfunction in Zucker obese rats is mediated by oxidative stress and protein kinase C. *Diabetes* 53:1352-1359, 2004

[66] Fergus DJ, Martens JR, and England SK. Kv channel subunits that contribute to voltage-gated K+ current in renal vascular smooth muscle. *Pflugers Arch.* 445:697-704, 2003

[67] Forestier C, Pierrard J, and Vivaudou M. Mechanism of action of K channel openers on skeletal muscle KATP channels. Interactions with nucleotides and protons. *J Gen Physiol* 107:489-502, 1996

[68] Frank RN. Diabetic retinopathy: current concepts of evaluation and treatment. *Clin.Endocrinol.Metab.* 15:933-969, 1986

[69] Frisbee JC. Impaired dilation of skeletal muscle microvessels to reduced oxygen tension in diabetic obese Zucker rats. *Am.J.Physiol Heart Circ.Physiol* 281:H1568-H1574, 2001

[70] Frisbee JC, Maier KG, and Stepp DW. Oxidant stress-induced increase in myogenic activation of skeletal muscle resistance arteries in obese Zucker rats. *Am.J.Physiol Heart Circ.Physiol* 283:H2160-H2168, 2002

[71] Fujii K, Heistad DD, and Faraci FM. Effect of diabetes mellitus on flow-mediated and endothelium-dependent dilatation of the rat basilar artery. *Stroke* 23:1394-1498, 1992

[72] Giles TD, Ouyang J, Kerut EK, Given MB, Allen GE, McIlwain EF, and Greenberg SS. Changes in protein kinase C in early cardiomyopathy and in gracilis muscle in the BB/Wor diabetic rat. *Am J Physiol* 274:H295-H307, 1998

[73] Giugliano D, Ceriello A, and Paolisso G. Oxidative stress and diabetic vascular complications [see comments]. *Diab.Care* 19:257-267, 1996

[74] Given MB, Greenberg SS, and Giles TD. Coronary vasodilator responses to bradykinin in euglycemic and diabetic rats. *Am.J.Hypertens.* 14:446-454, 2001

[75] Gribble FM, Reimann F. Pharmacological modulation of K(ATP) channels. *Biochem.Soc.Trans.* 30:333-339, 2002

[76] Gschwend S, Henning RH, de Zeeuw D, and Buikema H. Coronary myogenic constriction antagonizes EDHF-mediated dilation: role of KCa channels. *Hypertens.* 41:912-918, 2003

[77] Guzik TJ, Mussa S, Gastaldi D, Sadowski J, Ratnatunga C, Pillai R, and Channon KM. Mechanisms of increased vascular superoxide production in human diabetes mellitus: role of NAD(P)H oxidase and endothelial nitric oxide synthase. *Circ.* 105:1656-1662, 2002

[78] Hanner M, Schmalhofer WA, Munujos P, Knaus HG, Kaczorowski GJ, and Garcia ML. The beta subunit of the high-conductance calcium-activated potassium channel

contributes to the high-affinity receptor for charybdotoxin. *Proc.Natl.Acad.Sci.U.S.A* 94:2853-2858, 1997

[79] Harrison DG. The endothelial cell. *H.D.S.* 1:95-100, 1992

[80] Hathaway CA, Heistad DD, Piegors DJ, and Miller FJ, Jr. Regression of atherosclerosis in monkeys reduces vascular superoxide levels. *Circ.Res.* 90:277-283, 2002

[81] Hayashi K, Kanda T, Homma K, Tokuyama H, Okubo K, Takamatsu I, Tatematsu S, Kumagai H, and Saruta T. Altered renal microvascular response in Zucker obese rats. *Metabolism* 51:1553-1561, 2002

[82] Hink U, Li H, Mollnau H, Oelze M, Matheis E, Hartmann M, Skatchkov M, Thaiss F, Stahl RA, Warnholtz A, Meinertz T, Griendling K, Harrison DG, Forstermann U, and Munzel T. Mechanisms underlying endothelial dysfunction in diabetes mellitus. *Circ.Res.* 88:E14-E22, 2001

[83] Hirai N, Kawano H, Hirashima O, Motoyama T, Moriyama Y, Sakamoto T, Kugiyama K, Ogawa H, Nakao K, and Yasue H. Insulin resistance and endothelial dysfunction in smokers: effects of vitamin C. *Am.J.Physiol Heart Circ.Physiol.* 279:H1172-H1178, 2000

[84] Hirashima O, Kawano H, Motoyama T, Hirai N, Ohgushi M, Kugiyama K, Ogawa H, and Yasue H. Improvement of endothelial function and insulin sensitivity with vitamin C in patients with coronary spastic angina: possible role of reactive oxygen species. *J Am Coll.Cardiol.* 35:1860-1866, 2000

[85] Hoak JC, Czervionke RL, Fry GL, Haycraft DL, and Brotherton AA. Role of the vascular endothelium. *Philos.Trans.R.Soc.Lond.Biol.* 294:331-338, 1981

[86] Holmuhamedov EL, Jovanovic S, Dzeja PP, Jovanovic A, and Terzic A. Mitochondrial ATP-sensitive K^+ channels modulate cardiac mitochondrial function. *Am.J.Physiol.* 275:H1567-H1576, 1998

[87] Hulme JT, Coppock EA, Felipe A, Martens JR, and Tamkun MM. Oxygen sensitivity of cloned voltage-gated K(+) channels expressed in the pulmonary vasculature. *Circ.Res.* 85:489-497, 1999

[88] Hunt JV, Wolff SP. Oxidative glycation and free radical production: a causal mechanism of diabetic complications. *Free Radic. Res. Commun.* 12-13 Pt 1:115-123, 1991

[89] Ichinari K, Kakei M, Matsuoka T, Nakashima H, and Tanaka H. Direct activation of the ATP-sensitive potassium channel by oxygen free radicals in guinea-pig ventricular cells: its potentiation by MgADP. *J.Mol.Cell Cardiol.* 28:1867-1877, 1996

[90] Iida Y, Katusic ZS. Mechanisms of cerebral arterial relaxations to hydrogen peroxide. *Stroke* 31:2224-2230, 2000

[91] Inagaki N, Gonoi T, Clement JP, Namba N, Inazawa J, Gonzalez G, Aguilar-Bryan L, Seino S, and Bryan J. Reconstitution of IKATP: an inward rectifier subunit plus the sulfonylurea receptor. *Science* 270:1166-1170, 1995

[92] Inagaki N, Gonoi T, Clement JP, Wang CZ, Aguilar-Bryan L, Bryan J, and Seino S. A family of sulfonylurea receptors determines the pharmacological properties of ATP-sensitive K+ channels. *Neuron* 16:1011-1017, 1996

[93] Inagaki N, Seino S. ATP-sensitive potassium channels: structures, functions, and pathophysiology. *Jpn.J.Physiol.* 48:397-412, 1998

[94] Inoguchi T, Battan R, Handler E, Sportsman JR, Heath W, and King GL. Preferential elevation of protein kinase C isoform beta II and diacylglycerol levels in the aorta and heart of diabetic rats: differential reversibility to glycemic control by islet cell transplantation. *Proc.Natl.Acad.Sci.U.S.A* 89:11059-11063, 1992

[95] Inoguchi T, Li P, Umeda F, Yu HY, Kakimoto M, Imamura M, Aoki T, Etoh T, Hashimoto T, Naruse M, Sano H, Utsumi H, and Nawata H. High glucose level and free fatty acid stimulate reactive oxygen species production through protein kinase C--dependent activation of NAD(P)H oxidase in cultured vascular cells. *Diabetes* 49:1939-1945, 2000

[96] Inoguchi T, Sonta T, Tsubouchi H, Etoh T, Kakimoto M, Sonoda N, Sato N, Sekiguchi N, Kobayashi K, Sumimoto H, Utsumi H, and Nawata H. Protein kinase C-dependent increase in reactive oxygen species (ROS) production in vascular tissues of diabetes: role of vascular NAD(P)H oxidase. *J.Amer.Soc.Nephrol.* 14:S227-S232, 2003

[97] Inoguchi T, Xia P, Kunisaki M, Higashi S, Feener EP, and King GL. Insulin's effect on protein kinase c and diaglycerol induced by diabetes and glucose in vascular tissues. *Am.J.Physiol.* 267:E369-E379, 1994

[98] Inoue T, Matsunaga R, Sakai Y, Yaguchi I, Takayanagi K, and Morooka S. Insulin resistance affects endothelium-dependent acetylcholine-induced coronary artery response. *Eur.Heart J.* 21:895-900, 2000

[99] Ishii H, Koya D, and King GL. Protein kinase C activation and its role in the development of vascular complications in diabetes mellitus. *J.Mol.Med.* 76:21-31, 1998

[100] Ishikawa T, Hume JR, and Keef KD. Modulation of K^+ and Ca^{2+} channels by histamine H1-receptor stimulation in rabbit coronary artery cells. *J.Physiol. (Lond)* 468:379-400, 1993

[101] Isomoto S, Kondo C, Yamada M, Matsumoto S, Higashiguchi O, Horio Y, Matsuzawa Y, and Kurachi Y. A novel sulfonylurea receptor forms with BIR (Kir6.2) a smooth muscle type ATP-sensitive K^+ channel. *J.Biol.Chem.* 271:24321-24324, 1996

[102] Jin JS, Bohlen HG. Non-insulin-dependent diabetes and hyperglycemia impair rat intestinal flow-mediated regulation. *Am.J.Physiol* 272:H728-H734, 1997

[103] Kamata K, Miyata N, and Kasuya Y. Functional changes in potassium channels in aortas from rats with streptozotocin-induced diabetes. *Eur.J.Pharmacol.* 166:319-323, 1989

[104] Katakam PV, Ujhelyi MR, Hoenig ME, and Miller AW. Endothelial dysfunction precedes hypertension in diet-induced insulin resistance. *Am.J.Physiol* 275:R788-R792, 1998

[105] Katakam PV, Ujhelyi MR, and Miller AW. EDHF-mediated relaxation is impaired in fructose-fed rats. *J.Cardiovasc.Pharmacol.* 34:461-467, 1999

[106] Kim YK, Lee MS, Son SM, Kim IJ, Lee WS, Rhim BY, Hong KW, and Kim CD. Vascular NADH oxidase is involved in impaired endothelium-dependent vasodilation in OLETF rats, a model of type 2 diabetes. *Diabetes* 51:522-527, 2002

[107] Koch RO, Trieb M, Koschak A, Wanner SG, Gauthier KM, Rusch NJ, Knaus HG: Design and use of antibodies for mapping K^+ channel expression in the cardiovascular system. In Potassium channels in cardiovascular biology. Archer SL, Rusch NJ, Eds. New York, Kluwer Academic/Plenum Publisher, 2001, p. 91-102

[108] Korovkina VP, England SK. Detection and implications of potassium channel alterations. *Vascul.Pharmacol.* 38:3-12, 2002

[109] Lacza Z, Puskar M, Kis B, Perciaccante JV, Miller AW, and Busija DW. Hydrogen peroxide acts as an EDHF in the piglet pial vasculature in response to bradykinin. *Am.J.Physiol Heart Circ.Physio.* 283:H406-H411, 2002

[110] Laight DW, Desai KM, Anggard EE, and Carrier MJ. Endothelial dysfunction accompanies a pro-oxidant, pro-diabetic challenge in the insulin resistant, obese Zucker rat in vivo. *Eur.J.Pharmacol.* 402:95-99, 2000

[111] Lamas S, Marsden PA, Li GK, Tempst P, and Michel T. Endothelial nitric oxide synthase: molecular cloning and characterization of a distinct constitutive enzyme isoform. *Proc.Natl.Acad.Sci.U.S.A* 89:6348-6352, 1992

[112] Lee TS, Saltsman KA, Ohashi H, and King GL. Activation of protein kinase C by elevation of glucose concentration: proposal for a mechanism in the development of diabetic vascular complications. *Proc.Natl.Acad.Sci.U.S.A* 86:5141-5145, 1989

[113] Lenaz G, Bovina C, D'Aurelio M, Fato R, Formiggini G, Genova ML, Giuliano G, Pich MM, Paolucci U, Castelli GP, and Ventura B. Role of mitochondria in oxidative stress and aging. *Ann.N.Y.Acad.Sci.* 959:199-213, 2002

[114] Li H, Chai Q, Gutterman DD, and Liu Y. Elevated glucose impairs cAMP-mediated dilation by reducing Kv channel activity in rat small coronary smooth muscle cells. *Am.J.Physiol Heart Circ.Physiol.* 285:H1213-H1219, 2003

[115] Li H, Gutterman DD, Rusch NJ, Bubolz A, and Liu Y. Nitration and functional loss of voltage-gated K^+ channels in rat coronary microvessels exposed to high glucose. *Diabetes* 53:2436-2442, 2004

[116] Li PL, Campbell WB. Epoxyeicosatrienoic acids activate K^+ channels in coronary smooth muscle through a guanine nucleotide binding protein. *Circ.Res.* 80:877-884, 1997

[117] Li PL, Zou AP, and Campbell WB. Regulation of potassium channels in coronary arterial smooth muscle by endothelium-derived vasodilators. *Hypertens.* 29:262-267, 1997

[118] Liu Q, Flavahan NA. Hypoxic dilatation of porcine small coronary arteries: role of endothelium and KATP-channels. *Br.J.Pharmacol.* 120:728-734, 1997

[119] Liu Y, Hudetz AG, Knaus HG, and Rusch NJ. Increased expression of Ca^{2+}-sensitive K^+ channels in the cerebral microcirculation of genetically hypertensive rats: evidence for their protection against cerebral vasospasm. *Circ.Res.* 82:729-737, 1998

[120] Liu Y, Sato T, O'Rourke B, and Marban E. Mitochondrial ATP-dependent potassium channels: novel effectors of cardioprotection? *Circ.* 97:2463-2469, 1998

[121] Liu Y, Terata K, Chai Q, Li H, Kleinman LH, and Gutterman DD. Peroxynitrite inhibits Ca2+-activated K+ channel activity in smooth muscle of human coronary arterioles. *Circ.Res.* 91:1070-1076, 2002

[122] Liu Y, Terata K, Rusch NJ, and Gutterman DD. High glucose impairs voltage-gated K^+ channel current in rat small coronary arteries. *Circ. Res.* 89:146-152, 2001

[123] Lonnqvist F, Thome A, Nilsell K, Hoffstedt J, and Arner P. A pathogenic role of visceral fat beta 3-adrenoceptors in obesity. *J.Clin.Invest.* 95:1109-1116, 1995

[124] Lu M, Wang W. Reaction of nitric oxide with superoxide inhibits basolateral K^+ channels in the rat CCD. *Am.J.Physiol.* 275:C309-C316, 1998

[125] MacMillan-Crow LA, Cruthirds DL. Invited review: manganese superoxide dismutase in disease. *Free Radic.Res.* 34:325-336, 2001

[126] Marshall JJ, Kontos HA. Endothelium-derived relaxing factors: a perspective from in vivo data. *Hypertens.* 16:371-386, 1990

[127] Martens JR, Gelband CH. Alterations in rat interlobar artery membrane potential and K+ channels in genetic and nongenetic hypertension. *Circ.Res.* 79:295-301, 1996

[128] Mathe D. Dyslipidemia and diabetes: animal models. *Diabete Metab.* 21:106-111, 1995

[129] Mayhan WG. Effect of diabetes mellitus on response of the basilar artery to activation of ATP-sensitive potassium channels. *Brain Res.* 636:35-39, 1994

[130] Mayhan WG, Faraci FM. Responses of cerebral arterioles in diabetic rats to activation of ATP- sensitive potassium channels. *Am.J.Physiol.* 265:H152-H157, 1993

[131] Mays DJ, Foose JM, Philipson LH, and Tamkun MM. Localization of the Kv1.5 K^+ channel protein in explanted cardiac tissue. *J.Clin.Invest.* 96:282-292, 1995

[132] McCobb DP, Fowler NL, Featherstone T, Lingle CJ, Saito M, Krause JE, and Salkoff L. A human calcium-activated potassium channel gene expressed in vascular smooth muscle. *Am.J.Physiol* 269:H767-H777, 1995

[133] Mellemkjaer S, Nielsen-Kudsk JE. Glibenclamide inhibits hypoxic relaxation of isolated porcine coronary arteries under conditions of impaired glycolysis. *Eur.J.Pharmacol.* 270:307-312, 1994

[134] Miller AW, Dimitropoulou C, Han G, White RE, Busija DW, and Carrier GO. Epoxyeicosatrienoic acid-induced relaxation is impaired in insulin resistance. *Am.J.Physiol Heart Circ.Physiol.* 281:H1524-H1531, 2001

[135] Miller AW, Katakam PV, and Ujhelyi MR. Impaired endothelium-mediated relaxation in coronary arteries from insulin-resistant rats. *J.Vasc.Res.* 36:385-392, 1999

[136] Miura H, Bosnjak JJ, Ning G, Saito T, Miura M, and Gutterman DD. Role for hydrogen peroxide in flow-induced dilation of human coronary arterioles. *Circ.Res.* 92:e31-e40, 2003

[137] Miura H, Liu Y, and Gutterman DD. Human Coronary Arteriolar Dilation to Bradykinin Depends on Membrane Hyperpolarization. *Circ.* 99:3132-3138, 1999

[138] Mohazzab H, Kaminski PM, and Wolin MS. Lactate and PO2 modulate superoxide anion production in bovine cardiac myocytes: potential role of NADH oxidase. *Circ.* 96:614-620, 1997

[139] Mohazzab-H KM, Kaminski PM, and Wolin MS. NADH oxidoreductase is a major source of superoxide anion in bovine coronary artery endothelium. *Am.J.Physiol.* 266:H2568-h2572, 1994

[140] Morales MJ, Castellino RC, Crews AL, Rasmusson RL, and Strauss HC. A novel beta subunit increases rate of inactivation of specific voltage-gated potassium channel alpha subunits. *J.Biol.Chem.* 270:6272-6277, 1995

[141] Najibi S, Cohen RA. Enhanced role of potassium channels in relaxation of hypercholesterolemic rabbit carotid artery to nitric oxide. *Am.J.Physiol.* 38:H805-H811, 1995

[142] Najibi S, Cowan CL, Palacino JJ, and Cohen RA. Enhanced role of potassium channels in relaxations to acetylcholine in hypercholesterolemic rabbit carotid artery. *Am.J.Physiol.* 266:H2061-H2067, 1994

[143] Nakhostine N, Lamontagne D. Adenosine contributes to hypoxia-induced vasodilation through atp-sensitive k+ channel activation. *Am.J.Physiol.* 265:H1289-H1293, 1993

[144] Nandi A, Kitamura Y, Kahn CR, and Accili D. Mouse models of insulin resistance. *Physiol Rev.* 84:623-647, 2004

[145] Ng TF, Lee FK, Song ZT, Calcutt NA, Lee AY, Chung SS, Chung SK, Ng DT, and Lee LW. Effects of sorbitol dehydrogenase deficiency on nerve conduction in experimental diabetic mice. *Diabetes* 47:961-966, 1998

[146] Node K, Kitakaze M, Kosaka H, Minamino T, and Hori M. Bradykinin mediation of Ca^{2+} activated K^+ channels regulates coronary blood flow in ischemic myocardium. *Circ.* 95:1560-1567, 1997

[147] Olivier M, Hsiung CA, Chuang LM, Ho LT, Ting CT, Bustos VI, Lee TM, De Witte A, Chen YD, Olshen R, Rodriguez B, Wen CC, and Cox DR. Single nucleotide polymorphisms in protein tyrosine phosphatase 1{beta} (PTPN1) are associated with essential hypertension and obesity. *Hum.Mol.Genet.* 13:1885-1892, 2004

[148] Oskarsson HJ, Hofmeyer TG, Coppey L, and Yorek MA. Effect of protein kinase C and phospholipase A2 inhibitors on the impaired ability of human diabetic platelets to cause vasodilation. *Br. J. Pharmacol.* 127:903-908, 1999

[149] Overturf KE, Russell SN, Carl A, Vogalis F, Hart PJ, Hume JR, Sanders KM, and Horowitz B. Cloning and characterization of a Kv1.5 delayed rectifier K^+ channel from vascular and visceral smooth muscles. *Am.J.Physiol.* 267:C1231-C1238, 1994

[150] Panes J, Kurose I, Rodriguez-Vaca MD, Anderson DC, Miyasaka M, Tso P, and Granger DN. Diabetes exacerbates inflammatory responses to ischemia-reperfusion. *Circ.* 93:161-167, 1996

[151] Pang BS, Wang C, Luo Q, Zhang LM, Zhu M, Mao YL, Huang XX, and Guo WJ. Study of the function of coagulation, fibrinolysis and pulmonary vascular endothelium before and after experimental pulmonary thromboembolism in rabbits. *Zhonghua Jie.He.He.Hu Xi.Za Zhi.* 27:381-384, 2004

[152] Park MK, Lee SH, Lee SJ, Ho WK, and Earm YE. Different modulation of Ca-activated K channels by the intracellular redox potential in pulmonary and ear arterial smooth muscle cells of the rabbit. *Pflugers Arch.* 430:308-314, 1995

[153] Pena AS, Wiltshire E, Gent R, Hirte C, and Couper J. Folic acid improves endothelial function in children and adolescents with type 1 diabetes. *J.Pediatr.* 144:500-504, 2004

[154] Perez-Martin A, Raynaud E, and Mercier J. Insulin resistance and associated metabolic abnormalities in muscle: effects of exercise. *Obes.Rev.* 2:47-59, 2001

[155] Pieper GM, Dondlinger L. Glucose elevations alter bradykinin-stimulated intracellular calcium accumulation in cultured endothelial cells. *Cardiovasc.Res.* 34:169-178, 1997

[156] Pleiner J, Schaller G, Mittermayer F, Bayerle-Eder M, Roden M, and Wolzt M. FFA-induced endothelial dysfunction can be corrected by vitamin C. *J.Clin.Endocrinol.Metab.* 87:2913-2917, 2002

[157] Pomposiello S, Rhaleb NE, Alva M, and Carretero OA. Reactive oxygen species: role in the relaxation induced by bradykinin or arachidonic acid via EDHF in isolated porcine coronary arteries. *J.Cardiovasc.Pharmacol.* 34:567-574, 1999

[158] Pongs O. Molecular biology of voltage-dependent potassium channels. *Physiol Rev* 72:S69-S88, 1992

[159] Post JM, Hume JR, Archer SL, and Weir EK. Direct role for potassium channel inhibition in hypoxic pulmonary vasoconstriction. *Am.J.Physiol.* 262:C882-C890, 1992

[160] Rajagopalan S, Kurz S, Munzel T, Tarpey M, Freeman BA, Griendling KK, and Harrison DG. Angiotensin II-mediated hypertension in the rat increases vascular superoxide production via membrane NADH/NADPH oxidase activation. Contribution to alterations of vasomotor tone. *J.Clin.Invest.* 97:1916-1923, 1996

[161] Rasmusson RL, Morales MJ, Wang S, Liu S, Campbell DL, Brahmajothi MV, and Strauss HC. Inactivation of voltage-gated cardiac K^+ channels. *Circ.Res.* 82:739-750, 1998

[162] Reimann F, Ashcroft FM, and Gribble FM. Structural basis for the interference between nicorandil and sulfonylurea action. *Diabetes* 50:2253-2259, 2001

[163] Reimann F, Gribble FM, and Ashcroft FM. Differential response of K_{ATP} channels containing SUR2A or SUR2B subunits to nucleotides and pinacidil. *Mol.Pharmacol.* 58:1318-1325, 2000

[164] Rettig J, Heinemann SH, Wunder F, Lorra C, Parcej DN, Dolly JO, and Pongs O. Inactivation properties of voltage-gated K^+ channels altered by presence of beta-subunit. *Nature* 369:289-294, 1994

[165] Roberts ES, Lin H, Crowley JR, Vuletich JL, Osawa Y, and Hollenberg PF. Peroxynitrite-mediated nitration of tyrosine and inactivation of the catalytic activity of cytochrome P450 2B1. *Chem.Res.Toxicol.* 11:1067-1074, 1998

[166] Rorsman P, Berggren PO, Bokvist K, and Efendic S. ATP-regulated K^+ channels and diabetes mellitus. *NIPS* 5:143-147, 1990

[167] Ross J, Armstead WM. Differential role of PTK and ERK MAPK in superoxide impairment of K_{ATP} and K_{Ca} channel cerebrovasodilation. *Am.J.Physiol. Regul.Integr.Comp Physiol.* 285:R149-R154, 2003

[168] Saigo M, Hsue PY, and Waters DD. Role of thrombotic and fibrinolytic factors in acute coronary syndromes. *Prog.Cardiovasc.Dis.* 46:524-538, 2004

[169] Schernthaner G. Cardiovascular mortality and morbidity in type-2 diabetes mellitus. *Diabetes Res.Clin.Pract.* 31 Suppl:S3-13:S3-13, 1996

[170] Shi G, Nakahira K, Hammond S, Rhodes KJ, Schechter LE, and Trimmer JS. Beta subunits promote K^+ channel surface expression through effects early in biosynthesis. *Neuron* 16:843-852, 1996

[171] Shiba T, Inoguchi T, Sportsman JR, Heath WF, Bursell S-E, and King GL. Correlation of diacylglycerol and protein kinase C activity in rat retina to retinal circulation. *Am.J.Physiol.* 265:E783-E793, 1993

[172] Shieh CC, Coghlan M, Sullivan JP, and Gopalakrishnan M. Potassium channels: molecular defects, diseases, and therapeutic opportunities. *Pharmacol.Rev.* 52:557-594, 2000

[173] Shinozaki K, Hirayama A, Nishio Y, Yoshida Y, Ohtani T, Okamura T, Masada M, Kikkawa R, Kodama K, and Kashiwagi A. Coronary endothelial dysfunction in the insulin-resistant state is linked to abnormal pteridine metabolism and vascular oxidative stress. *J. Am. Coll.Cardiol.* 38:1821-1828, 2001

[174] Standen NB, Quayle JM. K^+ channel modulation in arterial smooth muscle. *Acta Physiol. Scand.* 164:549-557, 1998

[175] Stassen JM, Arnout J, and Deckmyn H. The hemostatic system. *Curr.Med.Chem.* 11:2245-2260, 2004

[176] Studer RK, Craven PA, and DeRubertis FR. Role for protein kinase C in the mediation of increased fibronectin accumulation by mesangial cells grown in high-glucose medium. *Diabetes* 42:118-126, 1993

[177] Terzic A, Vivaudou M: Molecular pharmacology of ATP-sensitive K^+ channels: How and Why? In Potassium channels in cardiovascular biology. Archer SL, Rusch NJ, Eds. New York, Kluwer Academic, 2001, p. 257-277

[178] Tesfamarian B, Cohen RA. Free radicals mediate endothelial cell dysfunction caused by elevated glucose. *Am.J.Physiol.* 263:H321-H326, 1992

[179] Thengchaisri N, Kuo L. Hydrogen peroxide induces endothelium-dependent and -independent coronary arteriolar dilation: role of cyclooxygenase and potassium channels. *Am.J.Physiol Heart Circ.Physiol* 285:H2255-H2263, 2003

[180] Tiefenbacher CP, Kreuzer J. Nitric oxide-mediated endothelial dysfunction--is there need to treat? *Curr.Vasc.Pharmacol.* 1:123-133, 2003

[181] Tokube K, Kiyosue T, and Arita M. Openings of cardiac KATP channel by oxygen free radicals produced by xanthine oxidase reaction. *Am J Physiol* 271:H478-H489, 1996

[182] Tokube K, Kiyosue T, and Arita M. Effects of hydroxyl radicals on K_{ATP} channels in guinea-pig ventricular myocytes. *Pflugers Arch.* 437:155-157, 1998

[183] Trumpower BL. New concepts on the role of ubiquinone in the mitochondrial respiratory chain. *J.Bioenerg.Biomembr.* 13:1-24, 1981

[184] Trumpower BL. The protonmotive Q cycle. Energy transduction by coupling of proton translocation to electron transfer by the cytochrome bc1 complex. *J.Biol.Chem.* 265:11409-11412, 1990

[185] Turrens JF, Alexandre A, and Lehninger AL. Ubisemiquinone is the electron donor for superoxide formation by complex III of heart mitochondria. *Arch.Biochem.Biophys.* 237:408-414, 1985

[186] Wang J, Juhaszova M, Rubin LJ, and Yuan XJ. Hypoxia inhibits gene expression of voltage-gated K^+ channel alpha subunits in pulmonary artery smooth muscle cells. *J.Clin.Invest.* 100:2347-2353, 1997

[187] Weiger TM, Hermann A, and Levitan IB. Modulation of calcium-activated potassium channels. *J.Comp Physiol A Neuroethol.Sens.Neural Behav.Physiol.* 188:79-87, 2002

[188] Weik R, Neumcke B. ATP-sensitive potassium channels in adult mouse skeletal muscle: characterization of the ATP-binding site. *J.Membr.Biol.* 110:217-226, 1989

[189] Wolin MS. How could a genetic variant of the p22(phox) component of NAD(P)H oxidases contribute to the progression of coronary atherosclerosis?. *Circ.Res.* 86:365-366, 2000

[190] Wu X, Makynen H, Kahonen M, Arvola P, and Porsti I. Mesenteric arterial function in vitro in three models of experimental hypertension. *J.Hypertens.* 14:365-372, 1996

[191] Yamada M, Isomoto S, Matsumoto S, Kondo C, Shindo T, Horio Y, and Kurachi Y. Sulphonylurea receptor 2B and Kir6.1 form a sulphonylurea-sensitive but ATP-insensitive K^+ channel. *J.Physiol.* 499 (Pt 3):715-720, 1997

[192] Yasuda H, Sonobe M, Yamashita M, Terada M, Hatanaka I, Huitian Z, and Shigeta Y. Effect of prostaglandin e1 analogue tfc 612 on diabetic neuropathy in streptozocin-induced diabetic rats. *Diabetes* 38:832-838, 1989

[193] Yu W, Xu J, and Li M. NAB domain is essential for the subunit assembly of both alpha-alpha and alpha-beta complexes of shaker-like potassium channels. *Neuron* 16:441-453, 1996

[194] Zou M, Martin C, and Ullrich V. Tyrosine nitration as a mechanism of selective inactivation of prostacyclin synthase by peroxynitrite. *Biol.Chem.* 378:707-713, 1997

[195] Zou MH, Shi C, and Cohen RA. High glucose via peroxynitrite causes tyrosine nitration and inactivation of prostacyclin synthase that is associated with thromboxane/prostaglandin H(2) receptor-mediated apoptosis and adhesion molecule expression in cultured human aortic endothelial cells. *Diabetes* 51:198-203, 2002

[196] Zouali H, Velho G, and Froguel P. Polymorphism of the glycogen synthase gene and non-insulin-dependent diabetes mellitus. *N.Engl.J.Med.* 328:1568, 1993

In: Trends in Diabetes Research
Editor: Ashley M. Ford, pp. 107-129

ISBN: 1-59454-796-3

Chapter V

Pathogenesis of Testicular ALL

Hisham El Morsi[1], Kwee Lan Yong[2], Keith Patterson[2] and Andrew Jewell[1*]

[1] School of Life Sciences, Kingston University,
Penrhyn Road, Kingston-Upon-Thames, Surrey KT1 2EE. UK.
[2] Haematology Department, University College London,
98 Chenies Mews, London WC1E 6HX

Abstract

Treatment for childhood Acute Lymphoblastic Leukaemia (ALL) improved dramatically during the second half of the twentieth century, with four-year survival rates of up to 60% being recorded. Extramedullary relapse in the central nervous system (CNS) required the introduction of cranial irradiation and intrathecal methotrexate. The second most common extramedullary site to show ALL relapse is the testis. The development of more intensive treatment protocols has reduced the incidence of testicular relapse, but relapse in the testis may still occur 13 years after initial treatment. However the pathogenesis of testicular leukaemia remains unclear. It is not known whether malignant lymphoblasts survive long-term in the testicular interstitium, or spread into the testis from subclinical leukaemic involvement on the bone marrow. Animal models, and some clinical data, may provide a sanctuary site from chemotherapeutic agents. In addition, the local micro-environment in the testis may provide cytokines and growth factors which support the survival and proliferation of the malignant lymphoblasts. This review summarises the current state of our understanding of which of these factors may be important in the testis, and of the known effects on ALL cells.

* Correspondence: A. P. Jewell,School of Life Sciences, Kingston University, Penrhyn Road, Kingston-Upon-Thames, Surrey KT1 2EE. UK.Telephone 0208 547 2000 x2468; Fax 0208 547 7562, Email: a.jewell@kingston.ac.uk

Acute Lymphoblastic Leukaemia (All)

As recently as the 1960's, childhood ALL had a very bad prognosis, and most patients were destined to die within few weeks. The noticeable progress in the management of ALL resulted in the improvement of survival, and the 4-year survival rate had increased from around 0% during the sixties of the twentieth century to 60% today (Ritzen, 1990). This advance had led to the identification of a serious complication of the disease as it advances through the central nervous system (CNS) causing meningeal leukaemia in 50% of cases (Wong *et al*, 1980; Jackson *et al*, 1983; Jackson *et al*, 1984) which necessitated the introduction of CNS prophylaxis through cranial irradiation and the administration of intrathecal methotrexate (Ritzen, 1990).

Before the introduction of CNS prophylaxis, (1968-1972) the outcome for males and females was similar. However, between 1972-1978, with a better management of the disease, the addition of CNS prophylaxis, and the improvement of survival, the difference in prognosis in favour of females became evident (Sather *et al*, 1981a; Sather *et al*, 1981b). Ritzen, (1990) reported a 30-37% 5 years disease free survival rate for boys compared to 50-70 % for girls. Sather *et al*, 1981b reported 1.7 fold higher relapse rate in boys after discontinuation of the treatment, and Russo and Schiliro, (1986) in a critical review reported that cessation of treatment after 3 years carried a risk of relapse 10-20% higher in boys than girls. These observations placed females in the favourable prognostic groups, and males were found to have poorer prognosis. Not only did boys have a higher incidence of the disease, but also their rate of relapse was higher (Ritzen, 1990).

The reason for this apparent sex difference is not clear. However, among the children surviving the first 3 years, testicular relapse (TR) is still a major contributing factor for the different prognosis between boys and girls (Ritzen, 1990).

Childhood Testicular Leukaemia

The testis is the second most common extramedullary site to show ALL relapse after the central nervous system (CNS) (Jahnukainen *et al*, 1995a). Testicular ALL was described by Nies *et al*, (1965) and Finklestein *et al*, (1969), and the clinical problem behind childhood testicular leukaemia was first described by Stoffel *et al*, (1975). In studies of patients suffering from acute lymphoblastic leukaemia, 28-92% of testicular biopsies were positive for leukaemic infiltrations, while the ovaries showed much lower involvement rate of 11-24% (Aur *et al*, 1978; Furman *et al*, 1990; Hustu and Aur, 1978).

With the development of more intensive treatment protocols, the incidence of disease involvement in testicular biopsies dropped to 8.5-37% (Russo *et al*, 1990; Russo and Schiliro', 1986), and the more recent intensive treatment regimens reduced this to less than 5% in some centres (Miller *et al*, 1983a; Miller *et al*, 1983b; Miller *et al*, 1990; Miller and Miller, 1990; Sather *et al*, 1981b). Another interesting observation that emerged during the study of testicular leukaemia was the much lower rate of involvement in adults; only 1-2% may show manifestations of testicular leukaemia (Jahnukainen *et al*, 1993). These observations suggested that the testes in boys preferentially support the survival of leukaemic blasts and that the maturation changes of the individual somehow protect the testes in adults from the invading lymphoblasts.

Clinically, testicular leukaemia is often recognised as a unilateral painless firm scrotal/testicular swelling. However, it may be bilateral in 1-2 % and painful in 0.1-0.2% of cases (Eden *et al*, 1983). Ultrasound examination typically shows an enlarged hypoechoic testicular swelling +/- a small focus of normal appearing -echogenic- testicular tissue (Lupetin *et al*, 1983a; Lupetin *et al*, 1983b). At biopsy both testes are generally involved, although only one is affected clinically. Histological examination of the biopsied tissue classically reveals massive diffuse interstitial infiltration of a uniform population of leukaemic blast cells with variable degree of invasion and destruction of the seminiferous tubules (Gill *et al*, 1989; Wong *et al*, 1980).

According to the time of onset, testicular leukaemia is divided into two biologically distinct categories. Children presenting with overt testicular leukaemia at diagnosis or those developing testicular relapse early in the course the disease, typically after the first year of chemotherapy, are usually at a higher risk of developing multiple drug resistance and poorer prognosis, with an outcome similar to cases of early bone marrow relapse. Fortunately this group accounts for a minority of cases of about 1-5% (Gajjar *et al*, 1996; Russo and Schiliro', 1986).

On the other hand, testicular relapse that occurs shortly after cessation of treatment or discovered as an occult focus by elective biopsy at the end of treatment, occurs in 10-20% but has been reported to be as low as 0.9% and as high as 40% (Chessells *et al*, 1986a; Jahnukainen *et al*, 1998; Miller *et al*, 1983a; Miller *et al*, 1990; Nachman *et al*, 1990). This group has a good response to re-induction treatment and an excellent outcome of 70% 5-year disease free survival. Nevertheless, due to the testicular damage exerted by treatment, these patients require close follow up and endocrinological support as more than 80% of patients would require hormonal therapy through puberty and adult life (Grundy *et al*, 1997). Furthermore, the damage caused by irradiation, which results in endocrine failure, usually renders these children sterile, and important consequence of testicular leukaemia.

Prognostic Value of Testicular Leukaemia

In spite of the fact that evolving protocols in ALL treatment have led to a reduction in the incidence of testicular relapse to less than 5% (Lal *et al*, 1998; Miller *et al*, 1990; Miller and Miller, 1990), the testis can still represent a sanctuary for the malignant lymphoblasts for as long as 7-13 years (Franck *et al*, 1998; Wong *et al*, 1980). There are no reliable predictors of the likelihood of testicular relapse, even the prognostic criteria, including the most significant variables, i.e. the white blood count (WBC), age, sex and cytogenetics abnormalities, have very low predictive powers as they were found to correlate very weakly to anticipation of the outcome of treatment. In a statistical study of 1552 patients (Donadieu *et al*, 1998), these variables could explain no more than 4% of the variation of the outcome of the disease and could only identify a minority of patients among those suffering the long term risk of treatment failure.

More direct approaches attempting to identify boys at higher risk of developing testicular relapse employing presymptomatic testicular biopsy at the end of chemotherapy were unsuccessful. A proportion (10%) of patients with histologically negative biopsies relapsed subsequently and in many cases, the biopsies were difficult to interpret because of the presence of "suspicious" cells that could not be classified definitely as malignant or benign. Immunostaining for terminal deoxynucleotidyl transferase (TdT) positive cells produced 5% false –ve results and another 5% false +ve results, and was hence no better than conventional histology (Chessells *et al*, 1986b). Finally and most importantly the early detection and treatment of occult testicular relapse had no significant effect on long-term survival (Chessells *et al*, 1986a; Miller *et al*, 1990; Nachman *et al*, 1990). On the other hand, studies aiming at improving the detection of minimal residual disease (MRD) in the bone marrow and testicular tissues have failed to predict those patients likely to suffer extramedullary relapses (Brisco *et al*, 1994; Chessells *et al*, 1986a; Tiedemann *et al*, 1982). The bone marrow in several studies was free of MRD even at the time of extramedullary relapse (Brisco *et al*, 1994; Eden *et al*, 1983). However, in a more recent study, MRD detection in the testicular biopsies using the polymerase chain reaction (PCR) to detect clone specific antigen receptor genes have been tried and showed promising results. This technique may accurately identify unilateral testicular disease in boys with ALL and may be better than bone marrow samples to identify boys who will subsequently suffer a testicular relapse (Lal *et al*, 1998).

Pathogenesis of Testicular Leukaemia

Despite the clinical importance of testicular relapse in childhood ALL, the pathogenesis is still controversial. It is not known whether the leukaemic lymphoblasts escape the impact of chemotherapy in the testicular interstitium, or later spread into the testis from subclinical leukaemic involvement in bone marrow (O'Reilly *et al*, 1995). However, the problem in these studies is that the bone marrow is, in most cases, studied at the time of overt testicular relapse, and no information about the preceding minimal residual disease in the testicular tissue is provided. Sequential bone marrow samples taken before isolated testicular relapse have in many cases failed to show minimal residual leukaemia before isolated testicular relapses (O'Reilly *et al*, 1995). The marrow analysis has also proved to be a poor predictor of other isolated extramedullary relapses (Brisco *et al*, 1994; Eden *et al*, 1983;Tiedemann *et al*, 1982).

On the other hand studies using animal models of ALL have revealed that during the untreated course of disease, leukaemic lymphoblasts can spread into the interstitium of the premature testis. Testicular factors like testicular growth factors, testicular endothelium and testicular interstitial cells may be able locally to control the penetration of leukaemic cells into the testicular interstitium and the intratesticular proliferation of leukaemic lymphoblasts (Jahnukainen *et al*, 1993; Jahnukainen *et al*, 1995a; Jahnukainen *et al*, 2001; Russo and Schiliro', 1986).

Local Factors that May be Involved in the Pathogenesis of Testicular Leukaemia

In looking for factors responsible for the tendency of leukaemic cells to survive for long periods inside the testes, several factors may be involved, e.g.: the lower testicular temperature that is needed for optimal function of the testis, the vascular endothelial barrier that gradually develops, and the testicular interstitial cells that produce several cytokines and growth factors locally in the testes. It must be kept in mind as well that the 10th year of life is known to be a turning point in puberty, the time when adult-type Leydig cells start to develop, Sertoli cells change their secretory pattern, leading to the initiation of spermatogenesis, and the locally produced testicular cytokines reach their peak levels (Table 1 and Table 2). These maturational events and the lower testicular temperature and growth factors produced by the invading lymphoblasts may be related to the appearance of an increasing tendency for testicular relapses at pre- and early puberty and a sharp decline afterwards at the time of spermatogenesis.

Testicular Structure

The testes are paired organs located in the scrotum and are partially surrounded by the *tunica vaginalis*. The *tunica albuginea* penetrates deeply into the posterior aspect of the testis forming the mediastinum testis, in which the hilum is located. Through the hilar ducts, blood vessels, nerves and lymphatic vessels enter and leave. Connective tissue trabeculae project from the mediastinum into the interior of the testis, dividing it into several hundred lobules. Within each lobule are the seminiferous tubules, 500 million in each testis. The seminiferous tubules are lined by primitive germ cells and by Sertoli cells. The tight junctions between adjacent Sertoli cells form the blood testis barrier that prevents many large molecules from passing from the interstitial tissue. The interstitial tissue between the seminiferous tubules is filled with small vessels and lymphatics. Fibroblasts, macrophages, lymphocytes, and most importantly Leydig cells are found here, it is the interstitial space in which leukaemic infiltrates may be found.

Leydig Cells

The Leydig cells are the major components of the testicular interstitium. There is evidence from *in vitro* studies that the adult type Leydig cells bind normal lymphocytes to their surface and decrease their proliferation (Jahnukainen *et al*, 1995b). This antiproliferative activity is more likely to be due to the direct contact between the cells rather than the secretions of Leydig cells as cell culture supernatant did not inhibit lymphocyte proliferation. In an *in vivo* study (Jahnukainen *et al*, 1995b), electron microscopic studies of ALL blasts inside the premature and mature murine testes provided new insights to the interaction between the leukaemic cells and the microstructures of the immature testicular interstitium. The leukaemic cells were shown to attach to and disrupt the structure of Leydig cells and may use the low level of proliferation activity and tolerance to cytotoxic drugs as protection from the effect of the chemotherapeutic agents used in the treatment of ALL. The leukaemic cells were seen surrounded by Leydig cells, which appeared like a blockade between the leukaemic cell and the testicular blood capillaries.

Testicular Temperature

The male gonad requires a specialised temperature environment to produce spermatozoa, for not only does spermatogenesis occur most effectively at a relatively cool temperature (32-34°C), but also the core body temperature is lethal for the male germ cells (Morgentaler *et al*, 1999). Mammals, have a specialised extra-corporal pouch, (the scrotum), to sustain a cool testicular environment. Despite testicular temperature being similar in both children and adults, the lower testicular temperature represents the major difference in environment between testicles and ovaries. The ovaries are located intra-abdominally at body temperature (37-37.5°C), while the extra-abdominal location of the testes expose them to a lower temperature environment, which is needed for the optimal physiological function. The mean scrotal temperature is 32.5°C, which may lower the proliferation of leukaemic cells, thus causing them to be less sensitive to the cytotoxic drugs (Russo and Schiliro, 1986).

Mechanisms of Testicular Temperature Maintenance

In fact, maintaining the necessary testicular temperature environment is not only a matter of a simple passive scrotal presence of the testes, but five main anatomic features allow the testes to remain cool:

1. The dartos muscle.
2. The cremaster muscle.
3. The countercurrent heat exchange system around the testes.
4. An absent fatty skin layer of the scrotum.
5. Abundant scrotal skin sweat glands.

The dartos muscle lines the scrotum and relaxes when ambient temperature is warm, this cools the testes by causing them to lie further away from the body, which is the local heat source. The cremasteric fibres in the spermatic cord act similarly but more directly on testicular distance from the body. As warm blood in the testicular artery courses peripherally to the testes, some of its heat is transferred to the cooler returning blood in the surrounding veins of the pampiniform plexus. This is a counter current heat exchange system, causing blood in the testicular artery to become progressively cooler as it travels towards the testes. Finally, the absence of fat in scrotal skin allows ambient temperature to cool the testes without intervening insulation, and sweat glands contribute to heat loss by evaporative cooling (Kastelic *et al*, 1997a; Kastelic *et al*, 1997b).

Testicular Temperature and ALL

Regardless of the mechanisms and changes of the human testes to suit spermatogenesis, this lower testicular temperature adaptation besides the changes in cellular structure around puberty, may allow the leukaemic cells to survive for long periods inside the human testis (Jahnukainen *et al*, 1993; Jahnukainen *et al*, 1995a; Jahnukainen *et al*, 1995b; Russo and Schiliro', 1986).

A few observations suggest that temperature may be important in the control of ALL growth and survival.

1. The lower temperature is one of the differences between the ovaries and the testes, the ovaries are placed in the abdominal cavity at the same temperature as other organs, and the frequency of their involvement in ALL is much less than the testicular one (Aur *et al*, 1978; Furman *et al*, 1990; Hustu and Aur, 1978; Sather *et al*, 1981a; Sather *et al*, 1981b). The increased testicular incidence had led to the poorer outcome of males compared with females (Ritzen, 1990), with this difference in outcome becoming more significant with the discontinuation of the treatment, presumably at the time when a hypothermic low proliferating clone of leukaemic cells find a chance to re-grow and relapse (Ritzen, 1990).
2. The suggestion by several authors that the lower proliferation of malignant cells of solid and/or haematopoietic origin -when incubated at lower temperatures- may protect them from the cytotoxicity of chemotherapy (Auersperg, 1966; Cavaliere *et al*, 1967; Fondy *et al*, 1974; Gloria and George, 1980; Rao and Engelberg, 1965).

However, the effect of temperature on the leukaemic cells may not be restricted to the childhood acute lymphoblastic leukaemia, it may extend to affect the other types of childhood and adult leukaemias such as acute promyelocytic leukaemia APL (Forrest *et al*, 1997; Shaffer *et al*, 1992; Furman *et al*, 1990), acute monocytic leukaemia (Nishikawa *et al*, 1987a; Nishikawa *et al*, 1987b), and acute myeloid leukaemia (AML) (Lehmann *et al*, 1997).

Studies on Malignancies and Temperature

The interest in the effect of temperature on cancer started more than one and half centuries ago, when it was observed that temperatures above the physiologic value might have destructive effects on cancer. Several lines of evidence have since accumulated to suggest that cancer cells are selectively sensitive to hyperthermia both *in vivo* and *in vitro* than normal cells (Agostinelli *et al*, 1994; Auersperg, 1966; Bisht and Uma, 1996; Carper *et al*, 1997; Cavaliere *et al*, 1967; Giovanella and Mondovi, 1977; Mondovi *et al*, 1968; Mondovi *et al*, 1969a; Mondovi *et al*, 1969b; Moriyama *et al*, 1986; Muckle and Dickson, 1971; Muckle *et al*, 1971a; Muckle *et al*, 1971b; Palzer and Heidelberger, 1973; Storm *et al*, 1996; Turano *et al*, 1970). Giovanella *et al*, 1970 and Moriyama *et al*, 1986 showed that leukaemic cells were more sensitive to supranormal temperature (39-42°C) than normal cells, and that several aspects of the cell kinetics including survival, glycolysis, nucleic acids and protein synthesis and O_2 uptake were affected by higher temperature. Indeed, in ALL during chemotherapy, hyper-pyrexia is regularly caused by febrile neutropaenia and this may be one mechanism by which strong chemotherapy improves response in acute leukaemia

The effect of hypothermia on cancer cells, on the other hand, was not widely investigated. However, of the few *in vitro* experiments carried out on mammalian cells, Chinese hamster cells HA1 grown at 32°C had a lower proliferation and more resistance to X irradiation than control cells (Gloria and George, 1980) and the proliferation of HeLa cells was inhibited when the cells were incubated at lower culture temperature (32°C) (Rao and Engelberg, 1965).

The *in vivo* effect of testicular temperature on ALL cells in murine animal models was also studied by Jahnukainen *et al*, (1995b), and a lower proliferation rate of ALL cells was observed. However, if the lower temperature of the testis alone predisposes to leukaemic cell survival, we may expect to see relapse in the nose and ears. Apart from lower testicular temperature, Jahnukainen *et al*, (1993) studied the effect of blood testis barrier on the advancement of testicular leukaemia.

Blood Testis Barrier

Blood testis barrier, represented by the tight junctions between Sertoli cells is required for the physiological function of the testes, i.e. spermatogenesis. This barrier was shown to gradually develop during the maturation stages of the individual until it finally develops adult characteristics (Setchell *et al*, 1988). Riccardi *et al*, (1982) showed that the methotrexate level inside the adult seminiferous tubules was 18-50 times lower than the plasma level. This barrier structure was protected even from the effects of higher temperature when the testicles were made abdominal in experimental murine cryptorchidism studies (Holash *et al*, 1993a; Holash *et al*, 1993b; Holash and Stewart, 1993; Stewart *et al*, 1990; Stewart and Brown, 1990). On the other hand, the vascular endothelium of the testicular microvessels is known to undergo physiological changes during puberty to become selectively permeable. This selective permeability greatly facilitates the access of peptides and proteins from the vascular compartment to the interstitial tissue (Stewart *et al*, 1990). Holash *et al*, (1993a) showed that these testicular microvessels share the barrier features of the blood brain barrier, and that the barrier properties of the testicular microvessels were maintained by Leydig cells. The structure of the testicular microvessels is disrupted by the invading leukaemic cells (Jahnukainen *et al*, 1995b). The capillaries, arterioles and venules become hypertrophic, the endothelium becomes thickened and the lumen is occluded in many places. The endothelial tight junctions become closed, but in many places the endothelium surrounding the junctions become thinner than controls (Jahnukainen *et al*, 1995b).

It is unlikely, however, that this barrier would create a real concentration gradient between the blood and the testicular interstitium, even with the above-mentioned histological changes caused by the invading leukaemic cells. It may, however, slow down the passage of cytotoxic drugs used in the treatment of ALL. Methotrexate was shown to diffuse readily into the interstitial space and was only 2 times less than the corresponding methotrexate plasma level. Moreover, evidence of cytotoxic drugs affecting the structure of the testicular interstitium have been demonstrated as histological examinations of the testicular biopsies demonstrated testicular fibrosis following the administration of cytotoxic drugs (Kobayashi *et al*, 1996; Lendon *et al*, 1978; Riccardi *et al*, 1982; Shalet *et al*, 1981).

Nonetheless, the higher incidence of pre-adult testicular leukaemia may be attributed to the higher permeability of the immature testicular vascular endothelium, in the sense that it may allow the malignant lymphoblasts to accumulate inside the testes early in the course of the disease before the start of chemotherapy (Jahnukainen *et al*, 1993; Wong *et al*, 1980). Afterwards, these lymphoblasts may be protected from the effect of cytotoxic drugs by interacting with the testicular cells, and cytokines and growth factors produced by them (Jahnukainen *et al*, 1995a; Jahnukainen *et al*, 1995b; Jahnukainen *et al*, 2001; Ritzen, 1990;).

Testicular Cytokines, and Growth Factors that Might Be Involved in the Pathogenesis of Testicular Leukaemia

The testicular interstitium contains different types of cells, including Leydig cells, leukocytes, fibroblasts, and in patients with ALL, malignant ALL lymphoblasts during the course of the disease. These cells and their products of cytokines and growth factors may be involved in the penetrance of ALL both in the premature testes early in the course of the disease and the long periods of their survival afterwards (Jahnukainen *et al*, 1993; Jahnukainen *et al*, 1995a; Jahnukainen *et al*, 1995b Ritzen, 1990). Nonetheless, the mechanism by which the malignant cells migrate to the interstitial space and survive for long periods inside the testis are still undetermined.

The other observation that coincides with maturational events of the testes is the immune privileged characteristics of the testicular interstitium, where a graft of foreign tissue, that would be rejected promptly if placed at a conventional body sites, enjoys prolonged (perhaps even indefinite) survival without suffering the deleterious consequences of immune rejection. However, it is not known to what extent this immunosuppressive activity participates in the defence against overt testicular disease and ALL relapse. This immunosuppressive activity has been identified to be TGFβ related (Jahnukainen *et al*, 1995a; Letterio and Roberts, 1997; Letterio and Roberts, 1998). Extracts from adult testes, containing high molecular weight peptides (>5 KDa) were shown to contain a number of proteins that bind to specific receptors on the surface of lymphocytes and may inhibit their proliferation (Table 1 and Table 2). These include TGFβ (Pollanen *et al*, 1988; Pollanen *et al*, 1990; Pollanen *et al*, 1992; Sainio-Pollanen *et al*, 1991), IL-1 ((Stanton *et al*, 1986a; Stanton *et al*, 1986b), IGF-I (Hunt and Eardley, 1986), Activin and Inhibin (de Kretser *et al*, 1999; Hedger *et al*, 1998; Robertson *et al*, 1992; Tompkins *et al*, 1998).

Table 1. Cytokines produced locally at the testes

Factor	Molecular weight	Producing cells	Reference
IGF I	7.7 Kda	Sertoli and peritubular cells	Hunt and Eardley 1986
IL-1	17.5 KDa	Sertoli	Stanton *et al* 1986b
Inhibin	31KDa	Sertoli and Leydig	Hedger *et al* 1998
Activin	31KDa	Sertoli	Hedger *et al* 1998
TGF-β	25 KDa	Sertoli and peritubular cells	Pollanen *et al* 1988

The cell surface receptors for these cytokines have been detected in lymphocytes (Table 2)

Table 2. Lymphocyte receptors for, and immunoregulatory effects of peptides in the testis

Factor	Detected on	Effect	Reference
IGF-I	Lymphocytes	Inhibition of lymphocyte proliferation	(Hunt and Eardley, 1986)
		Stimulation of leukaemic cell proliferation	(Sinclair *et al*, 1988)
IL-1	T lymphoma cell line	Stimulation of thymocyte proliferation	(Sinclair *et al*, 1988)
		Stimulation of chemotaxis for lymphocytes.	(Stanton *et al*, 1986a)
TGFβ	Lymphocytes	Inhibition of B cell differentiation	(Pollanen *et al*, 1988)
Activin		Inhibition of mitogenesis of thymocyte	(Hedger *et al*, 1989)
Inhibin		Stimulation of mitogenesis of thymocyte	(Hedger *et al*, 1989)

Interleukin-1 (Il-1)

A wide range of cells including astrocytes, fibroblasts, hepatocytes, keratinocytes, monocytes, T-cells, testicular Sertoli cells and macrophages (Pollanen and Uksila, 1990) are known to produce IL-1. IL-1 plays a central role as a major mediator of inflammation and a key member coordinating many components of the cytokine network and has a wide range of biological effects. The basis for the variable biologic properties of IL-1 is the effect of this single molecule on the expression of various genes and/or expression of surface receptors. In general, IL-1 either initiates transcription or stabilises mRNA for a variety of genes; for example, IL-1 increases transcription for *IL-1Ra, IL-2*, and *IL-1* genes. Meanwhile, it stabilises and increases mRNA for GM-CSF, and IL-3, and initiates IGF-I and IL-6 via both mechanisms. Hence, in haematopoiesis it has the ability to increase the production of G-CSF, GM-CSF, and IL-3 and stem cell factor. It also increases surface receptors or receptor binding for GM-CSF, TFGβ on T cells, IGF on chondrocytes, and IL-2 and IL-4 on leukaemic cell lines (Crosier and Clark, 1992). On the other hand, it decreases gene expression for TGFβ_1 and IGF-I in Leydig cells, and it down regulate IL-1RI receptor via decreasing its mRNA half-life (Dinarello, 1996a).

Increased IL-1 production has been reported in patients with various diseases including solid tumours, leukaemias and other diseases and may play a role in regulating the behaviour of these diseases (Dinarello, 1996a). In leukaemia, several studies demonstrated spontaneous *IL-1* gene expression in AML, CML, adult T-cell leukaemia and ALL. AML blasts spontaneously expressing IL-1β, are mostly of the subtype M4 and M5, and it is significant that these two subtypes show a tendency to affect and/or relapse into the testis (Grier *et al*, 1987; Lehmann *et al*, 1997; Odom *et al*, 1990; Tobelem *et al*, 1980). In contrast to IL-1α, which induces lymphocytes infiltration into the skin, IL-1β was shown to cause an inflammatory like process in the testicular microvessels and thus induce lymphocyte infiltration into the testis (Bergh and Cajander, 1990; Bergh and Soder, 1990; Setchell, 1990).

In ALL, blasts positive for myeloid markers produce IL-1α, which increases the proliferation of these cells (Komada *et al*, 1993). IL-1 added to cultures of ALL cells stimulated proliferation that was not inhibited by neutralising antibodies to GM-CSF, TNFα, IL-3 or IL-6. In contrast the addition of IL-1 neutralising antibodies prevented IL-1 induced growth (Carter *et al*, 1994a; Carter *et al*, 1994b).

GMCSF, M-CSF, TNF, and IL-1 are among the cytokines that induce transcription and in many cases synthesis of IL-1 family. Depending on the stimulant, IL-1β mRNA levels increase rapidly within 15 minutes, but start to decrease after 4 hours, probably due to a decrease in mRNA half-life or synthesis of transcriptional repressor (Dinarello, 1996a). However, exogenous IL-1 stimulates production of both α and β forms of IL-1 stabilise IL-1 mRNA, and sustains IL-1 level for over 24 hours. Corticosteroids inhibit the transcription of most cytokines including IL-1. This reduction takes place without suppressing IL-1Ra production. TGF-β also suppresses gene expression and synthesis of IL-1 (Dinarello, 1996a).

Insulin Like Growth Factor-I (Igf-I)

Testicular IGF-I is produced by Sertoli cells and peritubular cells (Pollanen *et al*, 1988), and has been isolated from human serum, which is a rich source of IGFs (Hall *et al*, 1988b). Biological functions. According to the original somatomedin hypothesis, IGFs mediate the actions of growth hormone and indeed other agents, thus IGF-I molecules carry out important endocrine, autocrine and paracrine functions. IGFs play a pivotal role in the overall growth of the body as demonstrated by experiments on mice animal models. In the absence of IGF-I the body weight is usually 30% of normal adult body weight and low levels of IGF-I is associated with small body weight. Studies on mice embryos with a knockout of the IGFs/IGF receptor demonstrated the importance of IGF-1, as deletion of the IGF-I receptor alleles led to death shortly after birth (Burtscher *et al*, 1999).

A great number of studies have emphasised the effect of IGF-I on cell DNA synthesis and multiplication and others have drawn the attention to the differentiating effect of IGF-I on target cells (Skottner *et al*, 1988). One such study demonstrated the importance of IGF-I for the maturation of and steroid production by testicular Leydig cells (Chatelain *et al*, 1988; Saez *et al*, 1988).

Serum IGF-I levels display an age dependency. The serum levels are low at birth, rise during childhood with a peak during puberty, and decline thereafter with increasing age (Hall *et al*, 1988a). With regard to testicular functions, IGF-I is typically associated with growth maturation and steroidogenesis-promoting activities of Leydig cells; its level in the serum reaches a peak level during puberty (Chatelain *et al*, 1988; Saez *et al*, 1988).

IGFs and their receptors have attracted the attention as targets for mitogenesis and tumour progression enhancers. An abundance of experimental evidence now indicates that IGFs utilize several independent pathways that each by itself can advance tumour progression. IGFs have been shown as well to facilitate transformation of cells by oncogenes, to prevent the execution of apoptosis and, finally, to induce tumours cell invasion (Sinclair *et al*, 1988; Valentinis and Baserga, 1996; Valentinis *et al*, 1999; Baserga, 1999; Baserga, 1996). Although several studies have demonstrated that the proliferation of lymphoblasts in response to several hormones is mediated via IGF-I, there is still a disagreement about this observation (Geffner *et al*, 1996), and despite several studies showed that IGF-I stimulated growth and proliferation of leukaemic cells, some leukaemic cell lines failed to respond to the mitogenic effect of IGF-I, even though they were shown to express IGF-I receptors on their surfaces (Sinclair *et al*, 1988).

Granulocyte-Macrophage Colony Stimulating Factor (Gm-Csf)

GM-CSF is produced by the leukaemic blasts infiltrating the testes (Freedman *et al*, 1993). GM-CSF may induce proliferation of abnormal clonogenic cells in a variety of human leukaemias (Bradbury *et al*, Demetri, 1992; Demetri and Antman, 1992; Lange *et al*, 1987; 1992; Russell, 1992, Estrov et al 1996) In addition to these effects, there are several lines of evidence that ALL cells express functional cell surface receptors, and respond with a brisk augmentation of blast colony growth when exposed to exogenous GM-CSF (Freedman *et al*, 1993). Freedman *et al* 1993 showed that ALL cells support their own growth via GM-CSF production when the cells reach a threshold of concentration. Jahnukainen *et al*, (1993) observed a similar pattern of growth in testicular leukaemia in a rodent model of acute lymphocytic leukaemia. This autocrine growth mechanism, whereby a malignant cell elaborates a factor that supports its own growth, is an important concept that is emerging as a unifying theme in studies of the role of growth factors in malignancy (Sporn, 1997; Sporn and Roberts, 1985a; Sporn and Roberts, 1985b; Sporn and Todaro, 1980). Moreover, Lange *et al* 1987 showed that GMCSF-dependent ALL and AML cell lines could be established from some children with either disease.

Tgfβ1, Tgfβ2, Inhibin and Activin

The historical background to the Inhibin field began over 70 years ago, when it was noticed that experimental destruction of rat seminiferous tubules resulted in hypertrophy of the pituitary gland. This hypertrophy was suspected to be due to the lack of a circulating factor derived from the seminiferous tubules. As part of a feedback loop, hypertrophied pituitary cells were believed to be overproducing a factor that would normally induce the testes to produce a pituitary-targeted molecule. When it was noted that the development of hypertrophied cells following castration could be blocked or inhibited by the administration of an aqueous testicular extract, this water soluble substance was named Inhibin. (Knight, 1996; Muttukrishna and Knight, 1991).

The research that culminated in 1985/1986 resulted in the isolation and molecular characterization of this aqueous testicular extract component "Inhibin", during the purifying of which several surprises were revealed, including the discovery and molecular characterization of Activins, which share with Inhibin an ability to modulate pituitary FSH secretion. It has also emerged that (i) Inhibins and Activins are members of the diverse but structurally related disulfide-linked dimeric transforming growth factor beta, (TGF*β*), peptide family, (ii) Inhibins, and Activins function as intragonadal autocrine/paracrine regulators of follicle cell differentiation and steroidogenesis (iii) Inhibins, and Activins are expressed and have local regulatory roles in numerous extragonadal tissues, including brain, adrenal, bone marrow, placenta, and anterior pituitary.

Currently, Inhibin and Activin are still believed to be physiologically relevant in the regulation of pituitary gonadotrophin (FSH and LH) secretion. However, a number of aspects of the Inhibin story are being re-evaluated, including the physiological sources of Activin and Inhibin and the exact form(s) of the bioactive molecules. Furthermore, there is now some uncertainty regarding past measurements of circulating levels of Activin and Inhibin, making previous correlations with endocrine cycles difficult to interpret. Finally, the receptors for Activin (Inhibin receptors have not yet been identified) are now reported to bind a number of non-Activin/Inhibin molecules (Abe and Ibuki, 1996).

Transforming growth factor (TGF*β*) is the best-known physiological inhibitor of cell proliferation. Members of this family also play critical roles during embryogenesis in mammals, frogs, and flies and in many aspects of tissue repair and recycling.

TGF-*β* and related cytokines, e.g. bone morphogenetic proteins (BMPs), regulate cell fate in virtually all tissues by controlling proliferation, differentiation and apoptosis and are therefore important for the development and maintenance of most tissues. The effects of these factors are brought about by regulating the expression of genes encoding key determinants of cell phenotype, such as cell-cycle regulators, differentiation factors, cell-adhesion molecules and others.

The Relevance of the Tgfβ Family to Leukaemic Cells Survival in the Testis

The interest in the 4 members of the TGFβ superfamily of proteins, (TGFβ_1, TGFβ_2, Activin, and Inhibin) came from the earlier observations by (Pollanen *et al*, 1990) that the leukaemic cells are affected and controlled by high molecular weight proteins that are locally produced at the testes. These pleiotropic secreted signalling molecules possess potent immunoregulatory properties. TGFβ_1, for example, has been shown to be involved in immunological tolerance, whereby the immune system distinguishes self from nonself to prevent pathologic reactivity against self-antigens (Letterio and Roberts, 1997; Letterio and Roberts, 1998). Data also suggest that TGFβ maintains immune tolerance in peripheral tissues. Immune privileged features of the testes, for instance, have been shown to be TGFβ_2 related (Hedger *et al*, 1998), where it was shown that suppression of the immune response in the testis allows prolonged (possibly infinite) survival of a graft of foreign tissue and protects it from prompt immune rejection (Pollanen *et al*, 1988; Pollanen *et al*, 1990; Pollanen *et al*, 1992). However, the extent to which this immune suppression participates in supporting the survival of leukaemic cells in the testis is not known.

Activins and Inhibins share a few characteristics with TGFβs, including a similar molecular weight, latent structure, the multi and diverse functions, and a similar signal transduction pathway. Activin shares with TGFβ its ability to inhibit B and T lymphocytes, while Inhibin opposes the effect of Activin and TGFβ (de Jong *et al*, 1993; de Jong, 1997). Disruption of the signal transduction for both TGFβ and Activin has been shown to induce malignant transformation in solid tissues (Kitamura *et al*, 2000).

Moreover, new discoveries about this family of proteins and their diverse effects on cell kinetics and organ functions are emerging daily. For example the relation of Inhibin levels to spermatogenesis and male fertility is being reported recently, and may lead to the use of Inhibin B measurement as a routine assessment of male reproductive system together with the routine semen analysis.

Furthermore, the search for and characterisation of Inhibin receptors is currently being carried out, the success of which will lead to a major understanding of the functions of this protein.

Conclusion

There are a large number of candidate factors which may be implicated in testicular ALL, and one of the problems faced when trying to work out which are most important, is the technical difficulty in performing these experiments using conventional assay methodology. For example, in a traditional experimental design to compare seven independent variables at three different concentrations requires a large number of individual experiments (2187 experiments). We are therefore using a modification of the Taguchi methods in order to analyse multiple variables in a single experiemental setting. The Taguchi methods are widely used by quality engineering scientists to compare the effects of multiple variables, together with their interactions, with a simple and manageable experimental design. A study involving

7 factors at 3 different concentrations can be conducted with only 18 experimental runs by using orthogonal array distribution analysis. We anticipate that these experiments will generate insights into the pathogenesis of testicular ALL and may allow rational therapeutic intervention in the future.

References

Abe, Y. and Ibuki, Y. (1996) [Inhibin and activin]. *Nippon Sanka Fujinka Gakkai Zasshi*, 48, 708-720.

Agostinelli, E., Przybytkowski, E., Mondovi, B., and Averill-Bates, D.A. (1994) Heat enhancement of cytotoxicity induced by oxidation products of spermine in Chinese hamster ovary cells. *Biochem.Pharmacol.*, 48, 1181-1186.

Auersperg, N. (1966) Differential heat sensitivity of cells in tissue culture. *Nature*, 209, 415-416.

Aur, R.J., Simone, J.V., Verzosa, M.S., Hustu, H.O., Barker, L.F., Pinkel, D.P., Rivera, G., Dahl, G.V., Wood, A., Stagner, S., and Mason, C. (1978) Childhood acute lymphocytic leukemia: study VIII. *Cancer*, 42, 2123-2134.

Baserga, R. (1996) Controlling IGF-receptor function: a possible strategy for tumor therapy. *Trends Biotechnol.*, 14, 150-152.

Baserga, R. (1999) The IGF-I receptor in cancer research. *Exp.Cell Res.*, 253, 1-6.

Bergh, A. and Cajander,S. (1990) Immunohistochemical localization of inhibin-alpha in the testes of normal men and in men with testicular disorders. *Int.J Androl*, 13, 463-469.

Bergh, A. and Soder, O. (1990) Interleukin-1 beta but not interleukin-1 alpha, induces acute inflammation-like changes in the testicular microcirculation of adult rats. *J Reprod.Immunol.*, 17, 155-165.

Bisht, K.S. and Uma, D.P. (1996) Hyperthermia in cancer research: current status. *Indian J Exp.Biol.*, 34, 1183-1189.

Bradbury, D., Rogers, S., Reilly, I.A., Kozlowski, R., and Russell, N.H. (1992) Role of autocrine and paracrine production of granulocyte-macrophage colony-stimulating factor and interleukin-1 beta in the autonomous growth of acute myeloblastic leukaemia cells--studies using purified CD34-positive cells. *Leukemia*, 6, 562-566.

Brisco, M.J., Condon, J., Hughes, E., Neoh, S.H., Sykes, P.J., Seshadri, R., Toogood, I., Waters, K., Tauro,G., Ekert, H., and . (1994) Outcome prediction in childhood acute lymphoblastic leukaemia by molecular quantification of residual disease at the end of induction. *Lancet*, 343, 196-200.

Burtscher, I., Compagni, A., Lamm, G.M., and Christofori, G. (1999) An insulin-like growth factor-mediated, phosphatidylinositol 3' kinase- independent survival signaling pathway in beta tumor cells. *Cancer Res.*, 59, 3923-3926.

Carper, S.W., Rocheleau, T.A., Cimino, D., and Storm, F.K. (1997) Heat shock protein 27 stimulates recovery of RNA and protein synthesis following a heat shock. *J.Cell Biochem.*, 66, 153-164.

Carter, A., Haddad, N., Draxler, I., Israeli, E., Raz, B., and Tatarsky, I. (1994a) Respective effects of soluble interleukin-1 receptor and tumour necrosis factor receptor on IL-1 and

TNF-alpha-induced DNA synthesis of common acute lymphoblastic leukaemia blasts in vitro. *Br.J.Haematol.*, 86, 22-29.

Carter, A., Haddad, N., Draxler, I., and Tatarsky, I. (1994b) Effects of soluble interleukin-1 receptor and tumor-necrosis factor receptor, respectively, on the IL-1- and TNF-alpha-induced DNA synthesis of acute myeloblastic leukemia blasts in vitro. *Eur.J.Haematol.*, 53, 38-45.

Cavaliere, R., Ciocatto, E.C., Giovanella, B.C., Heidelberger, C., Johnson, R.O., Margottini,M., Mondovi,B., Moricca,G., and Rossi-Fanelli,A. (1967) Selective heat sensitivity of cancer cells. Biochemical and clinical studies. *Cancer*, 20, 1351-1381.

Chatelain, P., Penhoat, A., Perrard-Sapori, M.H., Jaillard, C., Naville, D., and Saez, J. (1988) Maturation of steroidogenic cells: a target for IGF-I. *Acta Paediatr.Scand.Suppl*, 347, 104-109.

Chessells, J.M., Durrant, J., Hardy, R.M., and Richards, S. (1986a) Medical Research Council leukaemia trial--UKALL V: an attempt to reduce the immunosuppressive effects of therapy in childhood acute lymphoblastic leukemia. Report to the Council by the Working Party on Leukaemia in Childhood. *J.Clin.Oncol.*, 4, 1758-1764.

Chessells, J.M., Pincott, J.R., and Daniels-Lake, W. (1986b) Terminal transferase positive cells in testicular biopsy specimens from boys with acute lymphoblastic leukaemia. *J.Clin.Pathol.*, 39, 1236-1240.

Crosier, P.S. and Clark, S.C. (1992) Basic biology of the hematopoietic growth factors. *Semin.Oncol.*, 19, 349-361.

de Jong, F.H. (1997) Testicular activin--too hot to handle? *Eur.J Endocrinol.*, 137, 448-449.

de Jong, F.H., de Winter,J.P., Wesseling,J.G., Timmerman,M.A., van Genesen,S., Van den Eijnden-van Raaij AJ, and van Zoelen,E.J. (1993) Inhibin subunits, follistatin and activin receptors in the human teratocarcinoma cell line Tera-2. *Biochem.Biophys.Res.Commun.*, 192, 1334-1339.

de Kretser, D.M., Hedger,M.P., and Phillips,D.J. (1999) Activin A and follistatin: their role in the acute phase reaction and inflammation. *J Endocrinol.*, 161, 195-198.

Demetri, G.D. (1992) Hematopoietic growth factors: current knowledge, future prospects. *Curr.Probl.Cancer*, 16, 177-259.

Demetri, G.D. and Antman,K.H. (1992) Granulocyte-macrophage colony-stimulating factor (GM-CSF): preclinical and clinical investigations. *Semin.Oncol.*, 19, 362-385.

Dinarello, C.A. (1996a) Biologic basis for interleukin-1 in disease. *Blood*, 87, 2095-2147.

Dinarello, C.A. (1996b) Thermoregulation and the pathogenesis of fever. *Infect.Dis.Clin.North Am.*, 10, 433-449.

Donadieu, J., Auclerc, M.F., Baruchel, A., Leblanc, T., Landman-Parker, J., Perel, Y., Michel, G., Cornu, G., Bordigoni, P., Sommelet, D., Leverger, G., Hill, C., and Schaison, G. (1998) Critical study of prognostic factors in childhood acute lymphoblastic leukaemia: differences in outcome are poorly explained by the most significant prognostic variables. Fralle group. French Acute Lymphoblastic Leukaemia study group. *Br.J.Haematol.*, 102, 729-739.

Eden, O.B., Rankin, A., and Kay, H.E. (1983) Isolated testicular relapse in acute lymphoblastic leukaemia of childhood. Report on behalf of the Medical Research Council's working party on leukaemia in childhood. *Arch.Dis.Child*, 58, 128-132.

Estrov, Z., Talpaz, M., Zipf, T.F., Kantarjian, H.M., Ku, S., Ouspenskaia, M.V., Hirsch-Ginsberg, C., Huh, Y., Yee, G., and Kurzrock, R. (1996) Role of granulocyte-macrophage colony-stimulating factor in Philadelphia (Ph1)-positive acute lymphoblastic leukemia: studies on two newly established Ph1-positive acute lymphoblastic leukemia cell lines (Z-119 and Z-181). *J.Cell Physiol*, 166, 618-630.

Finklestein, J.Z., Dyment, P.G., and Hammond, G.D. (1969) Leukemic infiltration of the testes during bone marrow remission. *Pediatrics*, 43, 1042-1045.

Fondy, T.P., Karker, K.L., Calcagnino, C., and Emlich, C.A. (1974) Effect of reserpine (NSC-59272)-induced hypothermia on lifespan in mouse L1210 leukemia. *Cancer Chemother.Rep.*, 58, 317-324.

Forrest, D.L., Dalal, B.I., Naiman, S.C., Horsman, D.E., Berry, B.R., Parslow, M.I., Singh, C.P., Benny, W.B., and Barnett, M.J. (1997) Testicular relapse of acute promyelocytic leukemia after allogeneic BMT. *Bone Marrow Transplant*, 20, 689-690.

Franck, P., Duffner, U., Schulze-Seemann, W., Riede, U., Dordelmann, M., and Niemeyer, C.M. (1998) Testicular relapse after 13 years of complete remission of acute lymphoblastic leukemia. *Urol.Int.*, 60, 239-241.

Freedman, M.H., Grunberger, T., Correa, P., Axelrad, A.A., Dube, I.D., and Cohen, A. (1993) Autocrine and paracrine growth control by granulocyte-monocyte colony-stimulating factor of acute lymphoblastic leukemia cells. *Blood*, 81, 3068-3075.

Furman, W.L., Fontanesi, J., Hustu, O., Dahl, G.V., Kalwinsky, D.K., and Pui, C.H. (1990) Testicular relapse in children with acute nonlymphoblastic leukemia. *Cancer*, 66, 2095-2098.

Gajjar, A., Ribeiro, R.C., Mahmoud, H.H., Sandlund, J.T., Liu, Q., Furman, W.L., Santana, V.M., Crist, W.M., Rivera, G.K., and Pui, C.H. (1996) Overt testicular disease at diagnosis is associated with high risk features and a poor prognosis in patients with childhood acute lymphoblastic leukemia. *Cancer*, 78, 2437-2442.

Geffner, M.E., Bersch, N., Scott, M., Bailey, R.C., and Golde, D.W. (1996) IGF-I does not mediate T-lymphoblast colony formation in response to estradiol, testosterone, 1,25(OH)2 vitamin D3, and triiodothyronine: studies in control and pygmy T-cell lines. *Biochem.Mol.Med.*, 59, 72-79.

Gill, B., Kogan, S., Rossman, B., Santorineou, M., Radel, E., Reda, E., and Levitt, S. (1989) Needle biopsy in the diagnosis of testicular leukemia in children. *J.Urol.*, 141, 1169-1171.

Giovanella, B.C., Lohman, W.A., and Heidelberger, C. (1970) Effects of elevated temperatures and drugs on the viability of L1210 leukemia cells. *Cancer Res.*, 30, 1623-1631.

Giovanella, B.C. and Mondovi, B. (1977) Selective heat sensitivity of cancer cells: Introduction. *Recent Results Cancer Res.*, 1-6.

Gloria, C.LI. and George, M.H. (1980) Adaptation to different growth temperatures modifies some mammalian cell survival responses. *Experimental Cell Research*, 128, 475-479.

Grier, H.E., Gelber, R.D., Camitta, B.M., Delorey, M.J., Link, M.P., Price, K.N., Leavitt, P.R., and Weinstein, H.J. (1987) Prognostic factors in childhood acute myelogenous leukemia. *J Clin.Oncol*, 5, 1026-1032.

Grundy, R.G., Leiper, A.D., Stanhope, R., and Chessells, J.M. (1997) Survival and endocrine outcome after testicular relapse in acute lymphoblastic leukaemia. *Arch.Dis.Child*, 76, 190-196.

Hall, K., Brismar, K., and Thoren, M. (1988a) Update on somatomedin. *Acta Paediatr.Scand.Suppl*, 347, 87-92.

Hall, K., Lundin, G., and Povoa, G. (1988b) Serum levels of the low molecular weight form of insulin-like growth factor binding protein in healthy subjects and patients with growth hormone deficiency, acromegaly and anorexia nervosa. *Acta Endocrinol.(Copenh)*, 118 , 321-326.

Hedger, M.P., Drummond, A.E., Robertson, D.M., Risbridger, G.P., and de Kretser, D.M. (1989) Inhibin and activin regulate [3H]thymidine uptake by rat thymocyte and 3T3 cells in vitro. *Mol.Cell Endocrinol.*, 61, 133-138.

Hedger,M.P., Nikolic-Paterson,D.J., Hutchinson,P., Atkins,R.C., and de Kretser,D.M. (1998) Immunoregulatory activity in adult rat testicular interstitial fluid: roles of interleukin-1 and transforming growth factor beta. *Biol.Reprod.*, 58, 927-934.

Holash, J.A., Harik, S.I., Perry, G., and Stewart, P.A. (1993a) Barrier properties of testis microvessels. *Proc.Natl.Acad.Sci.U.S.A*, 90, 11069-11073.

Holash, J.A., Noden, D.M., and Stewart, P.A. (1993b) Re-evaluating the role of astrocytes in blood-brain barrier induction. *Dev.Dyn.*, 197, 14-25.

Holash, J.A. and Stewart, P.A. (1993) The relationship of astrocyte-like cells to the vessels that contribute to the blood-ocular barriers. *Brain Res.*, 629, 218-224.

Hunt, P. and Eardley, D.D. (1986) Suppressive effects of insulin and insulin-like growth factor-1 (IGF1) on immune responses. *J Immunol.*, 136, 3994-3999.

Hustu, H.O. and Aur, R.J. (1978) Extramedullary leukaemia. *Clin.Haematol.*, 7, 313-337.

Jackson, H., Bock, M., Jackson, N.C., and Lendon, M. (1983) The testis. A protected environment for leukaemic cells against cyclophosphamide in a mouse model. *Cancer Chemother.Pharmacol.*, 11, 200-202.

Jackson, H., Jackson, N.C., Bock, M., and Lendon, M. (1984) Testicular relapse in acute lymphoblastic leukaemia: studies with an experimental mouse model. *Br.J.Cancer*, 49, 73-78.

Jahnukainen, K., Attermo, P., Saari, T., Salmi, T.T., von Euler, M., Pollanen, P., and Soder, O. (1995a) Effects of testicular cytokines on proliferation of rat T-leukaemic lymphoblasts in vitro. *J.Reprod.Immunol.* , 28, 263-273.

Jahnukainen, K., Hou, M., Petersen, C., Setchell, B., and Soder, O. (2001) Intratesticular transplantation of testicular cells from leukemic rats causes transmission of leukemia. *Cancer Res.*, 61, 706-710.

Jahnukainen, K., Morris, I., Roe, S., Salmi, T.T., Makipernaa, A., and Pollanen, P. (1993) A rodent model for testicular involvement in acute lymphoblastic leukaemia. *Br.J.Cancer*, 67, 885-892.

Jahnukainen, K., Saari, T., Salmi, T.T., Pollanen, P., and Pelliniemi, L.J. (1995b) Reactions of Leydig cells and blood vessels to lymphoblastic leukemia in the rat testis. *Leukemia*, 9, 908-914.

Jahnukainen, K., Salmi, T.T., Kristinsson, J., Muller, J., Madsen, B., and Gustafsson, G. (1998) The clinical indications for identical pathogenesis of isolated and non- isolated testicular relapses in acute lymphoblastic leukaemia. *Acta Paediatr.*, 87, 638-643.

Kastelic, J.P., Cook, R.B., and Coulter, G.H. (1997a) Contribution of the scrotum, testes, and testicular artery to scrotal/testicular thermoregulation in bulls at two ambient temperatures. *Anim. Reprod.Sci.*, 45, 255-261.

Kastelic, J.P., Cook, R.B., and Coulter, G.H. (1997b) Scrotal/testicular thermoregulation and the effects of increased testicular temperature in the bull. *Vet.Clin.North Am.Food Anim Pract.*, 13, 271-282.

Kitamura, K., Aota, S., Sakamoto, R., Yoshikawa, S.I., and Okazaki, K. (2000) Smad7 selectively interferes with different pathways of activin signaling and inhibits erythroid leukemia cell differentiation. *Blood*, 95, 3371-3379.

Kobayashi, H., Urashima, M., Hoshi, Y., Uchiyama, H., Fujisawa, K., Akatsuka, J., Maekawa, K., and Hurusato, M. (1996) Testicular morphological changes in children with acute lymphoblastic leukemia following chemotherapy. *Acta Paediatr.Jpn.*, 38, 640-643.

Komada, Y., Zhou, Y.W., Zhang, S.L., Azuma, E., and Sakurai, M. (1993) Role in growth regulation of cytokines and cytokine receptors in acute lymphoblastic leukaemia expressing myeloid markers. *Br.J. Haematol.*, 84, 408-415.

Lal, A., Kwan, E., al Mahr, M., Zhou, L., Ferrara, D., Tobias, V., O'Gorman, H.D., Haber, M., Norris, M.D., and Marshall, G.M. (1998) Molecular detection of acute lymphoblastic leukaemia in boys with testicular relapse. *Mol.Pathol.*, 51, 277-281.

Lange, B., Valtieri, M., Santoli, D., Caracciolo, D., Mavilio, F., Gemperlein, I., Griffin, C., Emanuel, B., Finan, J., Nowell, P., and . (1987) Growth factor requirements of childhood acute leukemia: establishment of GM-CSF-dependent cell lines. *Blood*, 70, 192-199.

Lehmann, L.E., Guinan, E.C., Halpern, S.L., Donovan, M.J., Bierer, B.E., and Parsons, S.K. (1997) Isolated testicular relapse in an adolescent 5 years following allogeneic bone marrow transplantation for acute myelogenous leukemia. *Bone Marrow Transplant*, 19, 849-851.

Lendon, M., Hann, I.M., Palmer, M.K., Shalet, S.M., and Jones, P.H. (1978) Testicular histology after combination chemotherapy in childhood for acute lymphoblastic leukaemia. *Lancet*, 2, 439-441.

Letterio, J.J. and Roberts, A.B. (1997) TGF-beta: a critical modulator of immune cell function. *Clin.Immunol.Immunopathol.*, 84, 244-250.

Letterio, J.J. and Roberts, A.B. (1998) Regulation of immune responses by TGF-beta. *Annu.Rev.Immunol.*, 16, 137-161.

Lupetin, A.R., King, W., Rich, P., and Lederman, R.B. (1983a) The ultrasound diagnosis of testicular leukemia. *Ultrasound Med.Biol.*, Suppl 2, 423-426.

Lupetin, A.R., King, W., Rich, P., and Lederman, R.B. (1983b) Ultrasound diagnosis of testicular leukemia. *Radiology*, 146, 171-172.

Miller, D.R., Leikin, S., Albo, V., Sather, H., Karon, M., and Hammond, D. (1983a) Prognostic factors and therapy in acute lymphoblastic leukemia of childhood: CCG-141. A report from childrens cancer study group. *Cancer*, 51, 1041-1049.

Miller, D.R., Leikin, S.L., Albo, V.C., Palmer, N.F., Sather, H.N., and Hammond, G.D. (1990) The prognostic value of testicular biopsy in childhood acute lymphoblastic leukemia: a report from the Childrens Cancer Study Group. *J.Clin.Oncol.*, 8, 57-66.

Miller, D.R. and Miller, L.P. (1990) Acute lymphoblastic leukemia in children: an update of clinical, biological, and therapeutic aspects. *Crit Rev.Oncol.Hematol.*, 10, 131-164.

Miller, D.R., Steinherz, P.G., Feuer, D., Sather, H., and Hammond, D. (1983b) Unfavorable prognostic significance of hand mirror cells in childhood acute lymphoblastic leukemia. A report from the childrens Cancer Study Group. *Am.J.Dis.Child*, 137, 346-350.

Knight, P.G. (1996) Roles of inhibins, activins, and follistatin in the female reproductive system. *Front Neuroendocrinol.*, 17, 476-509.

Mondovi, B., Finazzi, A.A., Rotilio, G., Strom, R., Moricca, G., and Rossi, F.A. (1969a) The biochemical mechanism of selective heat sensitivity of cancer cells. II. Studies on nucleic acids and protein synthesis. *Eur.J.Cancer*, 5, 137-146.

Mondovi, B., Rotilio, G., Strom, R., Finazzi-Agro, A., Cavaliere, R., Moricca, G., and Rossi, F.A. (1968) Biochemical mechanism of selective heat sensitivity of tumour cells: preliminary results. *Ital.J.Biochem.*, 17, 101-106.

Mondovi, B., Strom, R., Rotilio, G., Finazzi, A.A., Cavaliere, R., and Rossi, F.A. (1969b) The biochemical mechanism of selective heat sensitivity of cancer cells. I. Studies on cellular respiration. *Eur.J.Cancer* , 5, 129-136.

Morgentaler, A., Stahl, B.C., and Yin, Y. (1999) Testis and temperature: an historical, clinical, and research perspective. *J.Androl*, 20, 189-195.

Moriyama, Y., Narita, M., Sato, K., Urushiyama, M., Koyama, S., Hirosawa, H., Kishi, K., Takahashi, M., Takai, K., and Shibata, A. (1986) Application of hyperthermia to the treatment of human acute leukemia: purging human leukemic progenitor cells by heat. *Blood*, 67, 802-804.

Muckle, D.S. and Dickson, J.A. (1971) The selective inhibitory effect of hyperthermia on the metabolism and growth of malignant cells. *Br.J.Cancer*, 25, 771-778.

Muckle, D.S., Dickson, J.A., and Johnston, I.D. (1971a) High fever and cancer. *Lancet*, 1, 972.

Muckle, D.S., Dickson, J.A., and Johnston, I.D. (1971b) The adjuvant effect of hyperthermia on the response of the VX2 carcinoma in rabbits to methotrexate or radiotherapy. *Br.J.Surg.*, 58, 869.

Muttukrishna, S. and Knight, P.G. (1991) Inverse effects of activin and inhibin on the synthesis and secretion of FSH and LH by ovine pituitary cells in vitro. *J.Mol.Endocrinol.*, 6, 171-178.

Nachman, J., Palmer, N.F., Sather, H.N., Bleyer, W.A., Coccia, P.F., Lukens, J.N., Siegel, S.E., and Hammond,G.D. (1990) Open-wedge testicular biopsy in childhood acute lymphoblastic leukemia after two years of maintenance therapy: diagnostic accuracy and influence on outcome--a report from Children's Cancer Study Group. *Blood*, 75, 1051-1055.

Nies, B.A., Malmgren, R.A., Chu, E.W., Del Vecchio, P.R., Thomas, L.B., and Freireich, E.J. (1965) Cerebrospinal fluid cytology in patients with acute leukemia. *Cancer*, 18, 1385-1391.

Nishikawa, A., Nakamura, Y., Nobori, U., Aoki, T., Higashino, H., Matsui, T., Kobayashi, Y., Yamashita, M., and Unishi, G. (1987a) Acute monocytic leukemia in children. Response to VP-16-213 as a single agent. *Cancer*, 60, 2146-2149.

Nishikawa, A., Nobori, U., Higashino, H., and Kobayashi, Y. (1987b) Occult testicular leukemia in a patient with acute monocytic leukemia [letter]. *Pediatr. Hematol. Oncol*, 4, 349-351.

O'Reilly, J., Meyer, B., Baker, D., Herrmann, R., Cannell, P., and Davies, J. (1995) Correlation of bone marrow minimal residual disease and apparent isolated extramedullary relapse in childhood acute lymphoblastic leukaemia. *Leukemia*, 9, 624-627.

Odom, L.F., Lampkin, B.C., Tannous, R., Buckley, J.D., and Hammond, G.D. (1990) Acute monoblastic leukemia: a unique subtype--a review from the Childrens Cancer Study Group. *Leuk.Res.*, 14, 1-10.

Palzer, R.J. and Heidelberger, C. (1973) Influence of drugs and synchrony on the hyperthermic killing of HeLa cells. *Cancer Res.* , 33, 422-427.

Pollanen, P., Soder, O., and Uksila, J. (1988) Testicular immunosuppressive protein. *J.Reprod.Immunol.*, 14, 125-138.

Pollanen, P. and Uksila, J. (1990) Activation of the immune system in the testis. *J.Reprod.Immunol.*, 18, 77-87.

Pollanen, P., von Euler, M., Sainio-Pollanen, S., Jahnukainen, K., Hakovirta, H., Soder, O., and Parvinen, M. (1992) Immunosuppressive activity in the rat seminiferous tubules. *J.Reprod.Immunol.*, 22, 117-126.

Pollanen, P., von Euler, M., and Soder, O. (1990) Testicular immunoregulatory factors. *J.Reprod.Immunol.*, 18, 51-76.

Rao, N.P. and Engelberg, J. (1965) HeLa Cells: Effects of Temperature on the Life Cycle. *Science*, 148, 1091-1094.

Riccardi, R., Vigersky, R.A., Barnes, S., Bleyer, W.A., and Poplack, D.G. (1982) Methotrexate levels in the interstitial space and seminiferous tubule of rat testis. *Cancer Res.*, 42, 1617-1619.

Ritzen, E.M. (1990) Testicular relapse of acute lymphoblastic leukemia (ALL). *J.Reprod.Immunol.*, 18 , 117-121.

Robertson, D.M., Foulds, L.M., Prisk, M., and Hedger, M.P. (1992) Inhibin/activin beta-subunit monomer: isolation and characterization. *Endocrinology*, 130, 1680-1687.

Russell, N.H. (1992) Autocrine growth factors and leukaemic haemopoiesis. *Blood Rev.*, 6, 149-156.

Russo, A., Russo, I., Nuciforo, G., Marcello, M.F., Palumbo, G., and Schiliro, G. (1990) Histologic and hormonal evaluation of the ovarian function in leukemic girls after successful treatment. *Pediatr.Hematol.Oncol.*, 7, 301-306.

Russo, A. and Schiliro', G. (1986) The enigma of testicular leukemia: a critical review. *Med.Pediatr.Oncol.*, 14, 300-305.

Saez, J.M., Chatelain, P.G., Perrard-Sapori, M.H., Jaillard, C., and Naville, D. (1988) Differentiating effects of somatomedin-C/insulin-like growth factor I and insulin on Leydig and Sertoli cell functions. *Reprod.Nutr.Dev.*, 28, 989-1008.

Sainio-Pollanen, S., Pollanen, P., and Setchell, B.P. (1991) Testicular immunosuppressive activity in experimental hypogonadism and cryptorchidism. *J.Reprod.Immunol.*, 20, 59-72.

Sather, H., Coccia, P., Nesbit, M., Level, C., and Hammond, D. (1981a) Disappearance of the predictive value of prognostic variables in childhood acute lymphoblastic leukemia: a report from Childrens Cancer Study Group. *Cancer*, 48, 370-376.

Sather, H., Miller, D., Nesbit, M., Heyn, R., and Hammond, D. (1981b) Differences in prognosis for boys and girls with acute lymphoblastic leukaemia. *Lancet*, 1, 739-743.

Setchell, B.P. (1990) Local control of testicular fluids. *Reprod.Fertil.Dev.*, 2, 291-309.

Setchell, B.P., Pollanen, P., and Zupp, J.L. (1988) Development of the blood-testis barrier and changes in vascular permeability at puberty in rats. *Int.J.Androl*, 11, 225-233.

Shaffer, D.W., Burris, H.A., and O'Rourke, T.J. (1992) Testicular relapse in adult acute myelogenous leukemia. *Cancer*, 70, 1541-1544.

Shalet, S.M., Hann, I.M., Lendon, M., Morris Jones, P.H., and Beardwell, C.G. (1981) Testicular function after combination chemotherapy in childhood for acute lymphoblastic leukaemia. *Arch.Dis.Child*, 56, 275-278.

Skottner, A., Kanje, M., Jennische, E., Sjogren, J., and Fryklund, L. (1988) Tissue repair and IGF-I. *Acta Paediatr.Scand.Suppl*, 347, 110-112.

Sinclair, J., McClain, D., and Taetle, R. (1988) Effects of insulin and insulin-like growth factor I on growth of human leukemia cells in serum-free and protein-free medium. *Blood*, 72 , 66-72.

Sporn, M.B. (1997) The importance of context in cytokine action. *Kidney Int.*, 51, 1352-1354.

Sporn, M.B. and Roberts,A.B. (1985a) Autocrine growth factors and cancer. *Nature*, 313, 745-747.

Sporn, M.B. and Roberts, A.B. (1985b) Autocrine, paracrine and endocrine mechanisms of growth control. *Cancer Surv.*, 4, 627-632.

Sporn, M.B. and Todaro, G.J. (1980) Autocrine secretion and malignant transformation of cells. *N.Engl.J.Med.*, 303, 878-880.

Stanton, T., Stevens, T.L., Ledbetter, J.A., and Wofsy, D. (1986a) Anti-Ly-1 antibody induces interleukin 2 release from T cells. *J. Immunol.*, 136, 1734-1737.

Stanton, T.H., Maynard, M., and Bomsztyk, K. (1986b) Effect of interleukin-1 on intracellular concentration of sodium, calcium, and potassium in 70Z/3 cells. *J Biol.Chem.*, 261, 5699-5701.

Stewart, R.J., Boyd, S., Brown, S., and Toner, P.G. (1990) The blood-testis barrier in experimental unilateral cryptorchidism. *J.Pathol.*, 160, 51-55.

Stewart, R.J. and Brown, S. (1990) Unilateral cryptorchidism: an animal model. *Aust.N.Z.J.Surg.*, 60, 905-906.

Stoffel, T.J., Nesbit, M.E., and Levitt, S.H. (1975) Extramedullary involvement of the testes in childhood leukemia. *Cancer*, 35, 1203-1211.

Storm, F.K., Mahvi, D.M., and Gilchrist, K.W. (1996) Heat shock protein 27 overexpression in breast cancer lymph node metastasis. *Ann.Surg.Oncol.*, 3, 570-573.

Strom, R., Crifo, C., Rossi-Fanelli, A., and Mondovi, B. (1977) Biochemical aspects of heat sensitivity of tumour cells. *Recent Results Cancer Res.*, 7-35.

Tiedemann, J., Chessells, J.M., and Sandland, R.M. (1982) Isolated testicular relapse in boys with acute lymphoblastic leukaemia: treatment and outcome. *Br.Med.J.(Clin.Res.Ed)*, 285, 1614-1616.

Tobelem, G., Jacquillat, C., Chastang, C., Auclerc, M.F., Lechevallier, T., Weil, M., Daniel, M.T., Flandrin, G., Harrousseau, J.L., Schaison, G., Boiron, M., and Bernard, J. (1980) Acute monoblastic leukemia: a clinical and biologic study of 74 cases. *Blood*, 55, 71-76.

Tompkins, A.B., Hutchinson, P., de Kretser, D.M., and Hedger, M.P. (1998) Characterization of lymphocytes in the adult rat testis by flow cytometry: effects of activin and transforming growth factor beta on lymphocyte subsets in vitro. *Biol.Reprod.*, 58, 943-951.

Turano, C., Ferraro, A., Strom, R., Cavaliere, R., and Fanelli, A.R. (1970) The biochemical mechanism of selective heat sensitivity of cancer cells. 3. Studies on lysosomes. *Eur.J Cancer*, 6, 67-72.

Valentinis, B. and Baserga, R. (1996) The IGF-I receptor protects tumor cells from apoptosis induced by high concentrations of serum. *Biochem.Biophys.Res.Commun.*, 224, 362-368.

Valentinis, B., Morrione, A., Peruzzi, F., Prisco, M., Reiss, K., and Baserga, R. (1999) Anti-apoptotic signaling of the IGF-I receptor in fibroblasts following loss of matrix adhesion. *Oncogene*, 18, 1827-1836.

Wong, K.Y., Ballard, E.T., Strayer, F.H., Kisker, C.T., and Lampkin, B.C. (1980) Clinical and occult testicular leukemia in long-term survivors of acute lymphoblastic leukemia. *J.Pediatr.*, 96, 569-574.

In: Trends in Diabetes Research
Editor: Ashley M. Ford, pp. 131-162

ISBN: 1-59454-796-3

Chapter VI

Experimental Approaches for Transplantation of Islets in the Absence of Immunosuppression

Bart J. de Haan, Marijke M. Faas, Albert F. Hamel and Paul de Vos*

Transplantation biology and Immunoendocrinology,
Department of Pathology and Laboratory Medicine,
section of Medical Biology, University of Groningen,
Hanzeplein 1, 9700 RB Groningen, The Netherlands.

Abstract

Transplantation of insulin producing cells in diabetic patients requires technologies to transplant tissues in the absence of immunosuppression since the side effect of immunosuppression can never be an acceptable alternative for insulin therapy. Much effort has been put into the development of immunomodulating technologies to transplant genetically or otherwise modified islet tissue in order to decrease the immunogenicity of the islet tissue. A number of these approaches have been shown to be effective in small rodents and to allow for life-long survival of islet grafts[1,2]. In spite of some successes it has not yet come to clinical application. Another approach is immunoisolation of tissue by encapsulation of pancreatic islets to protect the tissue from the host immune system by an artificial membrane. Basically, there are three major approaches of encapsulation. These include intravascular macrocapsules, which are anastomosed to the vascular system as AV shunt, extravascular macrocapsules, which are mostly diffusion chambers transplanted at different sites, and extravascular microcapsules transplanted in the peritoneal cavity. All systems have been shown to be successful in preclinical studies. These studies also showed that not all approaches meet

---

* Address correspondence to:. De Vos, Ph.D.Pathology and Laboratory Medicine, Section of Medical Biology, University of Groningen, Hanzeplein 19700 RB Groningen, The Netherlands, Phone: (31) (50) 3611045, Fax: (31) (50) 3619911, e-mail: B.J.DE.HAAN@MED.RUG.NL

the technical or physiological requirements for application in men. The extravascular approach provides advantages over the intravascular systems since it is associated with fewer complications such as thrombosis and infection. Microcapsules, due to their spatial characteristics, offer better diffusion capacity than macrocapsules. Recent progress in biocompatibility of microcapsules has brought this technology near clinical application. Critical issues such as limitations in the functional performance and survival are being discussed. The latest results show that both issues can be solved by transplantation of microencapsulated islets near blood vessels in prevascularized solid supports. Also, latest insights will be presented into the composition of the membranes for immuoisolating devices and the associated biocompatibility.

Introduction

The general goal in the treatment of insulin dependent diabetes mellitus (IDDM) is the prevention of late complications, and thereby improvement of the quality of patient life. There is no dispute that euglycemia is of essential importance to reach that goal. Euglycemia may be achieved by intensified insulin treatment, and the results of the Diabetes Control and Complications trial clearly demonstrate that this approach is effective since it delays the onset and reduces the progression of diabetic complications [3]. Intensified treatment, however, is not a simple achievement since it requires multiple daily injections, frequent monitoring, dosage adaptations and, thus, patient compliance. Also, it is associated with frequent episodes of severe hypoglycemia and with glycemic unawareness. A principally different approach to achieve euglycemia is to provide the diabetic patient with an endogenous rather than an exogenous source of insulin by the transplantation of endocrine pancreatic tissue. Pancreatic organ transplantation is now an established mode of treatment with a worldwide experience of more than 15.000 cases [4,5]. Results have substantially improved during the past two decades and present patient and one-year graft survival rates almost equal to those of kidney transplantation (respectively 98% and 85%). A successful pancreas transplant provides almost normal glucose homeostasis, but it requires life-long immunosuppressive medication. Since it is still unclear whether the advantage of a pancreas transplant over continued insulin treatment outweighs the disadvantage of obligatory immunosuppression, most transplant centers still restrict themselves to combined pancreas and kidney transplantation in diabetic patients with end-stage renal failure [4,6].

Islet transplantation, in contrast to pancreas transplantation, requires no major surgery.

Recent improvements in the technology are the administration of non-glucocorticoid immunosuppression (sirolimus, tacrlimus, daclizumab) by the Edmonton-group which is associated with one-year graft survival of 100% of the transplanted diabetic patients [7]. These advances have led to a tremendous growth in the number of research groups involved in human islet transplantation. Unfortunately, not all these groups have achieved the same level of success, which is usually attributed to different degrees in 'experiences' in efficacious isolation of functional islets. However, in spite of the inability of many groups to fully reproduce the Edmonton results, the general impression is that recent advances of the Edmonton group have brought islet-transplantation close to widespread clinical application.

Another pertinent advantage of islet transplantation over whole pancreas transplantation is that successful islet transplantation without immunosuppression might be achieved by relatively simple methods such as immunomodulation, genetic engineering of islets and immunoisolation. These experimental approaches will be discussed in the present paper in view of future clinical applications.

Immunomodulation

An attractive feature of free isolated islets is the ability to immunomodulate the tissue before transplantation in order to reduce the immunogenicity. During the past two decades various technical approaches have been tested to delete antigen-presenting cells in islets and to reduce the presentation of immunogenic peptides on islet cells. These approaches include culture at low temperatures[8] or under ultraviolet light [9,10], pretreatment with neutralizing or deleting antibodies [11], immunosuppressive drug pretreatment such as cyclophosphamide or deoxyguanosine pretreatment [12], cryopreservation [13,14], or irradiation [15]. All these technologies have proven successful in small rodents with graft survival rates for periods up to a year. Unfortunately, however, when applied in large animal models only temporary instead of prolonged survival of islet tissue was observed. Although the reasons for the difference in success of immunomodulation between rodents and large mammals remain to be studied it has been suggested that a plausible difference is the more complex and still not well understood biochemistry of human islets.

A very promising approach of immunomodulation is targeting the donor-derived costimulatory activity. It has been shown that coating of murine islet allografts with antibodies against co-stimulatory molecules CTLA4-Ig facilitates engraftment and induces permanent tolerance in 50% of the recipients [16]. This blockade of co-stimulatory molecules is also the basis of many genetic approaches to overcome graft rejection and will be discussed in more detail in the next section.

Genetic Engineering of Islets

In the past decade, islets have been genetically modified in order to block costimulatory molecules, to induce expression of Fas ligand (FasL) or immunosuppressive cytokines, and to inhibit gene transcription of regulatory proteins, such as nuclear factor-B [17-19]. However, the majority of present experimental strategies to reduce rejection of islet allografts by genetic engineering are aiming on blockade of the costimulatory pathway. This approach will be discussed in more detail in the next sections.

After transplantation of 'foreign' islets T-cell activation occurs which causes the upregulation of at least two essential co-stimulatory molecules. One of the molecules, CTLA4, binds B7 with a high affinity and provides a negative signal to the T cell. The other molecule, ICOS, binds B7H/B7RP-1, and is required for an adequate humoral immune response and induction of cytokine production such as interleukin 4. Many groups involved in genetic engineering of islet-tissue have focussed in the past decade on the potential application of CTLA4-Ig for blockade of the costimulatory pathway. The main reason for that is the observation that T cells involved in rejection and in autoimmunity express high levels of CD80 (B7.1) and CD86 (B7.2) antigens both in rodent and humans. CTLA4-lg is a genetically engineered fusion protein of human CTLA4 and the IgG 1 Fc region, and prevents T-cell activation by binding with high affinity to human B7.

There are several successful approaches for delivery of CTLA4-Ig in the vicinity of transplanted islets. Chahine et al. [20] observed that cotransplantation of myoblasts transfected with CTLA4-Ig cDNA and syngenic to the host, significantly prolonged murine islet allograft survival. This approach, however, did only induce permanent survival when CTLA4-Ig was combined with blockade of the leukocyte function-associated-1 pathway by applying an additional monoclonal antibody (Fig. 1). Gainer et al [21,22] transfected CTLA4-Ig cDNA directly into islets rather than cells in the vicinity of the tissue and showed prolonged allograft survival in 50% of the recipients. Unfortunately, this method did not provide full protection since the islets showed peri-insulitis. The reason for this peri-insulitis is probably related to the fact that transfection is not permanent: the level of CTLA4-Ig obtained in transfected islets does vary ninefold, and the constructs disappear after 21-28 days [22].

The success of genetic engineering of islet cells in large mammals and humans remains to be proven but an optimistic view is realistic since a single CTLA4-Ig bolus improved renal allograft survival in a series of five Cynomolgus monkeys for periods longer than 50 days [23]. This suggest that similar mechanism of co-stimulation occur in large mammals and plausibly also in humans.

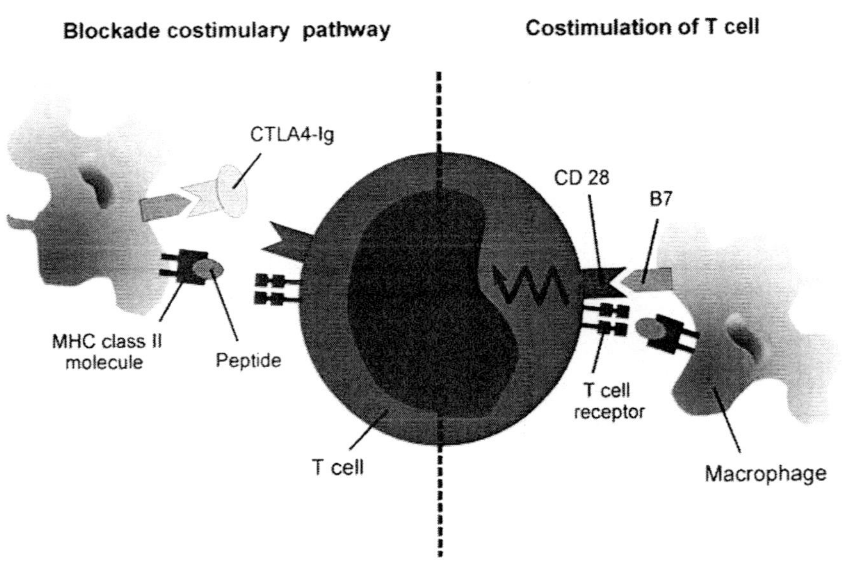

Figure 1. Schematic representation of T-cell stimulation after the presentation of a peptide by a macrophage. The macrophage presents the peptide to the T-cell receptor in context of MHC class 2. Simultaneously the CD28 receptor binds the macrophage co-stimulatory molecule B7 (right panel). Blocking the co-stimulatory pathway with CTLA4-Ig occurs by high affinity binding of this antibody to the B7 molecule thus preventing low affinity binding to CD28. As a result the peptide will not be presented to the T cell (left panel)

Immunoisolation

The possibility of transplanting cells in immunoprotective membranes for organ replacement dates back to 1933. At that time, Bisceglie [24] replaced the endogenous pancreas by transplanting insulin producing tissue encapsulated in a semipermeable but immunoprotective membrane to study the effects of absence of vascularization on the survival of tissues. It took, however, until 1943 before the concept of immunoisolation was established by Algire [25] who recognized that graft failure was delayed by encapsulating allo- and xenogenic tissues before transplantation. The group of Algire was also the first to illustrate the importance of biocompatibility since they found that graft failure was always accompanied by cellular overgrowth of the membranes. At present, transplantation of cells in immunoisolating devices is under study for the treatment of a wide variety of diseases, including Hemophilia B [26], anemia [27], dwarfism [28], kidney [29] and liver failure[30] pituitary [31] and central nervous system insufficiencies [32], and diabetes mellitus [33]. For diabetes mellitus research there are two major encapsulaton systems: macro- and microencapsulation (Fig. 2). The macrocapsules contain groups of islets enveloped together in one immunoisolating membrane that can be implanted as extravascular and intravascular device. With microencapsulation the islets are individually enveloped by their own capsule. These two approaches will be discussed in the next section.

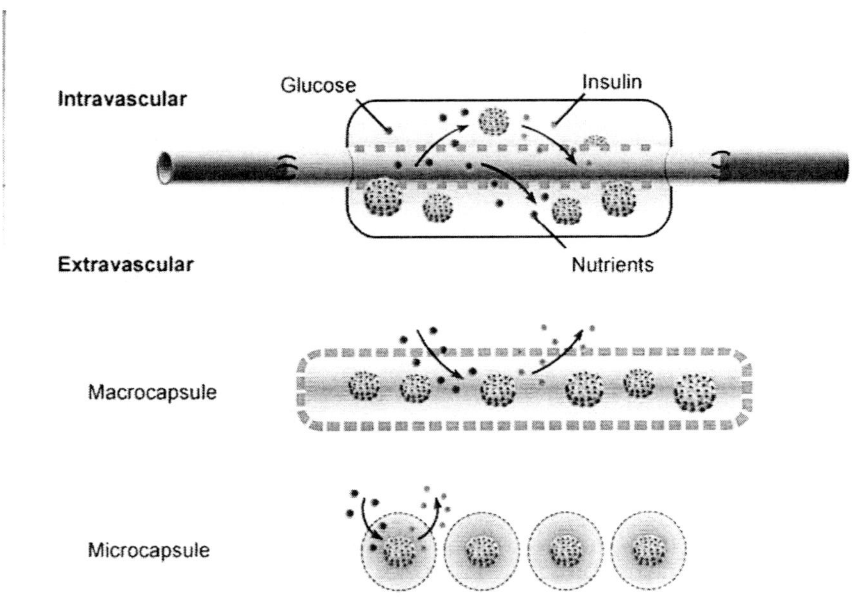

Figure 2. Immunoisolation in intravasculair and extravasculair devices.In immunoisolation with intravascular macrocapsule devices, islets are seeded on the outside of artificial capillaries, in close contact with the bloodstream. The extravascular capsules have a higher diffusion distance to the bloodstream due to the lack of vascularisation. Immunoisolation in extravascular macrocapsules there are several islets encapsulated in one capsule, while immunoisolation in extravascular microcapsules involves individual encapsulated islets.

Macrocapsules

Extravascular Macrocapsules

The extravascular macrocapsules can be implanted with minimal surgery in different sites such as the peritoneal cavity [34-37], the subcutaneous site [38-44], or the renal capsule [45]. The concept of extravascular devices does not require vascular anastomoses, since it is based on the principle of diffusion chambers [46]. The geometry may be planar in the form of a flat, circular double layer or tube-like as a so-called hollow fiber [46]. The surgical risks are much lower with extravascular than with the intravascular devices. Also, they can be readily retrieved, and they can be produced in a relatively simple way.

Many different biomaterials have been applied for the production of extravascular macrocapsules (Table 1). The hollow fiber geometry is usually preferred over the planar membranes for their smaller foreign body response [47]. Most studies on hollow fibers use fibers made of polyacrylonitrile and polyvinylchloride copolymer (PAN-PVC) [48,49]. They have been produced with a smooth or fenestrated outer skin with the same spongy matrix as applied in the intravascular. The design with the smooth outer skin proved to be the most successful since it provokes much less fibrosis than the rough fenestrated surface which allows host tissue to grow into the spongy matrix. Many modifications of this concept have been proposed in order to further improve the biocompatibility. One of those was the coating of the membranes with poly-ethyleenoxide to reduce protein adsorption [50]. Biocompatibility problems with extravascular macrocapsules are usually deleterious only to the function of the encapsulated tissue and have no or only minimal risk for the recipient. These biocompatibility problems are usually related to toxicity and activation of non-specific foreign body reactions resulting in fibrotic overgrowth with subsequent necrosis of the encapsulated tissue.

Table I. Main components of capsules proposed for macroencapsulation of pancreatic islets

Membrane Geometry Proposed by	Geometry	Proposed by
nitro-cellulose acetate	Planar	Algire 1943 [25]
polycarbonate	Planar	Strautz 1970 [187]
2-hydroxyethyl methacrylate (HEMA)	Planar	Klomp et al 1979 [57]
polytetrafluoroethylene	Planar	Rafael et al 1999
polyacrylonitrile and polyvinylchloride	Tubular	Archer et al 1980 [34] Zekorn
cellulose	Tubular	et al 1989
polyamide	Tubular	[188] Zekorn et al 1989 [188] Kessler
acrylonitrile and sodium-methallyl sulfonate(AN69)	Tubular	et al 1991 (59)
alginate-based		
polyvinyl alcohol (PVA)	Tubular	Lanza et al 1995 [189]
polyisobutylene	Tubular	Gamian et al 1999 [190]
	Tubular	Isayeva et al 2003 [191]

During the past few years, an interesting trend has been the growing number of groups applying hydrogels for extravascular macrocapsules. Hydrogels provide a number of features which are advantageous for the biocompatibility of the membranes. Firstly, as a consequence of the hydrophilic nature of the material, there is almost no interfacial tension with surrounding fluids and tissues, which minimizes the protein adsorption and cell adhesion. Furthermore, the soft and pliable features of the gel reduce the mechanical or frictional irritations to surrounding tissue. And, finally, they provide a high degree of permeability for low molecular weight nutrients and metabolites, which is required for the optimal functioning of living cells[51,52].

Many hydrogels have been applied, such as gels prepared of alginate [53-55], agarose [37,56], 2-hydroxyethyl methacrylate HEMA [57,58] and a copolymer of acrylonitrile and sodium-methallyl sulfonate, AN69 [59]. Primary attention has been focussed on the hydrogel membrane AN69, which induced only minimal fibrosis in the peritoneal cavity of rats [60,61] but had low permeability for insulin [60,61]. Kessler et al [60,61] have introduced corona discharge to obtain a membrane with a more hydrophobic surface. Less molecules adhered to the surface of such membranes, which improved not only the permeability for insulin but also its long-term biocompatibility. One year after implantation in rats, only few macrophages were found on the membrane's surface. Moreover, encouraging results were reported by Jain et al who demonstrated functional porcine islets transplanted in agarose macrobeads almost 200 days after intraperitoneal transplantation into BB rats [37].

Intravascular Macrocapsules

The intravascular device is usually composed of a microporous tube with blood flow through its lumen and with a housing on its outside containing the implanted tissue [62,63]. The device is implanted by vascular anastomoses to the vessels of the host. The most intensively studied intravascular device is the modified diffusion chamber of Chick et al [64]. It is technically advanced and has been tested extensively in small [65] as well as in large animals [65,66] The original device was composed of a number of small diameter artificial capillaries contained by one large diameter tube. The artificial capillaries were composed of fibers of polyacrylonitrile and polyvinylchloride copolymer (PAN-PVC) similar to those used in extravascular devices [48][49]. This PAN-PVC ultrafiltration capillary design [31] has a lumen loaded with islets at the outside of the artificial capillaries. The design permits for close contact between the islets and blood, separated only by the microporous walls of the capillaries. These devices were found to induce normoglycemia in diabetic rats [65], dogs [66] and monkeys [65] but required systemic anticoagulation. The duration of this normoglycemia was usually restricted to several hours and successes of a somewhat longer duration were exceptional. Clotting of the blood in the lumen of these small diameter artificial capillaries proved to be a major obstacle, in spite of anticoagulant medication in massive doses. This thrombus formation was an early sign of insufficient biocompatibility, and has led to the use of tubular membranes with larger diameters in the hope of minimizing or eliminating clot formation in the absence of systemic anticoagulation.

The latter large lumen device is composed of a single, coiled, and tubular membrane with an internal diameter of 5-6 mm. The membrane is somewhat modified but still composed of PAN-PVC with a nominal molecular weight cutoff of 50 kDa. This membrane was found to be rather successful, since these devices implanted as high flow arteriovenous fistulas could remain patent for periods of seven weeks in the absence of systemic anticoagulant therapy [67]. This success is in part explained by the high flow rates through the device which prevents adhesion of cells to the membranes or collection of those cells in the immediate vicinity [48].

Allo- and xenogenic islets in the high flow devices were successfully transplanted to diabetic dogs [68-73] but the efforts to improve the blood-compatibility have probably interfered with the efficacy of the device as an implantation site for islets. This view is derived from the following observations. First, two devices per recipient instead of one were required to achieve adequate secretion capacity while maintaining the same numbers of islets per device [74]. Furthermore, it has not been possible to load the space between the membranes and the housing with an islet-tissue density higher than 5-10% of the volume [31], in spite of the fact that the large lumen is exposed to arterial blood with optimal concentrations of nutrients and oxygen. It is quite plausible that the high flow rates through the device, which are required to keep the device patent, do not allow sufficient exchange of glucose, insulin and nutrients to permit long term survival and adequate function of the islets.

There are also indications that the materials applied in this kind of devices are not only thrombogenic but also insufficiently compatible with long term functional survival of the islets. For example, the PTFE as used for vascular anastomosis of the device has been shown to induce IL-1β production by macrophages [75], which cytokine is lethal for islets [76,77]. It is quite plausible that IL-1β causes loss of high numbers of islets during the period between implantation and complete integration of the prothesis since macrophages are usually the first cells to invade the implant [78-80]. This is another explanation for the fact that so many islets divided over two devices are required for maintaining normoglycemia in dogs.

Although the intravascular devices have shown some degree of success, the problems mentioned above should be solved if clinical application is considered. Even then, the complications associated with any type of vascular prosthetic surgery remain a serious threat, such as thrombosis, either primary or secondary to intimal hyperplasia at the venous anastomosis, defects of the device, or infection. This is a major drawback for wide application in large numbers of diabetic patients since any alternative to conventional insulin treatment should preferably carry no additional risk.

Microcapsules

Microencapsulation is the technique by which each islet is enveloped in its own, spherical semipermeable membrane. Several arguments favor microcapsules over macrocapsules. Their spherical shape offers better diffusion capacity because of a better surface/volume ratio. Microcapsules cannot be easily disrupted, they are mechanically stable, they do not require complex or expensive manufacturing procedure, and they can be implanted into the patient by a simple injection procedure.

Reportedly, the clinical experience is still restricted to one recipient [81], but several research groups are concentrating on transplantation of microencapsulated islets in the experimental setting [42,43,82,83,83-104]. Although successful encapsulated islet grafts do induce normoglycemia in streptozotocin diabetic rodents recipients, some authors have reported reduced functional performance in response to glucose challenge [51,95,105-107].

For several years, we have been concentrating on microencapsulation and we have directed our efforts to a step-wise analysis of the factors influencing performance of the microencapsulated grafts. To this end, we have been using only one technique of alginate-polylysine microencapsulation as initially introduced by Lim and Sun [33], instead of testing other materials in a trial and error approach. Our aim is to define the conditions, which must be met for successful transplantation of microencapsulated islets as a feasible treatment of insulin dependent diabetes mellitus.

The Principle of Microencapsulation

The vast majority of groups apply hydrogels for production of microcapsules since these hydrogels are associated with optimal survival of the enveloped cells. Table 2 lists the most commonly applied biomaterials for this technique. A major distinction exists between water-soluble polymers such as alginates and water insoluble polymers such as HEMA-MMA. Water insoluble polymers are preferred by a number of groups [58,108-110] since it is assumed that after implantation they are more stable than water soluble polymers. However, a major obstacle in using water insoluble polymers for encapsulation of cells is the use of an organic solvent, which usually interferes with cellular function [58,111].

Table 2. Main components of capsules proposed for microencapsulation of pancreatic islets

Main component of the capsule	Source	Initially proposed by
Alginate	Alga	Lim and Sun 1980 (33) Zielinski 1994
Chitosan	Alga	(192)
Agarose	Alga	Iwata et al 1989 (96) Dawson et al 1987
Poly(hydroxyethylmetacrylate-methyl	Synthetic	(193)
methacrylate)(HEMA-MMA)	Synthetic	Kessler et al 1991 (59)
Copolymers of acrylonitrile (AN69)	Synthetic	Shimizu et al 1996 (194)
Protamine-heparine	Synthetic	Tatarkiewicz 1994 (195)
N-isopropylacrylamide	Synthetic	Sefton et al 1997 (196)
Polyacryates	Synthetic	Cruise et al 1999 (84)
Polyethyleneglycol (PEG)	Synthetic	Boninsegna 2003 (197)
Silica		

We, like others [98,103,104,112-114], have concentrated on alginate based capsules since they have repeatedly been found not to interfere with cellular function. Despite of their solubility in aqueous solutions, they have been shown to be stable for years in small and large animals and recently also in men [72,81,115]. The encapsulation technique is based on entrapment of individual islets in an alginate droplet, which is transformed into a rigid bead by gelification in a divalent cation solution, mostly rich in Ca^{2+}. The droplets are formed by forcing an alginate/cell mixture through a needle, which is installed in a droplet generator. In principle we can distinguish three techniques of droplet generation (Fig. 3). The first and most commonly applied approach, is the air-driven droplet generator [116].

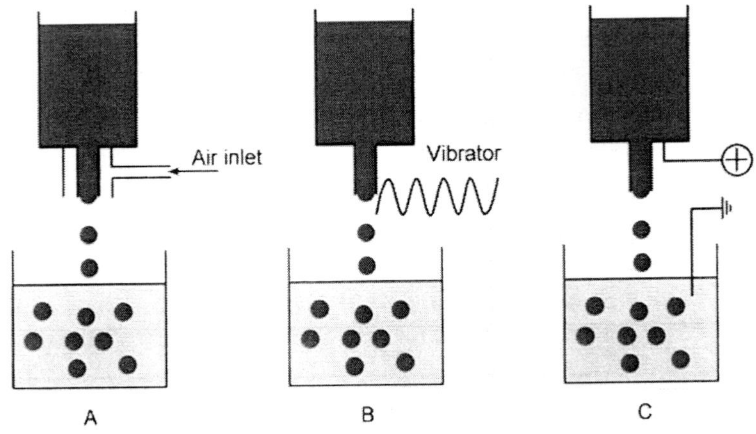

Figure 3. The basic principle of encapsulation is the formation of droplets by forcing an alginate/cell mixture through a needle, which is installed in a droplet generator. We can distinguish three techniques of droplet generation. The air-driven droplet generator (A) where droplets are formed by a co-axial airstream around the tip of a needle, which forces droplets of alginate to detach from the needle-tip. The size of the droplets can be decreased by increasing the airflow rate. With the vibration technique (B) detachment of the droplets from the needle is forced by substituting the airstream for vibration. With the latest technique, the voltage driven dropletgenerator (C), the dropletsize is controlled by a voltage difference between needle and gelification solution.

In these devices droplets are formed by a co-axial airstream around the tip of a needle which forces droplets of alginate to detach from the needle-tip. The size of the droplets can be decreased by increasing the airflow rate. In order to increase the production rate of droplets some groups have introduced a new approach by substituting the needle in de droplet generator for a vibration [117]. These devices do not need an airstream and by increasing the vibration frequency, the production rate can be increased while the droplet size decreases. Both the air-driven dropletgenerator and the vibration device have one major disadvantage, they do not allow for reproducible production of droplets with a size smaller than 500 μm [118]. Devices that produce capsules smaller than 500 μm may be mandatory since it has repeatedly been shown that small capsules are needed for optimal exchange of nutrients and metabolics as well as for adequate function of the enveloped cells. Therefore, a third category of devices has been introduced. These are the so-called voltage driven dropletgenerators. The technique of this device is based on administration of electrostatic forces to pull droplets off a needle-tip. The bead size can be varied by increasing the electrostatic potential between the gelling bath and the needle. Reportedly, this technique allows for reproducible production of droplets of 300 μm [103] but in our hands even smaller droplets of 175 μm can be readily obtained. Although the smallest capsule possible is prefered, it should be noted that the size of the capsules is not only limited by the technology applied but also by the size of the tissue to be encapsulated. With islet-encapsulation the size will be limited by the diameter of the islets which vary between 50 and 350 μm.

The next step in the encapsulation process is the gelification. Alginate-molecules are composed of mannuronic (M) and guluronic acids (G). The alginate-molecules are connected by Ca^{2+} through binding of consecutive blocks of G-molecules on each of both molecules.

The most commonly applied alginate-based capsule is the alginate-polylysine system. The beads are coated with a polylysine membrane by suspending the beads in a poly-L-lysine (PLL) solution. During this step PLL binds to mixed sequences of G and M in the alginate molecules [119,120]. This induces the formation of complexes at the capsule surface consisting of α-helical PLL surrounded by superhelically orientated polysaccharide chains [120]. The presence of these complexes decreases the porosity of the membrane. By varying the molecular weight, the concentration of the polylysine, and the incubation time one can modulate the porosity of the capsule membrane [94,121-126]. Usually, ten-minute incubation in 0.1 % polylysine with a molecular weight of 22 kDa is sufficient to form an immunoprotective membrane. However, it should be emphasized that the binding of polylysine does not only depend upon the incubation time and the molecular weight of the polylysine but also on the type and concentration of alginate [125,127] as well as on the incubation temperature [124,125,127]. In a final step, to provide biocompatibility, the capsules are suspended in a solution of alginate or other negatively charged molecules [124,127] to bind all positively charged polylysine residues still present at the capsule surface. We do not apply EGTA or citrate [111] to liquify the inner core of the capsule. The reason for this modification of the original Lim and Sun method [33] was, that we have observed many capsules loosing their integrity during the treatment.

A very important aspect of adequate biocompayibility, is a smooth and mechanically stable microcapsule. In our laboratory we have observed that high- rather than low-G alginates produce smooth beads with no obvious tails or strains. Moreover, we have found that after implantation, alginates with low-G concentrations had a tendency to swell with subsequent breakage of the PLL membrane followed by cellular overgrowth of the capsules. Therefore, for our studies we have chosen the alginate with an intermediate G-concentration.

The stability of the capsule is determined by stability of a membrane and stability of an alginate core. The stability of the membrane can be controlled by the PLL-step since shorter incubation time, lower PLL concentrations, and lower PLL molecular weight than described above, were associated with an increase of the number of capsules with broken membranes. Additionally, incubation at 4°C instead of room temperature led to less stable microcapsules. In spite of all the improvements in the stability of the capsules, tissue reactions still continued to interfere with longevity of the graft survival. We have found that other factors, not directly related to the production procedure per se, were responsible for the tissue reaction as a sign of insufficient biocompatibility of microcapsules.

Present Insights in Tissue Reponses Against Microcapsules

A major obstacle in the application of immunoisolation has been insufficient biocompatibility of the capsules which induced overgrowth of the capsules by inflammatory cells with necrosis of the enveloped therapeutic cells as a consequence [52,128]. It was shown that this insufficient biocompatibility of capsules is influenced by many factors. We found that the number of capsules that will be affected by cellular overgrowth is dependent on the chemical characteristics of the capsule-materials applied. We have shown that pure alginate rather than commercially available crude alginates should be applied for encapsulation [52]. Crude alginates are contaminated with several inflammatory substances such as polyphenols, which are associated with severe inflammatory reactions after implantation. When pure alginates are applied with an intermediate-G content we were able to reduce the overgrowth from 80-100% of the capsules to a portion of only 2-10% of the capsules. Also, it is important that there are no unbound PLL residues on the capsule surface. When PLL is not adequately bound by alginate it provokes a strong inflammatory response after implantation. The adequacy of binding of PLL depends on the composition of the alginate applied. Alginates are composed of blocks of guluronic acid (G-blocks), blocks of mannuronic acid (M-blocks), and alternating blocks of guluronic acid and mannuronic acid (G-M blocks). Adequate binding of PLL mainly depends on the amount of G-M blocks in the alginate. Small lower variations in the G-M content results in less efficient binding of PLL with overgrowth of the capsule surface as a consequence [119,120,129,130]. For adequate binding of PLL and neutralising the majority of its proinflammatory effects we have to apply a so-called intermediate-G alginate with 45% G and 30 % G-M blocks. Recently, our group has shown that, when adequately produced, empty capsules for cell-immunoisolation can survive for two years in the peritoneal cavity of rats [115].

It was found that the 2-10% overgrowth was caused by individual imperfections on a portion of the capsules such as protruding cells (Fig. 4) and incomplete bound PLL on the surface.

These imperfections are difficult to avoid in the current technological approach since we apply flexible alginates (with intermediate-G content) which is associated with some capsules with protruding cells. Also, the present technology is susceptible for small variations in G-M content in the alginate sources which cause tissue responses as the consequence of insufficient neutralisation of the proinflammatory PLL on the capsule surface [129,131-134]. In an attempt to solve the cell protrusion problem we have tested the biocompatibility of alginate-PLL capsules prepared of high-G alginates since from our *in vitro* studies follows that alginate with a high guluronic acid content (> 53%) provides stronger capsules with less protruding cells than capsules prepared of alginate with an intermediate guluronic acid content [52]. Unfortunately, these high-G alginates could not be applied for cell encapsulation since they were associated with severe tissue responses *in vivo* due to inefficacious binding of the proinflammatory polylysine.

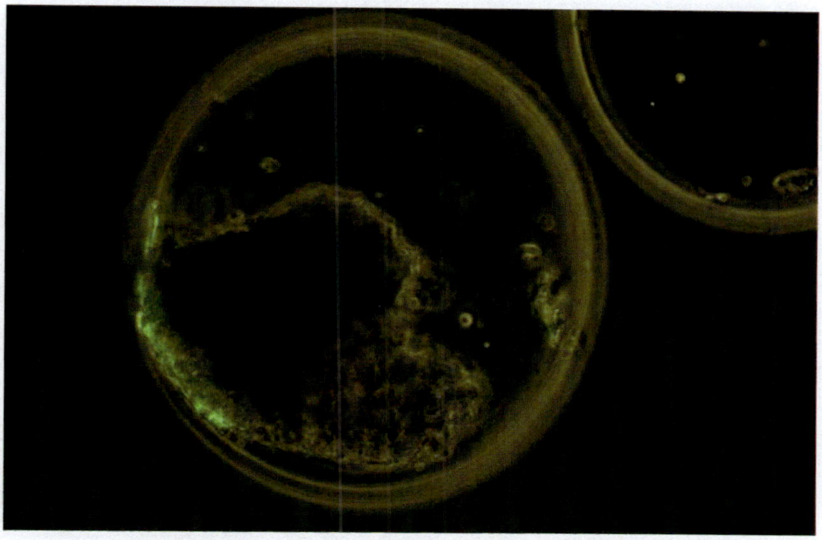

Figure 4. Inadequate encapsulation of pancreatic islets. The islet is incompletely encapsulated. Islet cells protruding from the capsule are specifically labeled by the FITC-labeled lectin RCA-I . (original magnification x 100).

In order to provide more insight in the structure of alginate-PLL capsules we have performed an physico-chemical analysis of the capsules by applying X-ray photoelectron spectroscopy [129,130,135]. This technique allows for identification of the chemical groups on the surface of the capsule on an atomic level. Up to now the capsule was assumed to be composed of a core of Ca-alginate which is enveloped by a membrane composed of two layers, *i.e.* an inner layer of alginate-PLL and an outer layer of Ca-alginate [33,136,137]. The data, which have lead to this model, were almost exclusively obtained by studying the chemical interactions of PLL with solved, non-Ca^{2+} bound and often individual components of alginate (*i.e* guluronic (G)-acid and mannuronic (M)-acid monomers) and not by studying the chemical structure of the capsules as such. In our studies on true capsules, we never observed Ca^{2+} in the membrane of the capsules, which has the following implications for the assumed structure of the capsules. First, the alginate-PLL layer is not composed of the combination of alginate-PLL and Ca^{2+}-alginate but of the alginate-PLL only. The absence of Ca^{2+} also implies that the outer Ca-alginate layer does not exist and, consequently, that the membrane is not composed of two but of one layer only. Finally, we found sodium in the membrane, which is bound by carboxyl groups on consecutive blocks of G- and M-molecules, which remain unbound between the complexes of PLL and mixed sequences of G and M. Figure 5 shows the actual structure of alginate-PLL capsules.

These findings have serious implications for biocompatibility issues associated with microcapsules since it implies that the proinflammatory PLL is always on the surface of the capsules in direct contact with the inflammatory cells. It suggests that, for optimal biocompatibility, we have to focus on understanding and improving the interaction of the inflammatory polycations with alginate rather than improving the second coating step with alginate. Alternatively, we can perform an additional envelopment step of the capsules to prevent direct contact between the polycation with the surrounding tissues in the implantation site.

Purified intermediate-alginates reduced the overgrowth from 80-100% to a portion of only 2-10% of the capsules. When tested with encapsulated rat pancreatic islet allografts we found that this reduction in overgrowth did bring about an increase in graft survival time from 3 to 6 months. This illustrated that improving the quality of the capsules is a successful strategy in order to increase the longevity of the grafts. At this point it was unclear what caused failure of the cells since it was generally assumed that the loss of 2-10% of capsules could not explain the failure of the remaining 90-98% of the capsules [138]. In search of factors contributing to graft failure we analysed in subsequent investigations the inflammatory responses against the grafts. This was done at various time points between implantation and graft failure. The first new finding was that the responses against the grafts were not static as generally assumed [132,139-142] but dynamic [135] with involvement of different cell types as will be discussed in detail in the following section.

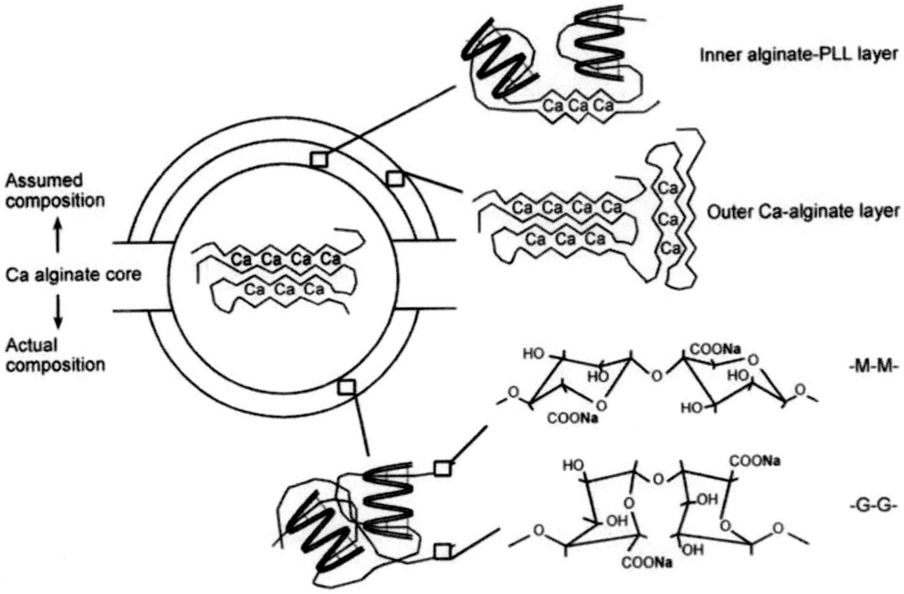

Figure 5. Schematic representation of the composition of the alginate-PLL membranes. In the assumed model the alginate core is surrounded with two layers. The inner layer of alginate-PLL is considered to be formed by two types of interactions. The first type is that of the interaction between the PLL and mixed sequences of guluronic acid (G) and manuronic acid (M) in the alginate molecules. This interaction reduces the permeability of the capsules by inducing the formation of complexes at the surface of α-helical PLL surrounded by superhelically orientated polysaccharide molecules. The other interaction is that between Ca^{2+} and alginate which is already formed in the gelation step in 100 mM $CaCl_2$. In the actual model the outer layer is composed of only one alginate-PLL layer containing PLL and Na^+ without the Ca-alginate. The Na^+ ions are bound by carboxyl groups present in the alginate.

The very first step in the tissue response is probably not related to the implantation of the 'foreign' capsules but to the required surgical procedure for implantation. Although it is only minor surgery, the procedure is associated with tissue damage as illustrated by the observation of erythrocytes in the peritoneal cavity at the first day after implantation. The bleedings and subsequent tissue repair is associated with the introduction of serum factors in the peritoneal cavity and release of bioactive proteins such as fibrinogen, trombin, and fibronectin[143]. These factors will have chemotactic effects on inflammatory cells which cells will subsequently migrate to the peritoneal site [144-147]. The bioactive proteins are adsorbed by the foreign polymers as of day 5 [135] resulting in adherence of cells at a portion of the capsules. These adherent cells were found to produce the cytokines IL-1β, TNF-α, and TGF-β, which further activate inflammatory cells in the vicinity of the foreign materials [143,147-149]. The observation of high numbers of basophils in the cellular infiltrate suggests that basophils play an important role in the host response against immunoisolated cells. Basophiles are strong producers of bioactive proteins and cytokines such as histamine [150-154], monocyte and macrophage chemoattractant proteins (MIP and MCP) [151,155], IL-4 [154,156,157], and IL-13 [154,158-160]. These cytokines are well known to have chemotactic and activating effects on inflammatory cells such as granulocytes, macrophages and fibroblasts. The above-described response is most severe during the first two weeks after implantation. In these two weeks, basophils and granulocytes gradually disappear from the graft site while macrophages and fibroblasts remain attached to a portion of 2-10% the capsules [135].

Recently, by performing both *in vitro* and *ex vivo* studies, we showed that even this small amount of overgrown capsules can have a pronounced effect on the functional survival of the encapsulated grafts. The macrophages on the 2-10% overgrown capsules stay activated (as indicated by upregulation of IL-1β and TNF-α mRNA) as of the moment of implantation until at least day 28 after implantation. This results in elevated apoptosis in the engrafted cells and release of graft-derived cytokines such as MCP-1 in the 90-98% nonovergrown capsules. The effect of this is a continuing circle of activation and loss of 40-80% of the cells in the graft (Fig. 6A) [161]. Therefore, we now consider this latter response and consequently the overgrowth on 2-10% of the capsules an important deleterious factor for adequate graft survival.

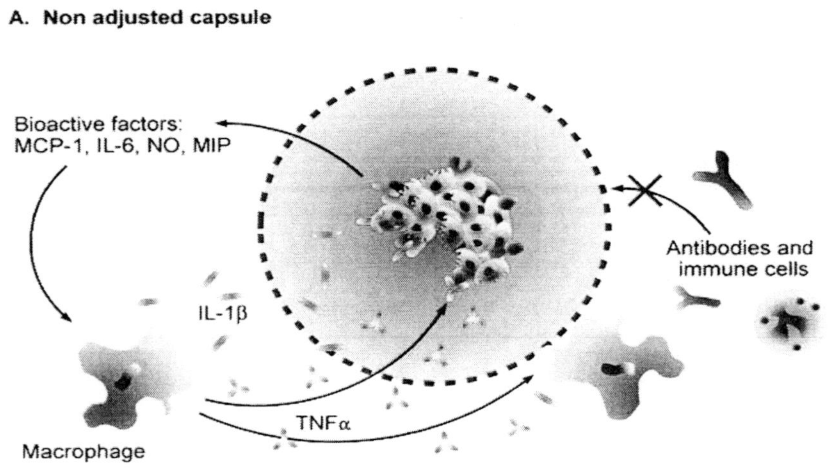

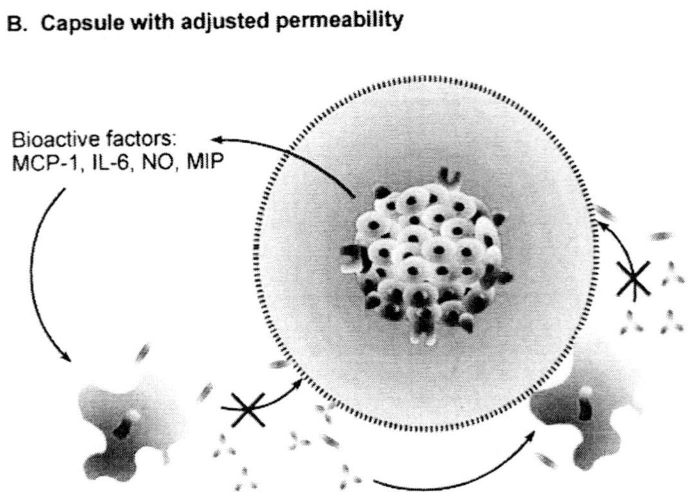

Figure 6. **A.** Schematic representation that a small amount of overgrowth on capsules can have a pronounced effect on the functional survival of the encapsulated grafts. The macrophages on the 2-10% overgrown capsules stay activated and the release of cytokines results in elevated apoptosis in the engrafted cells and release of graft-derived cytokines such as MCP-1 in the 90-98% nonovergrown capsules. The effect of this is a continuing circle of activation and loss of 40-80% of the cells in the graft [161]. **B.** Decreasing the permeability by chemical modification of the capsules prevents diffusion of large and multimeric cytokines such as TNF-α as well as small (e.g. IL-1β) cytokines, produced by the activated macrophages, into the capsules. The mechanism is that the chemical modifications for decreasing the permeability increased the negative charges of the alginate in the capsules, which induces repulsion of the negative charges on the tested cytokines-molecules.

Permeability of Capsules for Cytokines

As discussed in the preceding sections diffusion of graft-derived and inflammatory cell-derived cytokines is a major threat for the longevity of the encapsulated grafts. The permeability of the capsules for cytokines has always been a subject of debate. Scepticists have always assumed that the membranes of capsules can not adequately protect against deleterious cytokines with an approximate molecular weight of insulin or essential nutrients (5-15 kDa). Therefore, diffusion of cytokines into the capsules has always been the Achilles heel of immunoisolation. Recently, combined efforts of our group and that of Prof. Marchetti in Pisa have shown that this is not an insurmountable problem. It has been shown that the final effect of cytokines is dependent on the combined presence of different cytokines and on the concentration of cytokines [162]. We found *in vitro* that decreasing the permeability by chemical modification of the capsules prevents diffusion into the capsules of large and multimeric cytokines such as TNF-α. Also, diffusion of small cytokines (e.g. IL-1β) was reduced by changing the permeability of the membrane which was unexpected as the molecular weight of small cytokines such as IL-1β (17 kDa) was far below the molecular cut-off of the applied capsules (100 kDa) (Fig.6B). The mechanism is that the chemical modifications for decreasing the permeability increased the negative charges of the alginate in the capsules which induces repulsion of the negative charges on the tested cytokines-molecules. The observation that capsules can be selectively made impermeable for cytokines is very important since this can overcome the problem of the continuing circle of activation of cells in the overgrowth due the release of graft derived cytokines [163]

Also, we found evidence that cytokines may not interfere with islet function in case of xenografting of encapsulated islets in humans. We have observed that following exposure to a combination of human cytotoxic cytokines, a marked decrease in functional survival and a high percentage of apoptotic cells could be found in human islets but not in bovine islets [164]. Preliminary data show that this is due, at least in part, to the fact that xenogenic islet cells are less capable to bind and to take up human cytokines. This implies that, at least in some combinations, even when capsules are applied which are permeable for cytokines, the function and survival of xenogenic islet-sources will be less affected.

Metabolic Function of Encapsulated Islet Grafts

Adequate regulation of glucose levels by an encapsulated pancreatic islet graft requires a minute to minute regulation of blood glucose. In order to design such a transplant, it is mandatory to have sufficient insight in factors influencing the kinetics of insulin secretion by encapsulated islets. Functional performance of encapsulated grafts has mainly been studied with microencapsulated grafts. Therefore, in the next section we will mainly concentrate on the graft function of recipients of microencapsulated islets.

Insulin responses of encapsulated islets are influenced by the permeability of the capsule membrane and not by the islet-diameters or capsule diameter in the routinely applied 500-800 μm range. During our comparison of the glucose induced insulin responses of islets with different sizes, we surprisingly found no size-dependent differences in insulin secretion. This lack of effect of islet-size on insulin-secretion should probably be explained by the fact that in isolated islets the glucose is penetrating the islets by passive diffusion instead of by active transport to each, individual islet-cell by the bloodstream. This passive diffusion of glucose is predictably less efficient than active transport in normal, vascularized islets in the native pancreas [165,166]. Consequently, the glucose around large isolated islets will only stimulate islet-cells in the periphery rather than the more centrally located islet-cells.

The observation that encapsulated small, 90-120 μm islets show similar instead of lower glucose induced insulin responses than 150-180 and 210-300 μm islets suggests that the inclusion of only small islets in encapsulated grafts will have no consequences for the functional performance of the grafts. This is a pertinent consideration since small islets are associated with less protrusion [94,127,167] and, therefore, a lower rate of failing encapsulated islets. Another advantage of application of small islets is the reduction of problems associated with insufficient nutrition and central necrosis of the encapsulated islets with sizes larger than 150 μm [138]. This necrosis has been shown to be a major cause of failure of encapsulated grafts [52,138]. However, the effects of application of only the small rather than the large islets on longevity of encapsulated islet grafts requires some further research considerations since longevity of the graft is determined by the size of the graft volume [168,169] which volume is mainly determined by the number of large islets in the transplant [168,170,171].

Intraperitoneal transplantation of a microencapsulated islet graft restored normoglycemia in streptozotocin diabetic rat recipients within one week after transplantation. This normalization of blood glucose levels was associated with an evident metabolic improvement as illustrated by a normalization of body weight, normal HBAc1 levels and by a dramatic reduction in daily urine production. When functioning grafts were tested by oral or intravenous glucose challenge, glucose tolerance was found to be rather adequate as indicated by maximum glucose levels of 8.3 mM after the consumption of a glucose-rich meal but a rise in systemic insulin levels was never observed.

We have further substantiated this observation experimentally by assessing portal and systemic insulin responses and glucose levels after gradual infusion of low amounts of insulin into the peritoneal cavity, thereby mimicking the gradual release of insulin from the capsules of intraperitoneal graft. We found that the dose-dependent rise of insulin and decrease of glucose levels with intraperitoneal insulin infusion were strongly delayed and reduced as well as prolonged in comparison to intraportal insulin infusion [172][106]

The fact that the peritoneal cavity is not an optimal site for islet transplantation is also shown by the fact that the C-peptide level (which is released from islets in an equimolar concentration but not absorbed by abdominal organs and does not undergo hepatic extraction) is increased in the systemic circulation of an transplanted diabetic mice after an meal. However, this increase is delayed and decreased compared to normal mice[107]. The reason for the peritoneal cavity being less accommodating for transplanted islets is the lack of neovascularisation which also results in a relative hypoxia [31,173].

The absence of revascularization of the encapsulated islets interferes with both the functional performance and the longevity of the grafts [52,162,174]. Apparently, it is obligatory for clinical applications to find a site where encapsulated islets are in close contact with the blood stream. Unfortunately, it is difficult to find such a site since it should combine the capacity to bear a large graft volume in the immediate vicinity of blood vessels. Reported sites allowing for successful islet transplantation in mammals such as the liver [168,175-177], the spleen [168,178-180], and the renal capsule [40,169,181] do not meet these requirements since they can never carry the volumes of more than 100 ml of capsules required for transplantation in man [81,116,125]. To overcome this obstacle, we have recently introduced the concept of an intraperitoneally implanted solid support system for pancreatic islets [174]. This site allows for implantation of high numbers of islets, which can readily be retrieved and, theoretically, can be designed as such that it is highly vascularized.

This solid support system was developed of expanded polytetrafluoroethylene (ePTFE) since ePTFE have been shown to be biocompatible and to become neovascularized after implantation in the peritoneal cavity. Initially, we applied the concept of Thompson et al [182,183] in which solid supports are coated with collagen type IV (*i.e.* the collagen type predominantly present in the basal membrane) and acidic-fibroblast growth factors (a-FGF) to facilitate the ingrowth of blood vessels [174,182,183]. This solid support was shown to be very efficacious since normoglycemia was induced in all diabetic rats with islet transplants in the solid supports while this was only the case in 40% of the diabetic rats transplanted with islets in the unmodified peritoneal cavity without the solid support [174].

In our subsequent studies on vascularization of solid supports, we have focused on VEGF–165 [184-186], which is considered to have the greatest potential as angiogenic stimulus when compared to other angiogenic growth factors like acidic-fibroblast growth factor, basic-fibroblast growth factor, platelet derived growth factor, epidermal growth factor, epidermal growth factor, transforming growth factor alpha and beta, interleukines (IL-8 and TNF) or prostaglandines. Our present experimental approach is to stimulate vascularization of the solid supports applicable for encapsulated islets. These supports were prepared of flat sheet of ePTFE which were coated with collagen type IV and subsequently implanted in the peritoneal cavity in the immediate vicinity of the liver in order to promote portal drainage of insulin.

Concluding Remarks

It is clear that tremendous advances have been made in immunoisolation of pancreatic islets during the last few decades. It was shown that insufficient biocompatibility of capsules is influenced by many factors. When pure alginates are applied with an intermediate-G content we were able to reduce the overgrowth to a portion of only 2-10% of the capsules. This overgrowth in vivo on this small portion of the capsules is caused by individual imperfections on the capsule surface such as inadequate islet encapsulation, incomplete covering of the inflammatory PLL and the effect of the surgical procedure. Recent new insight has shown that these imperfections on the small portions of capsules are not without consequences. The imperfections attract inflammatory cells such as macrophages. These macrophages stay activated for prolonged periods of time since they remain activated by bioactive factors released by the islet-tissue in the capsules [161]. This is an important observation since it implies that for successful transplantation we should not only focus on finding adequate biomaterials but also delete the effects of the enveloped cells in sustaining the inflammatory response.

Another obstacle on the route to successful transplantation of encapsulated islets is the absence of an adequate islet source. Irrespective of the species (i.e. rat or human) we require multiple donors for a single transplantation. It is mandatory to gain sufficient insight in which factors determine success or failure of an islet isolation procedure. For islet-encapsulation it is of an additional importance that the islets are sufficiently 'clean', i.e. not contaminated with exocrine tissue since this holds the risk of protrusion of cells[94,167] and death of the encapsulated islets as a consequence.

Furthermore, the encapsulated islets should closely follow the kinetics of insulin release of a free, nonencapsulated islet. Therefore, we require the smallest capsule possible. However, decreasing the capsule diameter holds the risk of protrusion of cells. It has been shown that protrusion can be minimized by application of only the small islets in the graft rather than the larger islets. Whether application of only small islets has consequences for the functional performance of the grafts remains to be determined.

We have shown that lowering the permeability of the capsules by increasing the PLL incubation time can provide a mean to overcome the obstacle of diffusion of cytokines into the capsules. The efficacy of this approach for the blockade of the inflammatory responses induced by the islet in the capsules *in vivo* remains to be confirmed but it shows that obstacles which seem to be insurmountable can be solved by a step-wise analysis of factors determine success and failure of encapsulated grafts.

References

[1] Laumonier T, Potiron N, Boeffard F, Chagneau C, Brouard S, Guillot C, Soulillou JP, Anegon I, Le Mauff B: CTLA4Ig Adenoviral` Gene Transfer Induces Long-Term Islet Rat Allograft Survival, Without Tolerance, After Systemic but Not Local Intragraft Expression. *Hum.Gene Ther.* 14:561-575, 2003

[2] Demeterco C, Levine F: Gene therapy for diabetes. *Front Biosci.* 6:D175-D1912001

[3] The effect of intensive treatment of diabetes on the development and progression of long-term complications in insulin-dependent diabetes mellitus. The Diabetes Control and Complications Trial Research Group. *N.Engl.J.Med.* 329:977-986, 1993

[4] Robertson RP, Davis C, Larsen J, Stratta R, Sutherland DE: Pancreas and islet transplantation for patients with diabetes. *Diabetes Care* 23:112-116, 2000

[5] Sutherland DE, Gruessner AC, Gruessner RW: Pancreas transplantation: a review. *Transplant.Proc.* 30:1940-1943, 1998

[6] Kronson JW, Gillingham KJ, Sutherland DE, Matas AJ: Renal transplantation for type II diabetic patients compared with type I diabetic patients and patients over 50 years old: a single-center experience. *Clin.Transplant.* 14:226-234, 2000

[7] Shapiro AM, Lakey JR, Ryan EA, Korbutt GS, Toth E, Warnock GL, Kneteman NM, Rajotte RV: Islet transplantation in seven patients with type 1 diabetes mellitus using a glucocorticoid-free immunosuppressive regimen. *N.Engl.J.Med.* 343:230-238, 2000

[8] Faustman D, Lacy PE, Davie JM: Transplantation without immunosuppression. *Diabetes* 31 Suppl 4:11-16, 1982

[9] Hardy MA, Lau H, Weber C, Reemtsma K: Pancreatic islet transplantation. Induction of graft acceptance by ultraviolet irradiation of donor tissue. *Ann.Surg.* 200:441-450, 1984

[10] Lau H, Reemtsma K, Hardy MA: The use of direct ultraviolet irradiation and cyclosporine in facilitating indefinite pancreatic islet allograft acceptance. *Transplantation* 38:566-569, 1984

[11] Faustman DL, Steinman RM, Gebel HM, Hauptfeld V, Davie JM, Lacy PE: Prevention of rejection of murine islet allografts by pretreatment with anti-dendritic cell antibody. *Proc.Natl.Acad.Sci.U.S.A* 81:3864-3868, 1984

[12] Morris PJ, Finch DR, Garvey JF, Poole MD, Millard PR: Suppression of rejection of allogeneic islet tissue in the rat. *Diabetes* 29 Suppl 1:107-112, 1980

[13] Bowen KM, Andrus L, Lafferty KJ: Successful allotransplantation of mouse pancreatic islets to nonimmunosuppressed recipients. *Diabetes* 29 Suppl 1:98-104, 1980

[14] Zeng Y, Peterson L, Levisetti M, Torres M, Montag A, Thistlethwaite J-RJ: Immunomodulation of human islets results in prolonged in vivo islet graft survival. *Transplant.Proc.* 27:611-612, 1995

[15] Bhalla RK, Rich SJ, James RF, Bell PR, London NJ: The immunomodulation of cryopreserved pancreatic islets by gamma irradiation. A feasibility study. *Transplantation* 56:1045-1047, 1993

[16] Steurer W, Nickerson PW, Steele AW, Steiger J, Zheng XX, Strom TB: Ex vivo coating of islet cell allografts with murine CTLA4/Fc promotes graft tolerance. *J.Immunol.* 155:1165-1174, 1995

[17] Hsu PN, Lin HH, Tu CF, Chen NJ, Wu KM, Tsai HF, Hsieh SL: Expression of human Fas ligand on mouse beta islet cells does not induce insulitis but is insufficient to confer immune privilege for islet grafts. *J.Biomed.Sci.* 8:262-269, 2001

[18] Turvey SE, Gonzalez-Nicolini V, Kingsley CI, Larregina AT, Morris PJ, Castro MG, Lowenstein PR, Wood KJ: Fas ligand-transfected myoblasts and islet cell transplantation. *Transplantation* 69:1972-1976, 2000

[19] Takeda Y, Gotoh M, Dono K, Grochowiecki TR, Kimura F, Okuyama M, Shimizu J, Nagano H, Umeshita K, Sakon M, Miyasaka M, Monden M: Acceptance of islet allografts transplanted with Fas ligand expressing testicular allografts. *Transplant.Proc.* 31:624, 1999

[20] Chahine AA, Yu M, McKernan MM, Stoeckert C, Lau HT: Immunomodulation of pancreatic islet allografts in mice with CTLA4Ig secreting muscle cells. *Transplantation* 59:1313-1318, 1995

[21] Gainer AL, Suarez-Pinzon WL, Min WP, Swiston JR, Hancock-Friesen C, Korbutt GS, Rajotte RV, Warnock GL, Elliott JF: Improved survival of biolistically transfected mouse islet allografts expressing CTLA4-Ig or soluble Fas ligand. *Transplantation* 66:194-199, 1998

[22] Gainer AL, Korbutt GS, Rajotte RV, Warnock GL, Elliott JF: Expression of CTLA4-Ig by biolistically transfected mouse islets promotes islet allograft survival. *Transplantation* 63:1017-1021, 1997

[23] Kirk AD, Harlan DM, Armstrong NN, Davis TA, Dong Y, Gray GS, Hong X, Thomas D, Fechner J-HJ, Knechtle SJ: CTLA4-Ig and anti-CD40 ligand prevent renal allograft rejection in primates. *Proc.Natl.Acad.Sci.U.S.A* 94:8789-8794, 1997

[24] Bisceglie VV: Uber die antineoplastische Immunitat. *Krebsforsch* 40:141-158, 1933

[25] Algire GH: An adaption of the transparant chamber technique to the mouse. *J.Natl.Cancer Inst.* 4:1-11, 1943

[26] Liu HW, Ofosu FA, Chang PL: Expression of human factor IX by microencapsulated recombinant fibroblasts. *Hum.Gene.Ther.* 4:291-301, 1993

[27] Koo J, Chang TSM: Secretion of erythropoietin from microencapsulated rat kidney cells. *Int J Artif Organs* 16:557-560, 1993

[28] Chang PL, Shen N, Westcott AJ: Delivery of recombinant gene products with microencapsulated cells in vivo. *Hum.Gene.Ther.* 4:433-440, 1993

[29] Cieslinski DA, Humes HD: Tissue engineering of a bioartificial kidney. *Biotechnol.Bioeng.* 43:678-681, 1994

[30] Uludag H, Sefton MV: Metabolic activity and proliferation of CHO cells in hydroxyethyl methacrylate-methyl methacrylate (HEMA-MMA) microcapsules. *Cell Transplant.* 2:175-182, 1993

[31] Colton CK: Implantable biohybrid artificial organs. *Cell Transplantation* 4:415-436, 1995

[32] Aebischer P, Goddard M, Signore AP, Timpson RL: Functional recovery in hemiparkinsonian primates transplanted with polymer-encapsulated PC12 cells. *Exp.Neurol.* 126:151-158, 1994

[33] Lim F, Sun AM: Microencapsulated islets as bioartificial endocrine pancreas. *Science* 210:908-910, 1980

[34] Archer J, Kaye R, Mutter G: Control of streptozotocin diabetes in Chinese hamsters by cultured mouse islet cells without immunosuppression: a preliminary report. *J.Surg.Res.* 28:77-85, 1980

[35] Loudovaris T, Jacobs S, Young S, Maryanov D, Brauker J, Johnson RC: Correction of diabetic nod mice with insulinomas implanted within Baxter immunoisolation devices. *J.Mol.Med.* 77:219-222, 1999

[36] Lanza RP, Beyer AM, Chick WL: Xenogeneic humoral responses to islets transplanted in biohybrid diffusion chambers. *Transplantation* 57:1371-1375, 1994

[37] Jain K, Asina S, Yang H, Blount ED, Smith BH, Diehl CH, Rubin AL: Glucose control and long-term survival in biobreeding/Worcester rats after intraperitoneal implantation of hydrophilic macrobeads containing porcine islets without immunosuppression. *Transplantation* 68:1693-1700, 1999

[38] Lacy PE, Hegre OD, Gerasimidi Vazeou A, Gentile FT, Dionne KE: Maintenance of normoglycemia in diabetic mice by subcutaneous xenografts of encapsulated islets. *Science* 254:1782-1784, 1991

[39] Juang JH, Bonner-Weir S, Vacanti JP, Weir GC: Outcome of subcutaneous islet transplantation improved by a polymer device. *Transplant.Proc.* 27:3215-3216, 1995

[40] Juang JH, Bonner-Weir S, Wu YJ, Weir GC: Beneficial influence of glycemic control upon the growth and function of transplanted islets. *Diabetes* 43:1334-1339, 1994

[41] Scharp DW, Swanson CJ, Olack BJ, Latta PP, Hegre OD, Doherty EJ, Gentile FT, Flavin KS, Ansara MF, Lacy PE: Protection of encapsulated human islets implanted without immunosuppression in patients with type I or type II diabetes and in nondiabetic control subjects. *Diabetes* 43:1167-1170, 1994

[42] Suzuki K, Bonner-Weir S, Trivedi N, Yoon KH, Hollister-Lock J, Colton CK, Weir GC: Function and survival of macroencapsulated syngeneic islets transplanted into streptozocin-diabetic mice. *Transplantation* 66:21-28, 1998

[43] Suzuki K, Bonner-Weir S, Hollister-Lock J, Colton CK, Weir GC: Number and volume of islets transplanted in immunobarrier devices. *Cell Transplant.* 7:47-52, 1998

[44] Tatarkiewicz K, Hollister-Lock J, Quickel RR, Colton CK, Bonner-Weir S, Weir GC: Reversal of hyperglycemia in mice after subcutaneous transplantation of macroencapsulated islets. *Transplantation* 67:665-671, 1999

[45] Siebers U, Zekorn T, Bretzel RG, Planck H, Renardy M, Zschocke P, Federlin K: Histocompatibility of semipermeable membranes for implantable diffusion devices (bioartificial pancreas). *Transplant.Proc.* 22:834-835, 1990

[46] Scharp DW, Mason NS, Sparks RE: Islet immuno-isolation: the use of hybrid artificial organs to prevent islet tissue rejection. *World J.Surg.* 8:221-229, 1984

[47] Woodward SC: How fibroblasts and giant cells encapsulate implants: considerations in design of glucose sensors. *Diabetes Care* 5:278-281, 1982

[48] Colton CK, Avgoustiniatos ES: Bioengineering in development of the hybrid artificial pancreas. *J.Biomech.Eng.* 113:152-170, 1991

[49] Lanza RP, Borland KM, Lodge P, Carretta M, Sullivan SJ, Muller TE, Solomon BA, Maki T, Monaco AP, Chick WL: Pancreatic islet transplantation using membrane diffusion chambers. *Transplant.Proc.* 24:2935-2936, 1992

[50] Shoichet MS, Winn SR, Athavale S, Harris JM, Gentile FT: Poly(ethylene oxide)-grafted thermoplastic membranes for use as cellular hybrid bio-artificial organs in the central nervous system. *Biotech.Bioeng.* 43:563-572, 1994

[51] De Vos P, Van Schilfgaarde R. Biocompatibility Issues. In Kühtreiber WM, Lanza RP, Chick WL., eds. Cell encapsulation technology and therapeutics. Boston: Birkhäuser, 1999; 63-79.

[52] De Vos P, Tatarkiewicz K: Considerations for successful transplantation of encapsulated pancreatic islets. *Diabetologia* 45:159-173, 2002

[53] Lanza RP, Chick WL: Encapsulated Cell Therapy. *Scientific American Science and Medicine* 4:16-25, 1995

[54] Lanza RP, Hayes JL, Chick WL: Encapsulated cell technology. *BioTechnology* 14:1107-1111, 1996

[55] Lanza RP, Kuhtreiber WM, Ecker DM, Marsh JP, Staruk JE, Chick WL: A simple method for xenotransplanting cells and tissues into rats using uncoated alginate microreactors. *Transplant.Proc.* 28:8351996

[56] Iwata H, Takagi T, Amemiya H: Agarose microcapsule applied in islet xenografts (hamster to mouse). *Transplant.Proc.* 24:9521992

[57] Klomp GF, Ronel SH, Hashiguchi H, D'Andrea M, Dobelle WH: Hydrogels for encapsulation of pancreatic islet cells. *Trans.Am.Soc.Artif.Intern.Organs* 25:74-76, 1979

[58] Sefton MV: The good, the bd and the obvious: 1993 Clemson Award for Basic Research-Keynote Lecture. *Biomaterials* 14 (15):1127-1134, 1993

[59] Kessler L, Pinget M, Aprahamian M, Dejardin P, Damge C: In vitro and in vivo studies of the properties of an artificial membrane for pancreatic islet encapsulation. *Horm.metab.Res.* 23:312-317, 1991

[60] Kessler L, Legeay G, Jesser C, Damgé C, Pinget M: Influence of corona surface treatment on the properties of an artificial membrane used for Langerhans islets encapsulation: Permeability and biocompatibility studies. *Biomaterials* 16:185-191, 1995

[61] Kessler L, Legeay G, West R, Belcourt A, Pinget M: Physicochemical and biological studies of corona-treated artificial membranes used for pancreatic islets encapsulation: Mechanism of diffusion and interface modification. *J.Biomed.Mater.Res.* 34:235-245, 1997

[62] Knazek RA, Gullino PM, Kohler PO, Dedrick RL: Cell culture on artificial capillaries: an approach to tissue growth in vitro. *Science* 178:65-66, 1972

[63] Chick WL, Like AA, Lauris V: Beta cell culture on synthetic capillaries: an artificial endocrine pancreas. *Science* 187:847-849, 1975

[64] Chick WL, Like AA, Lauris V, Galletti PM, Richardson PD, Panol G, Mix TW, Colton CK: A hybird artifical pancreas. *Trans.Am.Soc.Artif.Intern.Organs* 21:8-15, 1975

[65] Sun AM, Parisius W, Healy GM, Vacek I, Macmorine HG: The use, in diabetic rats and monkeys, of artificial capillary units containing cultured islets of Langerhans (artificial endocrine pancreas). *Diabetes* 26:1136-1139, 1977

[66] Maki T, Lodge JP, Carretta M, Ohzato H, Borland KM, Sullivan SJ, Staruk J, Muller TE, Solomon BA, Chick WL, et al: Treatment of severe diabetes mellitus for more than one year using a vascularized hybrid artificial pancreas. *Transplantation* 55:713-717, 1993

[67] Galletti PM, Trudell LA, Panol G, Richardson PD, Whittemore A: Feasibility of small bore AV shunts for hybrid artificial organs in nonheparinized beagle dogs. *Trans.Am.Soc.Artif.Intern.Organs* 27:185-187, 1981

[68] Maki T, Mullon CJ, Solomon BA, Monaco AP: Novel delivery of pancreatic islet cells to treat insulin- dependent diabetes mellitus. *Clin.Pharmacokinet.* 28:471-482, 1995

[69] Maki T, O'Neil JJ, Porter J, Mullon CJP, Solomon BA, Monaco AP: Long-term function of porcine islets in xenogeneic hosts. *Transplant.Proc.* 28:8071996

[70] Maki T, Otsu I, O'Neil JJ, Dunleavy K, Mullon CJP, Solomon BA, Monaco AP: Treatment of diabetes by xenogeneic islets without immunosuppression - Use of a vascularized bioartificial pancreas. *Diabetes* 45:342-347, 1996

[71] Lanza RP, Chick WL: Transplantation of encapsulated cells and tissues. *Surgery* 121:1-9, 1997

[72] Lanza RP, Chick WL: Immunoisolation: At a turning point. *Immunology Today* 18:135-139, 1997

[73] Lanza RP, Lodge P, Borland KM, Carretta M, Sullivan SJ, Beyer AM, Muller TE, Solomon BA, Maki T, Monaco AP, et al: Transplantation of islet allografts using a diffusion-based biohybrid artificial pancreas: long-term studies in diabetic, pancreatectomized dogs. *Transplant.Proc.* 25:978-980, 1993

[74] Lanza RP, Sullivan SJ, Chick WL: Perspectives in diabetes. Islet transplantation with immunoisolation. *Diabetes* 41:1503-1510, 1992

[75] Krause TJ, Robertson FM, Liesch JB, Wasserman AJ, Grecos RS: Differential production of IL-1 on the surface of biomaterials. *Arch.Surg.* 125:1158-1160, 1990

[76] Sandler S, Eizirik DL, Sternesjo J, Welsh N: Role of cytokines in regulation of pancreatic B-cell function. *Biochem.Soc.Trans.* 22:26-30, 1994

[77] Cetkovic Cvrlje M, Eizirik DL: TNF-alpha and IFN-gamma potentiate the deleterious effects of IL- 1 beta on mouse pancreatic islets mainly via generation of nitric oxide. *Cytokine.* 6:399-406, 1994

[78] Remes A, Williams DF: Immune response in biocompatibility. *Biomaterials* 13:731-743, 1992

[79] Hunt JA, Flanagan BF, McLaughlin PJ, Strickland I, Williams DF: Effect of biomaterial surface charge on the inflammatory response: evaluation of cellular infiltration and TNF alpha production. *J.Biomed.Mater.Res.* 31:139-144, 1996

[80] Anderson JM, Langone JJ: Issues and perspectives on the biocompatibility and immunotoxicity evaluation of implanted controlled release systems. *J.Controlled Release.* 57:107-113, 1999

[81] Soon Shiong P, Heintz RE, Merideth N, Yao QX, Yao Z, Zheng T, Murphy M, Moloney MK, Schmehl M, Harris M, et al: Insulin independence in a type 1 diabetic patient after encapsulated islet transplantation. *Lancet* 343:950-951, 1994

[82] Calafiore R, Basta G, Luca G, Boselli C, Bufalari A, Cassarani MP, Giustozzi GM, Brunetti P: Transplantation of pancreatic islets contained in minimal volume microcapsules in diabetic high mammalians. *Ann.N.Y.Acad.Sci.* 875:vol1999

[83] Weber CJ, Safley S, Hagler M, Kapp J: Evaluation of graft-host response for various tissue sources and animal models. *Ann.N.Y.Acad.Sci.* 875:vol1999

[84] Cruise GM, Hegre OD, Lamberti FV, Hager SR, Hill R, Scharp DS, Hubbell JA: In vitro and in vivo performance of porcine islets encapsulated in interfacially photopolymerized poly(ethylene glycol) diacrylate membranes. *Cell Transplant.* 8:293-306, 1999

[85] Kulseng B, Skjak-Braek G, Ryan L, Andersson A, King A, Faxvaag A, Espevik T: Transplantation of alginate microcapsules: generation of antibodies against alginates and encapsulated porcine islet-like cell clusters. *Transplantation* 67:978-984, 1999

[86] Calafiore R, Basta G, Osticioli L, Luca G, Tortoioli C, Brunetti P: Coherent microcapsules for pancreatic islet transplantation: A new approach for bioartificial pancreas. *Transplant.Proc.* 28:812-813, 1996

[87] Grohn P, Klock G, Schmitt J, Zimmermann U, Horcher A, Bretzel RG, Hering BJ, Brandhorst D, Brandhorst H, Zekorn T, et al: Large-scale production of Ba(2+)-alginate-coated islets of Langerhans for immunoisolation. *Exp.Clin.Endocrinol.* 102:380-387, 1994

[88] Siebers U, Zekorn T, Horcher A, KlÖck G, Houben R, Frank H, Bretzel RG, Zimmermann U, Federlin K: Microencapsulated transplantation of allogeneic islets into specifically presensitized recipients. *Transplant.Proc.* 26:787-788, 1994

[89] Zimmermann U, KlÖck G, Federlin K, Hannig K, Kowalski M, Bretzel RG, Horcher A, Entenmann H, Sieber U, Zekorn T: Production of mitogen-contamination free alginates with variable ratios of mannuronic acid to guluronic acid by free flow electrophoresis. *Electrophoresis* 13:269-274, 1992

[90] Ar'Rajab A, Bengmark S, Ahren B: Insulin secretion in streptozotocin-diabetic rats transplanted with immunoisolated islets. *Transplantation* 51:570-574, 1991

[91] Basic D, Vacek I, Sun AM: Microencapsulation and transplantation of genetically engineered cells: A new approach to somatic gene therapy. *Artif.Cells Blood Substitutes Immobilization Biotechnol.* 24:219-255, 1996

[92] Chicheportiche D, Reach G: In vitro kinetics of insulin release by microencapsulated rat islets: effect of the size of the microcapsules. *Diabetologia* 31:54-57, 1988

[93] Crooks CA, Douglas JA, Broughton RL, Sefton MV: Microencapsulation of mammalian cells in a HEMA-MMA copolymer: effects on capsule morphology and permeability. *J.Biomed.Mater.Res.* 24:1241-1262, 1990

[94] De Vos P, De Haan BJ, Wolters GHJ, Van Schilfgaarde R: Factors influencing the adequacy of microencapsulation of rat pancreatic islets. *Transplantation* 62:888-893, 1996

[95] De Vos P, De Haan BJ, Wolters GHJ, Strubbe JH, Van Schilfgaarde R: Improved biocompatibility but limited graft survival after purification of alginate for microencapsulation of pancreatic islets. *Diabetologia* 40:262-270, 1997

[96] Iwata H, Amemiya H, Matsuda T, Takano H, Hayashi R, Akutsu T: Evaluation of microencapsulated islets in agarose gel as bioartificial pancreas by studies of hormone secretion in culture and by xenotransplantation. *Diabetes* 38 Suppl 1:224-225, 1989

[97] Korbutt GS, Elliott JF, Ao Z, Flashner M, Warnock GL, Rajotte RV: Microencapsulation of neonatal porcine islets: Long-term reversal of diabetes in nude mice and in vitro protection from human complement mediated cytolysis. *Transplant.Proc.* 29:21281997

[98] Sandler S, Andersson A, Eizirik DL, Hellerstrom C, Espevik T, Kulseng B, Thu B, Pipeleers DG, Skjak Braek G: Assessment of insulin secretion in vitro from microencapsulated fetal porcine islet-like cell clusters and rat, mouse, and human pancreatic islets. .*Transplantation* 63:1712-1718, 1997

[99] Stevenson WT, Sefton MV: Graft copolymer emulsions of sodium alginate with hydroxyalkyl methacrylates for microencapsulation. *Biomaterials* 8:449-457, 1987

[100] Sun AM: Advantages of microencapsulation as an immunoprotection method in the transplantation of pancreatic islets. *Ann.Transplant.* 2:55-62, 1997

[101] Yderstroede KB: Pancreatic islet transplantation. Experimental and clinical aspects. *Dan.Med.Bull.* 34:323-329, 1987

[102] Zhou M, Chen D, Yao Q, Xia Z, Wang C, Zhu H: Microencapsulation of rat islets prolongs xenograft survival in diabetic mice. *Chin.Med.J.Engl.* 111:394-397, 1998

[103] Halle JP, Leblond FA, Pariseau JF, Jutras P, Brabant MJ, Lepage Y: Studies on small (<300 microns) microcapsules: II--Parameters governing the production of alginate beads by high voltage electrostatic pulses. *Cell Transplant* 3:365-372, 1994

[104] Duvivier-Kali VF, Omer A, Parent RJ, O'Neil JJ, Weir GC: Complete protection of islets against allorejection and autoimmunity by a simple barium-alginate membrane. *Diabetes* 50:1698-1705, 2001

[105] De Vos P, Vegter D, Strubbe JH, De Haan BJ, Van Schilfgaarde R: Impaired glucose tolerance in recipients of an intraperitoneally implanted microencapsulated islet allograft is caused by the slow diffusion of insulin through the peritoneal membrane. *Transplant.Proc.* 29:756-757, 1997

[106] De Vos P, Vegter D, De Haan BJ, Strubbe JH, Bruggink JE, Van Schilfgaarde R: Kinetics of intraperitoneally infused insulin in rats: functional implications for the bioartificial pancreas. *Diabetes* 45:1102-1107, 1996

[107] Tatarkiewicz K, Garcia M, Omer A, Van Schilfgaarde R, Weir GC, De Vos P: C-peptide responses after meal challenge in mice transplanted with microencapsulated rat islets. *Diabetologia* 44:646-653, 2001

[108] Wells GD, Fisher MM, Sefton MV: Microencapsulation of viable hepatocytes in HEMA-MMA microcapsules: a preliminary study. *Biomaterials* 14:615-620, 1993

[109] Bartkowiak A, Canaple L, Ceausoglu I, Nurdin N, Renken A, Rindisbacher L, Wandrey C, Desvergne B, Hunkeler D: New multicomponent capsules for immunoisolation. *Ann.N.Y.Acad.Sci.* 875:vol1999

[110] Rihova B: Immunocompatibility and biocompatibility of cell delivery systems. *Adv.Drug Deliv.Rev.* 42:65-80, 2000

[111] Fritschy WM, Wolters GH, Van Schilfgaarde R: Effect of alginate-polylysine-alginate microencapsulation on in vitro insulin release from rat pancreatic islets. *Diabetes* 40:37-43, 1991

[112] Klock G, Frank H, Houben R, Zekorn T, Horcher A, Siebers U, Wohrle M, Federlin K, Zimmermann U: Production of purified alginates suitable for use in immunoisolated transplantation. *Appl.Microbiol.Biotechnol.* 40:638-643, 1994

[113] Kulseng B, Thu T, Espevik T, Skjåk-Bræk G: Alginate polylysine microcapsules as immune barrier: permeability of cytokines and immunoglobulins over the capsule membrane. *Cell Transplantation* 6:387-394, 1997

[114] Sawhney AS, Hubbell JA: Poly(ethylene oxide)-graft-poly(L-lysine)copolymers to enhance the biocompatibility of poly(L-lysine)-alginate micocapsules membranes. *Biomaterials* 13 (12):863-870, 1992

[115] De Vos P, Van Hoogmoed CG, van Zanten J, Netter S, Strubbe JH, Busscher HJ: Long-term biocompatibility, chemistry, and function of microencapsulated pancreatic islets. *Biomaterials* 24:305-312, 2003

[116] De Vos P, De Haan BJ, Van Schilfgaarde R: Upscaling the production of encapsulated islets. *Biomaterials* 18:1085-1090, 1997

[117] Serp D, Cantana E, Heinzen C, von Stockar U, Marison IW: Characterization of an encapsulation device for the production of monodisperse alginate beads for cell immobilization. *Biotechnol.Bioeng.* 70:41-53, 2000

[118] De Haan BJ, Faas MM, De Vos P: Factors influencing insulin secretion from encapsulated islets. *Cell Transplant.* 12:617-625, 2003

[119] Bystricky S, Malovikova A, Sticzay T: Interaction of acid polysaccharides with polylysine enantiomers, conformation probe in solution. *Carbohydrate Polymers* 15:299-308, 1991

[120] Bystricky S, Malovikova A, Sticzay T: Interaction of alginate and pectins with cationic polypeptides. *Carbohydr.Res.* 13:283-294, 1990

[121] King GA, Daugulis AJ, Faulkner P, Goosen MFA: Alginate-Polylysine Microcapsules of Controlled Membrane Molecular Weight Cutoff for Mammalian Cell Culture Engineering. *Biotechnol.Prog.* 3:231-240, 1987

[122] Vandenbossche GM, Van Oostveldt P, Remon JP: A fluorescence method for the determination of the molecular weight cut-off of alginate-polylysine microcapsules. *J.Pharm.Pharmacol.* 43:275-277, 1991

[123] Vandenbossche GM, Bracke ME, Cuvelier CA, Bortier HE, Mareel MM, Remon JP: Host reaction against alginate-polylysine microcapsules containing living cells. *J.Pharm.Pharmacol.* 45:121-125, 1993

[124] Vandenbossche GM, Bracke ME, Cuvelier CA, Bortier HE, Mareel MM, Remon JP: Host reaction against empty alginate-polylysine microcapsules. Influence of preparation procedure. *J.Pharm.Pharmacol.* 45:115-120, 1993

[125] De Vos P, Wolters GH, Fritschy WM, Van Schilfgaarde R: Obstacles in the application of microencapsulation in islet transplantation. *Int.J.Artif.Organs* 16:205-212, 1993

[126] Van Schilfgaarde R, De Vos P: Factors influencing the properties and performance of microcapsules for immunoprotection of pancreatic islets. *.J.Mol.Med.* 77:199-205, 1999

[127] Uludag H, de-Vos P, Tresco PA: Technology of mammalian cell encapsulation. *Adv.Drug Deliv.Rev.* 42:29-64, 2000

[128] Colton CK: Engineering challenges in cell-encapsulation technology. *Trends Biotechnol.* 14:158-162, 1996

[129] De Vos P, Van Hoogmoed CG, Busscher HJ: Chemistry and biocompatibility of alginate-PLL capsules for immunoprotection of mammalian cells. *J Biomed Mater Res.* 60:252-259, 2002

[130] Van Hoogmoed CG, Busscher HJ, De Vos P: Fourier transform infrared spectroscopy studies of alginate-PLL capsules with varying compositions. *J.Biomed.Mater.Res.* 67A:172-178, 2003

[131] De Vos P, De Haan B, Van Schilfgaarde R: Effect of the alginate composition on the biocompatibility of alginate-polylysine microcapsules. *Biomaterials* 18:273-278, 1997

[132] Strand BK, Ryan L, In 't Veld P, Kulseng B, Rokstad AM, Skjåk-Braek G, Espevik T: Poly-L-lysine induces fibrosis on alginate microcapsules via the induction of cytokines. *Cell Transplant* 10:263-277, 2001

[133] King A, Lau J, Nordin A, Sandler S, Andersson A: The effect of capsule composition in the reversal of hyperglycemia in diabetic mice transplanted with microencapsulated allogeneic islets. *Diabetes Technol.Ther.* 5:653-663, 2003

[134] Koch S, Schwinger C, Kressler J, Heinzen C, Rainov NG: Alginate encapsulation of genetically engineered mammalian cells: comparison of production devices, methods and microcapsule characteristics. *J.Microencapsul.* 20:303-316, 2003

[135] De Vos P, Van Hoogmoed CG, De Haan BJ, Busscher HJ: Tissue responses against immunoisolating alginate-PLL capsules in the immediate posttransplant period. *J.Biomed.Mater.Res.* 62:430-437, 2002

[136] Thu B, Bruheim P, Espevik T, Smidrod O, Soon-Shiong P, Skjak-Braek G: Alginate polycation microcapsules. I. Interaction between alginate and polycation. *Biomaterials* 17:1031-1040, 1996

[137] Dupuy B, Arien A, Perrot Minnot A.: FI-IR of membranes made with alginate-polylysine complexes. Variations with mannuronic or guluronic content of the polysaccharides. *Art.Cells., Blood subs., and Immob.Biotech.* 22:71-82, 1994

[138] De Vos P, van Straaten JF, Nieuwenhuizen AG, de Groot M, Ploeg RJ, De Haan BJ, Van Schilfgaarde R: Why do microencapsulated islet grafts fail in the absence of fibrotic overgrowth? *.Diabetes* 48:1381-1388, 1999

[139] Zhou D, Kintsourashvili E, Mamujee S, Vacek I, Sun AM: Bioartificial pancreas: alternative supply of insulin-secreting cells. *Ann.N.Y.Acad.Sci.* 875:208-218, 1999

[140] King A, Sandler S, Andersson A: The effect of host factors and capsule composition on the cellular overgrowth on implanted alginate capsules. *J. Biomed. Mater. Re.* 57:374-383, 2001

[141] Horcher A, Zekorn T, Siebers U, KlÖck G, Frank H, Houben R, Bretzel RG, Zimmermann U, Federlin K: Transplantation of microencapsulated islets in rats:

Evidence for induction of fibrotic overgrowth by islet alloantigens released from microcapsules. *Transplant.Proc.* 26:784-786, 1994

[142] Rafael E, Wu GS, Hultenby K, Tibell A, Wernerson A: Improved survival of macroencapsulated islets of Langerhans by preimplantation of the immunoisolating device: a morphometric study. *Cell Transplant.* 12:407-412, 2003

[143] Tang L, Eaton JW: Natural responses to unnatural materials: A molecular mechanism for foreign body reactions. *Mol.Med.* 5:351-358, 1999

[144] Tang L, Jennings TA, Eaton JW: Mast cells mediate acute inflammatory responses to implanted biomaterials. *Proc.Natl.Acad.Sci.U.S.A.* 95:8841-8846, 1998

[145] Hu WJ, Eaton JW, Tang L: Molecular basis of biomaterial-mediated foreign body reactions. *Blood* 98:1231-1238, 2001

[146] Tang L, Ugarova TP, Plow EF, Eaton JW: Molecular determinants of acute inflammatory responses to biomaterials. *J Clin.Invest.* 97:1329-1334, 1996

[147] Rihova B: Immunocompatibility and biocompatibility of cell delivery systems. *Adv.Drug Deliv.Rev.* 42:65-80, 2000

[148] Babensee JE, Anderson JM, McIntire LV, Mikos AG: Host response to tissue engineered devices. *Adv.Drug Deliv.Rev.* 33:111-139, 1998

[149] Hunt JA, McLaughlin PJ, Flanagan BF: Techniques to investigate cellular and molecular interactions in the host response to implanted biomaterials. *Biomaterials* 18:1449-1459, 1997

[150] Falcone FH, Haas H, Gibbs BF: The human basophil: a new appreciation of its role in immune responses. *Blood* 96:4028-4038, 2000

[151] Kobayashi H, Ishizuka T, Okayama Y: Human mast cells and basophils as sources of cytokines. *Clin.Exp.Allergy* 30:1205-1212, 2000

[152] Huntley JF: Mast cells and basophils: a review of their heterogeneity and function. *J.Comp.Pathol.* 107:349-372, 1992

[153] Schedle A, Samorapoompichit P, Fureder W, Rausch-Fan XH, Franz A, Sperr WR, Sperr W, Slavicek R, Simak S, Klepetko W, Ellinger A, Ghannadan M, Baghestanian M, Valent P: Metal ion-induced toxic histamine release from human basophils and mast cells. *J.Biomed.Mater.Res.* 39:560-567, 1998

[154] Schroeder JT, MacGlashan D-WJ, Lichtenstein LM: Human basophils: mediator release and cytokine production. *Adv.Immunol.* 77:vol 2001

[155] Tang L, Jennings TA, Eaton JW: Mast cells mediate acute inflammatory responses to implanted biomaterials. *Proc.Natl.Acad.Sci.U.S.A.* 95:8841-8846, 1998

[156] Brunner T, Heusser CH, Dahinden CA: Human peripheral blood basophils primed by interleukin 3 (IL-3) produce IL-4 in response to immunoglobulin E receptor stimulation. *J. Exp.Med.* 177:605-611, 1993

[157] Arock M, Merle-Beral H, Dugas B, Ouaaz F, Le-Goff L, Vouldoukis I, Mencia-Huerta JM, Schmitt C, Leblond-Missenard V, Debre P: IL-4 release by human leukemic and activated normal basophils. *J. Immunol.* 151:1441-1447, 1993

[158] Wedemeyer J, Galli SJ: Mast cells and basophils in acquired immunity. *Br.Med.Bull.* 56:936-955, 2000

[159] Li H, Sim TC, Alam R: IL-13 released by and localized in human basophils. *J Immunol.* 156:4833-4838, 1996

[160] Falcone FH, Haas H, Gibbs BF: The human basophil: a new appreciation of its role in immune responses. *Blood* 96:4028-4038, 2000

[161] De Vos P, Smedema I, van Goor H, Moes H, van Zanten J, Netters S, de Leij LF, de Haan A, De Haan BJ: Association between macrophage activation and function of micro-encapsulated rat islets. *Diabetologia* 46:666-673, 2003

[162] De Vos P, Marchetti P: Encapsulation of pancreatic islets for transplantation in diabetes: the untouchable islets. *Trends Mol.Med.* 8:363-366, 2002

[163] De Vos P, Smedema I, van Goor H, Moes H, van Zanten J, de Leij LFM, De Haan BJ: Association between macrophages activation and function of microencapsulated islets. *Diabetologia* 2003

[164] Piro S, Lupi R, Dotta F, Patane G, Rabuazzo MA, Marselli L, Santangelo C, Realacci M, Del-Guerra S, Purrello F, Marchetti P: Bovine islets are less susceptible than human islets to damage by human cytokines. *Transplantation* 71:21-26, 2001

[165] Monta~na E, Bonner-Weir S, Weir GC: Transplanted beta cell response to increased metabolic demand. Changes in beta cell replication and mass. *J.Clin.Invest.* 93:1577-1582, 1994

[166] Bonner Weir S: Regulation of pancreatic Beta-cell mass in vivo. *Recent Prog. Horm. Res.* 49:91-104, 1994

[167] De Vos P, De Haan BJ, Pater J, Van Schilfgaarde R: Association between capsule diameter, adequacy of encapsulation, and survival of microencapsulated rat islet allografts. *Transplantation* 62:893-899, 1996

[168] van Suylichem PT, Strubbe JH, Houwing H, Wolters GH, Van Schilfgaarde R: Rat islet isograft function. Effect of graft volume and transplantation site. *Transplantation* 57:1010-1017, 1994

[169] van Suylichem PT, Strubbe JH, Houwing H, Wolters GH, Van Schilfgaarde R: Insulin secretion by rat islet isografts of a defined endocrine volume after transplantation to three different sites. *Diabetologia* 35:917-923, 1992

[170] Wolters GH, van Suylichem PT, Van Deijnen JH, Van Schilfgaarde R: Factors influencing the isolation process of islets of Langerhans. *Horm.Metab.Res.Suppl.* 25:20-26, 1990

[171] Wolters GH, van Suylichem PT, Van Deijnen JH, Van Schilfgaarde R: Increased islet yield by improved pancreatic tissue dissociation: the effects of bovine serum albumin and calcium. *Transplant.Proc.* 21:2626-2627, 1989

[172] De Vos P, De Haan BJ, Vegter D, Hillebrands JL, Strubbe JH, Bruggink JE, Van Schilfgaarde R: Insulin levels after portal and systemic insulin infusion differ in a dose-dependent fashion. *.Horm.Metab.Res.* 30:721-725, 1998

[173] Avgoustiniatos ES, Colton CK: Effect of external oxygen mass transfer resistances on viability of immunoisolated tissue. *Ann NY Acad.Sci.* 31:145-167, 1997

[174] De Vos P, Hillebrands JL, De Haan BJ, Strubbe JH, Van Schilfgaarde R: Efficacy of a prevascularized expanded polytetrafluoroethylene solid support system as a transplantation site for pancreatic islets. *Transplantation* 63:824-830, 1997

[175] Gardemann A, Jungermann K, Grosse V, Cossel L, Wohlrab F, Hahn HJ, Blech W, Hildebrandt W: Reinnervation of pancreatic islets and regulation of insulin secretion by

hepatic sympathetic nerves after intraportal transplantation of islets into livers of diabetic rats. *Exp.Clin.Endocrinol.Diabetes* 103 Suppl. 2:107-111, 1995

[176] Andersson A, Korsgren O, Jansson L: Intraportally transplanted pancreatic islets revascularized from hepatic arterial system. *Diabetes* 38 Suppl 1:192-195, 1989

[177] Dunger A, Korsgren O, Andersson A: DNA replication in mouse pancreatic islets transplanted subcapsularly into the kidney or intraportally into the liver. Influence of unilateral nephrectomy or partial hepatectomy. *Transplantation* 49:686-689, 1990

[178] Kneteman NM, Warnock GL, Evans MG, Nason RW, Rajotte RV: Prolonged function of canine pancreatic fragments autotransplanted to the spleen by venous reflux. *Transplantation* 49:679-681, 1990

[179] Feldman SD, Hirshberg GE, Dodi G, Raizman ME, Scharp DW, Ballinger WF, Lacy PE: Intrasplenic islet isografts. *Surgery* 82:386-394, 1977

[180] Beattie GM, Hayek A: Islet cell mass and the longevity of islet grafts in diabetic rats. *Cell Transplant.* 2:119-122, 1993

[181] Ar'Rajab A, Ahren B, Alumets J, Logdberg L, Bengmark S: Islet transplantation to the renal subcapsular space improves late complications in streptozotocin-diabetic rats. *Eur.Surg.Res.* 22:270-278, 1990

[182] Thompson JA, Haudenschild CC, Anderson KD, DiPietro JM, Anderson WF, Maciag T: Heparin-binding growth factor 1 induces the formation of organoid neovascular structures in vivo. *Proc.Natl.Acad.Sci.U.S.A.* 86:7928-7932, 1989

[183] Thompson JA, Anderson KD, DiPietro JM, Zwiebel JA, Zametta M, Anderson WF, Maciag T: Site-directed neovessel formation in vivo. *Science* 241:1349-1352, 1988

[184] Trivedi N, Steil GM, Colton CK, Bonner-Weir S, Weir GC: Improved vascularization of planar membrane diffusion devices following continuous infusion of vascular endothelial growth factor. *Cell Transplant.* 9:115-124, 2000

[185] Neufeld G, Cohen T, Gengrinovitch S, Poltorak Z: Vascular endothelial growth factor (VEGF) and its receptors. *FASEB J.* 13:9-22, 1999

[186] Frelin C, Ladoux A, D'angelo G: Vascular endothelial growth factors and angiogenesis. *Ann.Endocrinol.Paris.* 61:70-74, 2000

[187] Strautz RL: Studies of hereditary-obese mice (obob) after implantation of pancreatic islets in Millipore filter capsules. *Diabetologia* 6:306-312, 1970

[188] Zekorn T, Siebers U, Filip L, Mauer K, Schmitt U, Bretzel RG, Federlin K: Bioartificial pancreas: the use of different hollow fibers as a diffusion chamber. *Transplant.Proc.* 21:2748-2750, 1989

[189] Lanza RP, Ecker D, Kühtreiber WM, Staruk JE, Marsh J, Chick WL: A simple method for transplanting discordant islets into rats using alginate gel spheres. *Transplantation* 59:1485-1487, 1995

[190] Gamian E, Kochman A, Rabczynski J, Burczak K: Badanie biokompatybilnosci i funkcjonowania protezy wewnatrzwydzielniczej czesci trzustki, wykonanej z zasiedlonych zywymi wyspami trzustki makrokapsulek PVA. [Biocompatibility testing and function of a pancreatic prosthesis consisting of viable pancreatic islets encapsulated in PVA macrocapsules]. *Polim.Med.* 29:3-20, 1999

[191] Isayeva IS, Kasibhatla BT, Rosenthal KS, Kennedy JP: Characterization and performance of membranes designed for macroencapsulation/implantation of pancreatic islet cells. *Biomaterials* 24:3483-3491, 2003
[192] Zielinski BA, Aebischer P: Chitosan as a matrix for mammalian cell encapsulation. *Biomaterials* 15:1049-1056, 1994
[193] Dawson RM, Broughton RL, Stevenson WT, Sefton MV: Microencapsulation of CHO cells in a hydroxyethyl methacrylate- methyl methacrylate copolymer. *Biomaterials* 8:360-366, 1987
[194] Shimizu S, Yamazaki M, Kubota S, Ozasa T, Moriya H, Kobayashi K, Mikami M, Mori Y, Yamaguchi S: In vitro studies on a new method for islet microencapsulation using a thermoreversible gelation polymer, N-isopropylacrylamide-based copolymer. *Artif.Organs* 20:1232-1237, 1996
[195] Tatarkiewicz K, Sitarek E, Fiedor P, Sabat M, Orlowski T: Protamine-heparin membrane for cell microencapsulation. *Transplant.Proc.* 26:35091994
[196] Sefton MV, Hwang JR, Babensee JE: Selected aspects of the microencapsulation of mammalian cells in HEMA-MMA. *Ann.N.Y.Acad.Sci.* 831260-70 *LHM:vol1997
[197] Boninsegna S, Bosetti P, Carturan G, Dellagiacoma G, Dal Monte R, Rossi M: Encapsulation of individual pancreatic islets by sol-gel SiO2: a novel procedure for perspective cellular grafts. *J.Biotechnol.* 100:277-286, 2003

In: Trends in Diabetes Research
Editor: Ashley M. Ford, pp. 163-190
ISBN: 1-59454-796-3

Chapter VII

Beneficial Effects of Eicosapentaenoic Acid Ethyl Ester (EPA-E) on Experimental Diabetic Rats

Lawrance Christopher, **L.N. Mathuram**, **G. Genitta*** **and S. Jayasundar***
Department of Pharmacology and Toxicology
Madras Veterinary College, Chennai-7
Lucknow, U.P., India

Abstract

We investigated the effect of chronic administration of highly purified eicosapentaenoic acid ethyl ester (EPA-E), an n-3 polyunsaturated fatty acid, on alloxan (ALL) induced diabetic Wistar rats. After four weeks of ALL (55 mg/kg, I.V.) administration, the diabetic animals were randomly divided into three groups. 1. Diabetic control, 2. EPA-E treated diabetic rats and 3. Verapamil treated diabetic rats. EPA-E and Verapamil were administered to the diabetic rats daily for three months. Age matched normal rats served as normal controls. During this study, plasma glucose, glycosylated hemoglobin, plasma triglycerides, cholesterol, LDL and HDL cholesterol. A significant increase in the plasma glucose, glycosylated hemoglobin, plasma triglycerides, cholesterol, and LDL and HDL ratio in diabetic control over normal control were noticed. EPA-E treatment significantly prevented the above parameters better than Verapamil. At the end of experiment, ECG, gravimetric ratio and myocardial enzyme markers were studied. In diabetic control group, diabetic cardiomyopathy was characterized by elevated CPK, gravimetric ratio, ST/R ratio in the ECG and bradycardia. EPA-E treatment significantly prevented the above parameters better than Verapamil. EPA-E may be considered as one of the treatment modalities for diabetic cardiomyopathy.

* Author for correspondence: Dr. C. Lawrance Christopher; Veterinary Scientist In-charge Experimental Animal Facility, Sanjay Gandhi Post Graduate Institute of Medical Sciences (SGPGIMS), Lucknow, U.P., India-226014Tel: 0522-2668700 ext 2278, 2790 Fax: 0522-2668017, E-mail: indiachrist99@yahoo.com

* Senior Research Fellow (Medical), Endocrinology, SGPGIMS, Lucknow, U.P., India

Keywords: EPA-E, Alloxan diabetic cardiomyopathy

1. Introduction

Diabetes mellitus is a group of metabolic diseases characterized by hyperglycemia resulting from defects in insulin secretion, insulin action, or both. The chronic hyperglycemia of diabetes is associated with long-term damage, dysfunction, and failure of various organs, especially the eyes, kidneys, nerves, heart, and blood vessels. [1]. Worldwide, there are about 143 million patients with diabetes, almost 5 times more than estimates of 10 years ago [2,3]. In India, more than 30 million people know that they have diabetes and the number is climbing steeply. Further India has the dubious distinction of having largest number of people with diabetes. Diabetes in turn, is the largest co-morbidity of patients with heart failure and adversely affects outcomes of cardiovascular disease [4]. The trend is unmistakable; both insulin resistance and heart failure have emerged as a major worldwide epidemic. It is therefore timely to take a fresh look at the effect of diabetes on heart and the treatment modalities for the cardiovascular complications associated with diabetes [5].

Although insulin deficiency is the primary cause for diabetes induced cardiac changes, insulin treatment alone insufficient to reverse these changes fully due to the altered myocardial energy metabolism [6,7]. Alterations in myocardial metabolism are the early consequences of experimental diabetes and had already been recognized by Starling and Evans nearly a centaury ago [8]. The early investigators made two important observation glucose uptake and the respiratory quotient (RQ) both decreased in the heart of diabetic animal and the metabolic abnormalities persist when the heart from diabetic animal perfused ex vivo with blood from a non diabetic animal. Despite these early observations, it took many decades to recognize that diabetes is as much a disease of dysregulatory fatty acid metabolism as it is a disease of dysregulatory glucose metabolism [9]. The normal reliance of the heart on fatty acid metabolism for energy production is increased in diabetes [10].

Over the past 20 years many studies and clinical investigations have been carried out on the metabolism of polyunsaturated fatty acids (PUFAs) in general and on n-3 fatty acids in particular (Figure 1). Omega-3-PUFA such as eicosapentaenoic acid and docosahexaenoic acid, the major components among the fatty acids, contained in the fish oil, have attracted much attention due to their wide range of biological activities. Today we know that these n-3 fatty acids are essential for normal growth and development of human being and animals and may play an important role in the prevention and management of coronary heart disease [11,12], hypertension [13-15], type 2 diabetes [16-17], renal disease [18-19], rheumatoid arthritis [20], ulcerative colitis [21], Crohn's disease [22] and chronic obstructive pulmonary disease [23].

On the basis of estimates from studies in Paleolithic nutrition and modern-day hunter-gatherer populations, it appears that human beings evolved consuming a diet that was much lower in saturated fatty acids than is today's diet [24]. Furthermore, the diet contained small and roughly equal amounts of n-6 and n-3 PUFAs (ratio of 1–2:1) and much lower amounts of trans fatty acids than does today's diet [24,25] and thus essential fatty acids, both n-6 (LA) and n-3 (ALA), have been part of our diet since the beginning of human life. Before the agricultural revolution about 10000 years ago human beings consumed about equal amounts of both.

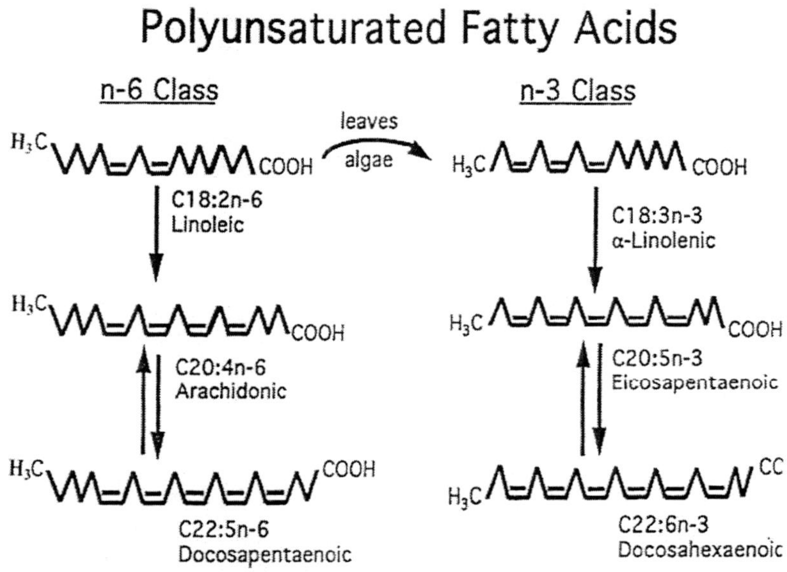

Figure 1.

However, over the past 100–150 y there has been an enormous increase in the consumption of n-6 fatty acids due to the increased intake of vegetable oils from corn, sunflower seeds, safflower seeds, cottonseed, and soybeans which in turn leads to the abnormal n-6 to n-3 ratio. n-6 and n-3 fatty acids are the parent moieties for the production of eicosanoids, e.g., prostaglandins, thromboxanes, and leukotrienes. Eicosanoids derived from n-6 fatty acids have opposing metabolic properties to those derived from n-3 fatty acids. A balanced intake of both n-6 and n-3 fatty acids is essential for health. There is competition among the enzymes involved in the elongation and desaturation of LA and ALA. A ratio of LA to ALA of 4:1 or less has been shown to be optimal for the elongation of 11 g of ALA to 1 g EPA. This is important for vegetarians because their diets are typically rich in LA and poor in ALA. Because EPA is biologically more active than ALA and high amounts of LA decrease the conversion of ALA to EPA, the optimal intake of LA relative to ALA is crucial for normal metabolism.

Further, recent studies delineate that a high intake of n-6 fatty acids shifts the physiologic state to one that is prothrombotic and proaggregatory, characterized by increased blood viscosity, vasospasm, and vasoconstriction and decreased bleeding time leads to a pathological state. n-3 Fatty acids, however, have antiinflammatory, antithrombotic, antiarrhythmic, hypolipidemic and vasodilatory properties which results in their beneficial effects on various pathological conditions.

It is interestingly observed and widely reported that a deficiency of essential fatty acid metabolism in both human and animal diabetes. Diabetes impairs essential fatty acid metabolism by decreasing activities of Δ 6 and Δ 5 desaturases, enzymes that convert dietary linoleic acid (LA) and α-linolenic acid to long-chain polyunsaturated fatty acids (PUFA), including γ-linolenic acid (GLA), arachidonic acid (AA), eicosapentaenoic acid (EPA), and docosahexaenoic acid (DHA) [26]. As a result, AA and DHA levels are reduced in membrane phospholipids of several tissues, including erythrocyte and sciatic nerve, in patients with type 1 diabetes and in diabetic animals [27-29].

By keeping all the above scientific facts in mind, this study is planned to investigate the effect of chronic administered EPA-ethyl ester on experimental diabetic rats in comparison with Verapamil a calcium channel blocker and known beneficial drug in cardiovascular complications associated with chronic diabetes.

2. Methodology

2.1. Experimental Animals and Diet

Age matched mature male Wistar rats weighing 180 ± 200 g were housed in a room illuminated daily from 0700 to 1900 hr (a 12:12-hr light: dark cycle) and maintained at 21° ± 1°C with a humidity of 55% ± 5%. The animals were allowed free access to standard solid rat chow (Lipton, Bangalore) and tap water, except where described otherwise. All studies were conducted in accordance with humane principles, which are based on the National Institutes of Health's Guide for the Care and Use of Laboratory Animals. All groups of animals were fed with the same commercial rat chow.

Table 1. Fatty acid composition of the rodent diet

Structure	Name	Quantity (g/kg)
Saturated fatty acid		
C12: 0	Lauric	0.26
C14: 0	Myristic	0.06
C16: 0	Palmitic	7.64
C18: 0	Stearic	1.50
C20: 0	Arachidic	0.10
C22: 0	Behenic	0.03
Mono-unsaturated		
C16: 1w7	Palmitoleic	0.07
C18: 1w9	Oleic	12.59
C20: 1w9	Gadoleic	0.17
C22: 1w9	Erucic	0.01
Poly-unsaturated		
C18: 2w6	Linoleic	31.35
C18: 3w3	Linolenic	2.76
C18: 4w3	Octadecatetraenoic	0.00
C20: 5w3	Eicosapentaenoic	0.00
C22: 6w3	Docosahexaenoic	0.00

Commercial rat chow composed of crude protein not less than 20.0%, crude fat not less than 4.5%, crude fiber not more than 5.5%, ash not more than 7.0%, added minerals not more than 2.5%. The details of fatty acid composition of these rodent diet are given in Table 1.

2.2. Experimental Design

2.2.1. Animal Selection

From all the experimental rats, under light ether anesthesia, 1–1.5 ml of blood was collected from the retro-orbital plexus of the eye as described in our previous studies [30,31] using heparinised capillary tube into heparinised eppendorf tubes. The blood glucose level was estimated to rule out spontaneous diabetes and animals having mean plasma sugar levels of about 50–70 mg/dl were selected for the present study.

2.2.2. Animal Model and Treatment Protocol

After a 24-h fasting period, three-quarters of the selected animals were injected with Alloxan (Sigma, USA. 55 mg/kg dissolved in normal saline PH 7) (0.5 ml) through tail vein, under light ether anesthesia, [32], whereas the rest, one-quarter of animals, labeled as Normal Control (NC), received the normal saline alone. After a gap of 4 weeks, only those alloxan-injected animals that showed fasting blood glucose above 200 mg/dl were selected for the study. Control and diabetic animal were randomly assigned to either untreated (or) treated groups four weeks after ALL (or) vehicle administration. This was taken as day 0 of the study.

EPA-E (90 mg/kg) [33] and Verapamil (25 mg/kg) [34] was administered to the rats via oral gavage with a 75 mm stainless tube. None of the animals treated by gavage demonstrated any apparent sign of discomfort/pain during the course of study. Both EPA-E and Verapamil treatment was initiated from four weeks after ALL (or) vehicle injection and was continued for a period of three months. Body weight, food and water consumption were recorded daily.

2.3. Plasma Analysis

The blood was collected from orbital plexus and rest of the sample was immediately centrifuged in micro centrifuge (Hetitech) at 3000 rpm, 15 minutes at 15°C. The clear supernatant plasma was retained; one aliquot was used for blood glucose estimation. Rest of the plasma was stored at -20°C for further analysis. All the samples were subjected to following estimations by using standard diagnostic kits (Reddy's Lab): plasma glucose by glucose oxidase method [35]; plasma cholesterol [36]; plasma triacylglycerol (triglycerides) [37]; LDL and HDL cholesterol [38].

2.4. Electro Cardio Graphy

ECG was recorded 4 weeks and 3 months after ALL (or) vehicle injection under light ether anesthesia in the same set of rats to avoid individual variation. The lead II ECG was recorded (by means of needle electrodes placed s.c. on the limbs ECG) in an ECG paper with a paper speed of 50 mm/second and sensitivity of 1 mV=10 mm in BPL -Cardiodart -ECG machine.

2.5. Serum Analysis

The blood was collected from heart. For each sample, an aliquot of whole blood was preserved for glycosylated hemoglobin estimation glycosylated hemoglobin by ion exchange resin method [39]. Serum creatinine phosphokinase levels were estimated colorimetrically by modified method of Hughes [40]. Serum LDH activity was estimated by UV kinetic method [41].

2.6. Morphometric Analysis

Animals were weighed before blood collection. They were then sacrificed by cervical dislocation and the heart was immediately removed. It was kept in normal saline then blotted on a filter paper to remove excess water before weighing. The heart weight (in milligrams) to body weight (in grams) ratio was calculated as described in the earlier reports [30,42].

2.7. Statistical Analysis

Data were expressed as means ± SE, as indicated in each Figure or Table. Statistical analyses were carried out using a computer program for randomized block design as well as complete randomized design and ANOVA has been performed to determine their significance between treatments [43].

3. Results

3.1. Effect of EPA-E and Verapamil on Body Weight, Feed and Water Intake

Table 2 describes the body weight, feed and water intake of normal, diabetic and diabetic treated animals. A statistical significant increase in feed and water intake and weight loss were noticed in the diabetic control group over normal control group ($p < 0.01$). Only EPA-E treated diabetic animal showed favorable effect on water intake and weight loss.

Table 2. Effect of EPA-E and Verapamil on feed intake, water intake and body weight

Variables	Normal Control	Diabetic Control	D+EPA-E	D+Verapamil
Feed intake (Grams/day)	32±3.5[a]	53±6.8[b]	45±3.8[b]	49±4.6[b]
Water intake (ml/day)	46±3.6[a]	110±7.5[c]	70±5.5[b]	100±6.5[c]
Body weight (in grams)	400±14.8[a]	258±8.8[c]	340±12.6[b]	275±9.2[c]

Data are mean ± SEM (n = 10). Values in the same row bearing different superscript differ significantly

3.2. Effect of EPA-E and Verapamil on Blood Glucose Level

A significant increase in blood glucose in the diabetic group over normal group was observed ($p < 0.01$). Among treatment group, only EPA-E treated group showed a favorable effect (Table 3).

Table 3. Effect of EPA-E and Verapamil on glycemic control

Variables	Normal Control	Diabetic Control	D+EPA-E	D+Verapamil
Glucose (mg/dl)	65±4.5[a]	330±10.2[c]	220±6.5[b]	310±8.8[c]
HbA1c (%)	4.5±0.3[a]	12±0.85[c]	6.9±0.45[b]	11±0.7[c]

Data are mean ± SEM (n = 10). Values in the same row bearing different superscript differ significantly

3.3. Effect of EPA-E and Verapamil on Glycosylated Hemoglobin

Table 3 describes the glycosylated hemoglobin level in various groups and the beneficial effect of EPA-E over Verapamil. A statistical significant increase in glycosylated haemoglobin level was noticed in the diabetic control group over normal control group ($p < 0.01$). How ever the EPA-E alone showed favorable effect.

3.4. Effect of EPA-E And Verapamil on Lipid Parameters

A significant increase in total cholesterol and triglycerides in the diabetic group over normal group was observed ($p < 0.01$). Among treatment group, both treated group showed a favorable effect. Between treatments, only EPA-E treated group showed a better effect than Verapamil treatment (Table 4).

Table 4. Effect of EPA-E and Verapamil on lipid parameters

Variables	Normal Control	Diabetic Control	D+EPA-E	D+Verapamil
Cholesterol (mg/dl)	60±4.5 [a]	152±8.2 [d]	90±5.8 [b]	112±7.2 [c]
Triglycerides (mg/dl)	65±5.3 [a]	165±9.8 [d]	88±5.6 [b]	115±6.8 [c]

Data are mean ± SEM (n = 10). Values in the same row bearing different superscript differ significantly

3.5. Effect of EPA-E and Verapamil on LDL/HDL Ratio

Fig. 2 explains the LDL/HDL ratio in all groups. A significant increase in LDL/HDL ratio in the diabetic group over normal group was observed ($p < 0.01$). Although both treatment able to show beneficial effect, EPA-E treated group showed a better beneficial effect than Verapamil treated group.

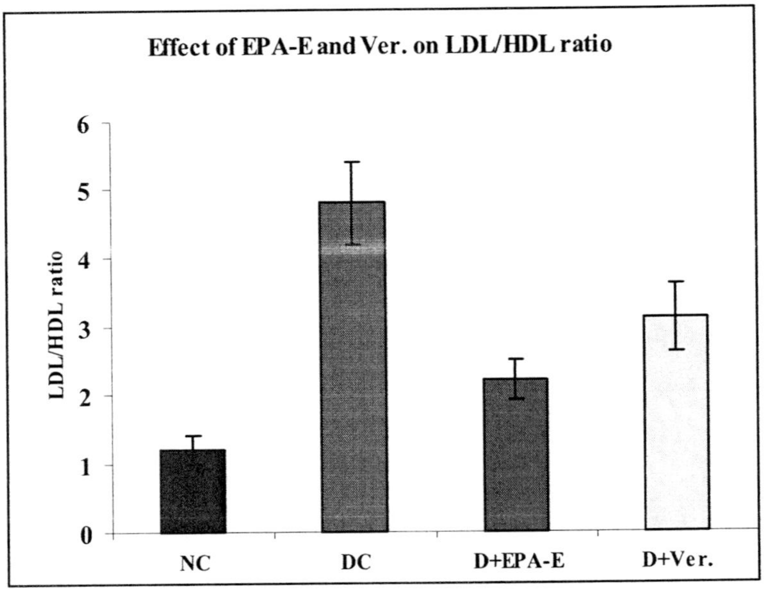

Figure 2.

3.5. Effect of EPA-E and Verapamil on Myocardial Enzyme Markers

There was no change in the LDH enzyme level in all the groups (Table 5). How ever CPK levels were significantly elevated the diabetic group over normal group ($p < 0.001$). Both treatments were able to show the cardio protective effect. How ever, EPA-E treated group completely reversed this elevation to the normal level (Fig 3).

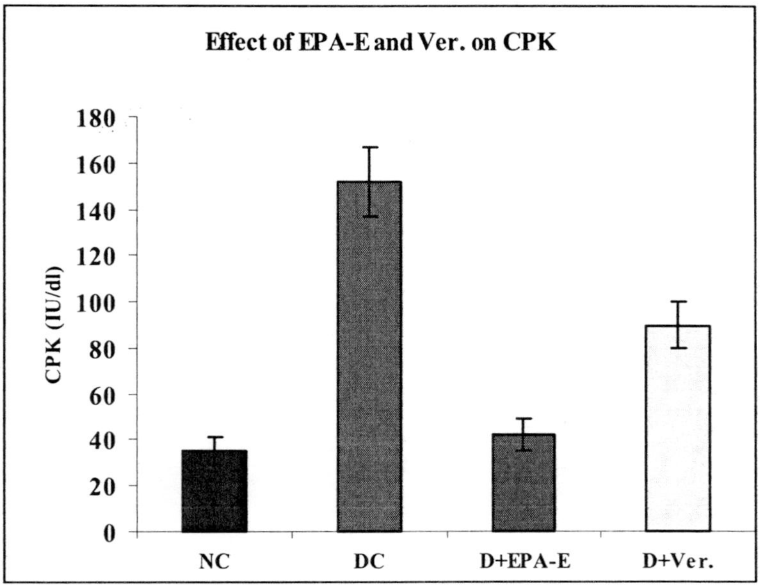

Bars bearing different superscripts differ significantly

Figure 3.

3.6. Effect of EPA-E and Verapamil on Gravimetric Ratio

Table 5 explains the gravimetric ratio in the different groups. A significant increase in gravimetric ratio in the diabetic group over normal group was observed ($p < 0.001$). Both treatments were able to inhibit this gravimetric ratio. How ever, EPA-E treated group completely reversed this elevation to the normal level.

Table 5. Effect of EPA-E and Verapamil on myocardial parameters

Variables	Normal Control	Diabetic Control	D+EPA-E	D+Verapamil
LDH (IU/dl)	155±14.8 [a]	169±16.4 [a]	165±15.7 [a]	170±17.8 [a]
Gravimetric ratio	2.21±0.05 [a]	2.88±0.09 [c]	2.31±0.06 [a]	2.65±0.08 [b]

Data are mean ± SEM (n = 10). Values in the same row bearing different superscript differ significantly

3.7. Effect of EPA-E and Verapamil on ECG

3.7.1. Effect of EPA-E and Verapamil on Bradycardia

Fig 4 explains the heart rate in all groups. A significant decrease in the heart rate in the diabetic group over normal group was observed ($p < 0.001$). Although both treatment able to show beneficial effect, EPA-E treated group showed a better beneficial effect than Verapamil treated group.

3.7.1. Effect of EPA-E and Verapamil on ST/R Ratio

A significant decrease in the ST/R ratio in the diabetic group over normal group was observed ($p < 0.001$). Although both treatment able to show beneficial effect, EPA-E treated group showed a better beneficial effect than Verapamil treated group (Fig 5).

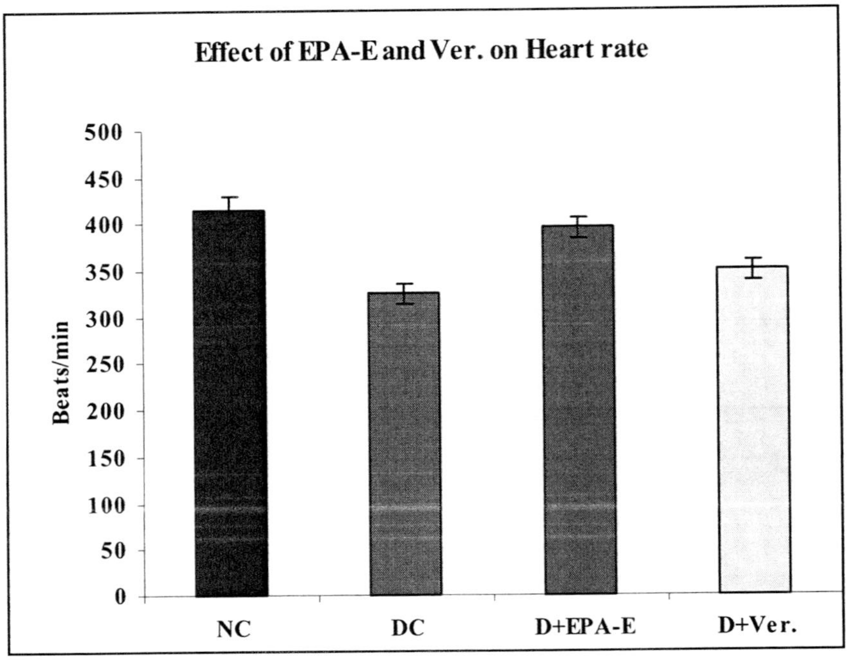

Figure 4.

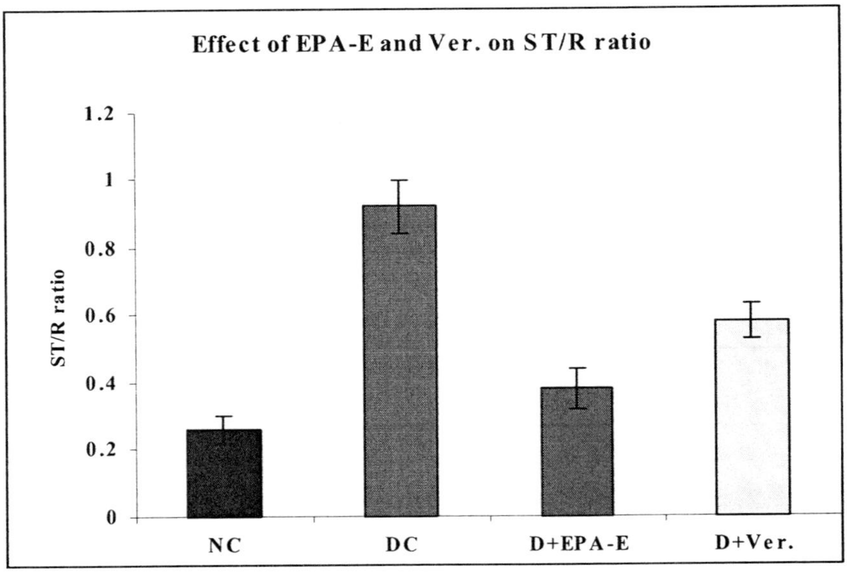

Figure 5.

4. Discussion

Experimental animal models have contributed extensive information about diabetes mellitus. Much of our present knowledge concerning the etiopathogenesis, treatment and prevention of human diabetes would never have been acquired without the study of animal models of diabetes [44]. Alloxan (or) Streptozotocin injected rodents exhibit hyperglycemia and other classical symptoms of IDDM such as hyperlipidemia, hypoinsulinemia, polyphagia, polydipsia and reduced body weight in spite of the fact still they have low insulin levels and they may survive for months [32]. Further ALL (or) STZ are the most commonly used specific diabetogenic agent and equally effective in producing cardiovascular complications associated with diabetes [45].

Alloxan causes diabetes through its selective destruction of insulin-producing beta cells of the pancreas [46,47]. Further, *in vitro* studies have also shown that alloxan is selectively toxic to pancreatic beta cells, leading to the induction of cell necrosis [48]. The cytotoxic action of alloxan is mediated by reactive oxygen species, with a simultaneous massive increase in cytosolic calcium concentration, leading to a rapid destruction of beta cells [49].

4.1. Effect of EPA-E and Verapamil on Body Weight, Feed and Water Intake

Polyuria, polydipsia and polyphagia are the most common characteristic sign of diabetes mellitus, where as weight loss is the typical sign of insulin dependent diabetes mellitus (IDDM). Alloxan induced diabetic rats are closely resemble the IDDM, that's why in this study all the diabetic rats showed the above characteristic symptoms. When the capacity of the kidneys to absorb glucose is surpassed, glucosuria ensues. Glucose is an osmotic diuretic and an increase in renal loss of glucose is accompanied by loss of water and electrolytes, termed polyuria. The result of the loss of water (and overall volume) leads to the activation of the thirst mechanism (polydipsia). The negative caloric balance, which results from, the glucosuria and tissue catabolism leads to an increase in appetite and food intake (polyphagia).

Verapamil did not have any effect on these parameters, but the EPA-E treatment significantly inhibited the polydipsia and weight loss associated with chronic diabetes. This beneficial effect may be due to the favorable effect on glycemic control thereby reducing the urinary glucose/energy loss. This in turn helpful in alleviating polydipsia, polyuria and weight loss associated with the diabetes mellitus.

4.2. Effect of EPA-E and Verapamil on Blood Glucose Level

Uncontrolled IDDM leads to increased hepatic glucose output. First, liver glycogen stores are mobilized then hepatic gluconeogenesis is used to produce glucose. Insulin deficiency also impairs non-hepatic tissue utilization of glucose. In particular, in adipose tissue and skeletal muscle, insulin stimulates glucose uptake. This is accomplished by insulin-mediated movement of glucose transporter proteins to the plasma membrane of these tissues. Reduced glucose uptake by peripheral tissues in turn leads to a reduced rate of glucose metabolism. In addition, the level of hepatic glucokinase is regulated by insulin. Therefore, a reduced rate of glucose phosphorylation in hepatocytes leads to increased delivery to the blood. Other enzymes involved in anabolic metabolism of glucose are affected by insulin (primarily through covalent modifications). The combination of increased hepatic glucose production and reduced peripheral tissues metabolism leads to elevated plasma glucose levels.

Although insulin deficiency is the primary defect in IDDM, in patients/animals with poorly controlled IDDM there is also a defect in the ability of target tissues to respond to the administration of insulin. There are multiple biochemical mechanisms that account for this impairment of tissues to respond to insulin. Deficiency in insulin leads to elevated levels of free fatty acids in the plasma as a result of uncontrolled lipolysis in adipose tissue. Free fatty acids suppress glucose metabolism in peripheral tissues such as skeletal muscle. This impairs the action of insulin in these tissues, i.e. the promotion of glucose utilization. Additionally, insulin deficiency decreases the expression of a number of genes necessary for target tissues to respond normally to insulin -- such as glucokinase in liver and the GLUT 4 class of glucose transporters in adipose tissue.

Hence, hyperglycemia is the common feature of both clinical as well as experimental diabetes, were noticed in the diabetic control group. Among treatment group, EPA-E significantly reduced blood glucose level, verapamil treated group showed neither favorable effect nor any adverse effect. Recent clinical studies in human diabetic patients documented that verapamil do not interfere the glycemic control, unlike the beta blockers [50]. The present research results fully support these findings

Conflicting results have been published about the effects of fish oil on glucose homeostasis [51-53]. Some [51-53] but not all [54,55] studies have reported that fish oil has detrimental effects on glycemic control in glucose-intolerant persons and in persons with type 2 diabetes. Although the reason given for the above controversy is the limitations in the earlier study design, still the controversy exist even in the well planned study design [56].

Although, the results of supplementing omega-3-PUFA in patients of IDDM give rise to some optimism [57], but in NIDDM it has been found omega-3-PUFA administration bring about a rapid reversible deterioration of blood glucose balance [51-53]. Previous investigators have provided no obvious explanation for these contradicting findings. How ever, previous study from our lab, we have reported a novel drug interaction between omega-3-PUFA and glibenclamide in STZ-diabetic wistar rat [31]. This gives a very good explanation for the all above controversies. Since IDDM treatment does not involve the use of glibenclamide to induce endogenous insulin release, omega-3-PUFA intake in IDDM gives promising result, where as NIDDM patients with glibenclamide/ without glibenclamide intake of omega-3-PUFA leads to contradictory results in the earlier reports. Further, the present animal model is IDDM, that's why EPA-E showed favorable effect on glycemic control of these diabetic rats. These results are in support of our previous findings [58]. This beneficial action may due to increased insulin sensitivity [59] through the peroxisome proliferator-activated receptor gamma (PPARgamma), a nuclear hormone receptor. EPE-E is the natural ligand and agonist of the peroxisome proliferator-activated receptor gamma

(PPARgamma) [60]. It also increases the expression of GLUT-4 receptor, which is responsible for the glucose transport into the cell [61].

4.3. Effect of EPA-E and Verapamil on Glycosylated Hemoglobin

The HbA1c test measures the amount of glucose sticking to the hemoglobin and the values are expressed in percentages. It is well known that hemoglobin is a protein susceptible to nonenzymatic glycosylation depending on the time of RBC's exposure to glucose and on the blood glucose concentration. The higher the level of blood sugar, the more glucose attaches to red blood cells. Further, once the glucose is attached to the hemoglobin, it stays there for the life of the RBC's, which is about 120 days and it gives an average amount of glucose that has been in a human's/animal's blood over the last 2 to 3 months. Thus the measurement of HbA1c provides an objective retrospective index of glycemic control for monitoring long-term diabetes [62].

The findings of a major diabetes study, the Diabetes Control and Complications Trial (DCCT), have shown that lowering the HbA1c value can delay or prevent the development of serious eye, kidney, and nerve disease in people with diabetes. Further, it also showed that lowering HbA1c levels by any amount improves a person's chances of staying healthy. Complications associated with diabetes were related to either the duration of diabetes or degree of hyperglycemia, which is measured by the level of HbA1c and hence HbA1c is the pre-eminent factor for quantifying the risk of complications in patients with diabetes and for monitoring glycemic control [63].

In this present study, only EPA-E showed beneficial effect in reducing HbA1c. This results are well correlated with blood glucose level, further EPA-E proved its beneficial effect in controlling blood glucose level over period of time. This beneficial effect is due to its action on peroxisome proliferator-activated receptor gamma (PPARgamma), a nuclear hormone receptor [60] leads to the increased insulin sensitivity [59] and through increased expression of GLUT-4 receptors [61].

4.4. Effect of EPA-E and Verapamil on Lipid Parameters

Hypercholesterolemia and hypertriglyceridemia are known to exist in both clinical and experimental diabetes [56,58]. These are all the factors, which determine cardio vascular complications associated with diabetes. One major role of insulin is to stimulate the storage of food energy following the consumption of a meal. This energy storage is in the form of glycogen in hepatocytes and skeletal muscle. Additionally, insulin stimulates hepatocytes to synthesize triglycerides and storage of triglycerides in adipose tissue. In opposition to increased adipocyte storage of triglycerides is insulin-mediated inhibition of lipolysis. Normally, the levels of malonyl-CoA are high in the presence of insulin.

These high levels of malonyl-CoA inhibit carnitine palmitoyltransferase I, the enzyme required for the transport of fatty acyl-CoA's into the mitochondria where they are subject to oxidation for energy production. Thus, in the absence of insulin, malonyl-CoA levels fall and transport of fatty acyl-CoA's into the mitochondria increases. Normally, plasma triglycerides are acted upon by lipoprotein lipase (LPL), an enzyme on the surface of the endothelial cells lining the blood vessels. In particular, LPL activity allows fatty acids to be taken from circulating triglycerides for storage in adipocytes. The activity of LPL requires insulin and in its absence a hypertriglyceridemia results.

Both verapamil as well as EPA-E showed beneficial effect, but EPA-E showed better results than verapamil. Verapamil is known to decrease triglycerides [64]. Fish oils are known to reduce cholesterol and triglycerides level in diseased conditions, but unable to show any effect in normal individual even though high dose has been tried unlike other cholesterol lowering drugs. The hypolipidemic effects of n-3 fatty acids are similar to those of n-6 fatty acids, provided that they replace saturated fats in the diet. n-3 Fatty acids have the added benefit of consistently lowering serum triacylglycerol concentrations, whereas the n-6 fatty acids do not and may even increase them [65].

Furthermore, Nestel [66] reported that consumption of high amounts of fish oil blunted the expected rise in plasma cholesterol concentrations in humans. Furthermore, fish oil reduces cholesterol absorption in humans [67] and monkeys [68], cholesterol synthesis in the liver is reduced and cholesterol secretion within VLDLs is lowered [67].

Although there is agreement that chylomicron assembly and secretion are reduced in isolated intestinal cells incubated with EPA, the interpretations of results differ. The mechanisms appear to include the reduction of apolipoprotion B formation and the diversion of EPA from triacylglycerols to phospholipids [69].

Studies in humans have shown that fish oils reduce the rate of hepatic secretion of VLDL triacylglycerol [70-74]. In normolipidemic subjects, n-3 fatty acids prevent and rapidly reverse carbohydrate-induced hypertriglyceridemia [72]. There is also an evidence from kinetic studies that fish oil increases the fractional catabolic rate of VLDL [71, 73, 74].

This hypotriacylglycerolemic effect of n-3 PUFAs may be mediated through reduced endogenous TRL synthesis, increased TRL removal, or a combination of both. Diminished endogenous TRL production has been shown in kinetic studies, in which the protein moiety of VLDLs was radio labeled and n-3 PUFAs reduced VLDL synthesis [75]. Chylomicrons and VLDLs compete for LPL-mediated removal from the circulation [76]. Therefore, reduced VLDL synthesis would promote chylomicron removal, thus reducing the postprandial triacylglycerolemic response. The presence of n-3 PUFAs in a meal also promotes removal of TRL from the circulation [77], and postprandial LPL activity is significantly greater after an n-3 PUFA meal compared with a saturated fatty acid–rich test meal [78]. Experimental studies have shown that fish oil consumption leads to significantly higher expression of adipose tissue LPL m RNA [79], which suggests that n-3 PUFA supplementation increases LPL-mediated TRL clearance. It is probable that n-3 PUFAs mediate their effect on plasma triacylglycerol concentrations by both reducing endogenous VLDL production and increasing TRL removal.

Studies have confirmed that fish oil increases oxidation of fatty acids by peroxisomal as well as mitochondrial routes [80], which may be mediated by peroxisome proliferator in the liver [81]; fish oil reduces fatty acid synthesis (owing to suppression of key enzymes) and diverts fatty acids to phospholipids [68]; although, fish oil reduces plasma fatty acids, this may be due to increased hepatic uptake through a transporter protein [81]; within the liver, triacylglycerol assembly is impaired through down regulation of esterifying enzymes [82].

4.5. Effect of EPA-E and Verapamil on LDL/HDL Cholesterol Ratio

Altered metabolism of triglyceride-rich lipoproteins is crucial in the pathophysiology of the atherogenic dyslipidemia of diabetes. Alterations include both increased hepatic secretion of VLDL and impaired clearance of VLDL and intestinally derived chylomicrons. An important consequence of retarded clearance is prolonged plasma retention of both VLDL and postprandial chylomicrons as partially lipolyzed remnant particles. These remnants, which include cholesterol-enriched intermediate-density lipoproteins (IDLs), are particularly atherogenic in humans and in a number of animal models [83,84].

Increased hepatic production and/or retarded clearance from plasma of large VLDL also result in increased production of precursors of small dense LDL particles. As many as seven distinct LDL subspecies, which differ in their metabolic behavior and pathological roles, have been identified [85]. Plasma VLDL levels correlate with increased density and decreased size of LDL [86,87]. In addition, LDL size and density are inversely related to plasma levels of HDL, especially the HDL2 subclass [88]. Small dense LDL particles appear to arise from the intravascular processing of specific larger VLDL precursors through a series of steps, including lipolysis [85]. Further triglyceride enrichment of the lipolytic products through the action of cholesteryl ester transfer protein, together with hydrolysis of triglyceride and phospholipids by hepatic lipase, leads to increased production of small dense LDL particles [83and84]. Plasma residence time of these LDL particles may be prolonged because of their relatively reduced affinity for LDL receptors [85].

HDL particles are heterogeneous, and multiple subclasses differing in diameter and density have been identified, ranging from the small dense HDL3c, HDL3b, and HDL3a to the larger HDL2a and HDL2b [89]. The reductions in HDL associated with diabetes and insulin resistance are multifactorial, but a major factor appears to be increased transfer of cholesterol from HDL to triglyceride-rich lipoproteins, with reciprocal transfer of triglyceride to HDL. Triglyceride-rich HDL particles are hydrolyzed by hepatic lipase and, as a result, are rapidly catabolized and cleared from plasma [90]. Typically, the reduced HDL levels in plasma of patients with type 2 diabetes are manifest as reductions in the HDL2b subspecies and relative or absolute increases in smaller, denser HDL3b and HDL3c.

The effects of fish oil on LDL metabolism represent the more controversial aspects of the n-3 fatty acid effects. Why does fish oil cause LDL-cholesterol concentrations to sometimes rise, at least in humans, when all the evidence suggests it should not? Fish oil depresses cholesterol synthesis and may reduce cholesterol absorption [67]. This focuses attention on LDL removal and particularly on the LDL (apolipoprotein B/E) receptor. There is evidence that fish oil down-regulates the receptor in hepatic cells [91,92]. Abnormal LDL binding to the receptor in human monocytes [92] and to skin fibroblasts has been ascribed to abnormalities in the LDL itself [93]. Changes in the LDL particles are minor, but tend towards larger, cholesterol-enriched LDLs [94,95]. LDL size relates to the exchange of lipids between LDL, VLDL, and HDL. Fish oil would reduce such exchanges through suppression of cholesterol ester transfer protein and thus favor larger LDL particles [94]. Reduced LDL synthesis has been reported with large amounts of fish oil [96].

Most reports indicate a favorable effect of fish oil on HDLs. The number of larger cholesterol-rich HDLs (in the HDL2 range) increases at the expense of HDL3 [94]. However, very high intake of fish oil may lower HDL concentrations [67]. The major effect of fish oil on HDL metabolism is mediated by a reduction in activity of cholesterol ester transfer protein [94], which transfers cholesterol esters from HDLs to VLDLs and LDLs, largely in exchange for VLDL triacylglycerols. Because triacylglycerol concentrations are also reduced, exchange is further diminished, favoring large cholesterol-rich HDL (and LDL) particles over the formation of triacylglycerol-enriched HDLs (and LDLs), which are more susceptible to catabolism.

4.6. Effect of EPA-E and Verapamil on Diabetic Cardiomyopathy

Diabetic cardiomyopathy is one of the chronic complications of diabetes mellitus and is characterized by decreased contractility of the left ventricle, diminished ventricular compliance [97-99] even in the absence of associated coronary disease or hypertension [97]. Accumulating data from experimental, pathological, epidemiological, and clinical studies have shown that diabetes mellitus results in cardiac functional and structural changes, independent of hypertension, coronary artery disease, or any other known cardiac disease, which support the existence of diabetic cardiomyopathy as a distinct clinical entity. The development of diabetic cardiomyopathy is likely to be multifactorial. Putative mechanisms include metabolic disturbances, myocardial fibrosis, small vessel disease, autonomic dysfunction, and insulin resistance. The most important mechanisms of diabetic cardiomyopathy are metabolic disturbances (depletion of glucose transporter 4, increased free fatty acids, carnitine deficiency, changes in calcium homeostasis), myocardial fibrosis (association with increases in angiotensin II, IGF-I, and inflammatory cytokines), small vessel disease (microangiopathy, impaired coronary flow reserve, and endothelial dysfunction), cardiac autonomic neuropathy (denervation and alterations in myocardial catecholamine levels), and insulin resistance (hyperinsulinemia and reduced insulin sensitivity).The mechanisms of metabolic disturbances, myocardial fibrosis, microvascular disease, CAN, and insulin resistance in diabetic cardiomyopathy imply that various treatments might be effective for preventing or delaying the development of diabetic cardiomyopathy and its complications. These include improving diabetic control; use of calcium blockers, angiotensin-converting enzyme (ACE) inhibitors, or related drugs; exercise training; lipid-lowering therapy; and antioxidant and insulin-sensitizing drugs, although there is no specific therapeutic strategies for diabetic cardiomyopathy exist at present. Hence research is urgently required into the molecular basis of diabetic cardiomyopathy such that more appropriate therapies may be formulated and tested [100].

4.6.1. Effect of EPA-E and Verapamil on Gravimetric Ratio

Myocardial fibrosis and myocyte hypertrophy are the most frequently proposed mechanisms to explain cardiac changes in diabetic cardiomyopathy. Studies in dogs, monkeys, and rabbits have shown that experimentally induced diabetes causes defects in cellular calcium transport [101], defects in myocardial contractile proteins [102], and an increase in collagen formation [103], which result in anatomic and physiological changes in the myocardium. Stimulation of α-adrenergic receptors causes myocyte hypertrophy and may exert an antiapoptotic action [104]. Overexpression of ß1-adrenergic receptors causes marked myocyte hypertrophy, interstitial fibrosis, and reduced contractile function, which was accompanied by increased myocyte apoptosis [105]. A study using phenylephrine or isoproterenol in streptozotocin-induced diabetic rats has demonstrated that the in vivo response to ß-adrenoceptor stimulation is well preserved, whereas the effects of α-stimulation are markedly reduced, especially in the left ventricle and systemic circulation [106], suggesting that the antiapoptotic effect may be also reduced in diabetes. There was a significant increase in heart-to-body weight ratio in DC group over NC group. This finding is in accordance with previous findings [30, 42,107]. EPA-E is able to show beneficial effect better than verapamil by acting through the above stated mechanism.

Verapamil is also showed some beneficial effect. This may be explained by the following way. Intracellular retention of calcium in diabetes is always associated with depletion of high-energy phosphate stores and a derangement of ultra structure and cardiac dysfunction. Calcium channel blockers are capable of reversing the intracellular calcium defects and preventing diabetes-induced myocardial changes. Verapamil has been shown to significantly improve the depressed rate of contraction and rate of relaxation, lower peak LV systolic pressure, and elevate LV diastolic pressure [108], as well as to improve the altered myofibrillar ATP^{ase} activity, myosin ATP^{ase}, myosin isoenzyme distribution, and sarcoplasmic reticular Ca^{2+}-pump activities in streptozocin-induced diabetic rats [109]. Diltiazem has been shown to suppress interstitial fibrotic changes in type II diabetic mice [110], and nifedipine increases insulin sensitivity and prevents the increase in cholesterol and triglyceride levels in streptozotocin-induced diabetic rats [111].

4.6.2. Effect of EPA-E and Verapamil on Myocardial Enzyme Markers

Serum CPK level is one of the enzyme markers for the cardiac muscle damage. Squadrito et al. observed that elevated serum CPK level, 10 times more than that of normal control in myocardial infarction [112]. In our study, the DC group had significant elevation of serum CPK levels, i.e. 2-2.5 times than that of normal, which is indicative of cardiomyopathy. This finding is in close agreement with the result of Cubria et al. and Lawrance Christopher in which they observed serum CPK levels to rise by two to three times that of normal in polyamine-induced cardiac hypertrophy and in diabetic cardiomyopathy [113,107]. EPA-E treatment completely blunted this elevation. This is in conformation with the earlier observation [30,107, 114], whome observed that Omega-3 PUFA treatment prevented the elevation of CPK in diabetic as well as ischemic myocardium.

Verapamil treatment partially abolished the elevation serum CPK. This beneficial effect may be due to the improvement of the altered myofibrillar ATP^{ase} activity, myosin ATP^{ase}, myosin isoenzyme distribution, sarcoplasmic reticular Ca^{2+}-pump activities in diabetic ventricular tissue [109] and inhibition of abnormal activation of cardiac PKC in diabetes [115]. There was no significant elevation of serum LDH as observed in acute myocardial infarction [116]. Elevated CPK with normal LDH, however, may only be indicative of presence of primary myocardial dysfunction, which is known to exist in diabetic cardiomyopathy [6, 7, and 30,107].

4.6.3. Effect of EPA-E and Verapamil on ECG

Bradycardia has frequently been reported in experimental diabetic rats [117,118]. This effect may have been due to changes in cardiac electrical properties [119and120], calcium handling [101,121,122], myocardial metabolism [123] and hypothyroidism [124]. ECG abnormalities like changes in the QT interval and T wave is frequently seen in clinical diabetic cardiomyopathy [125,126] as well as experimental diabetes [127]. Nearly all these changes are related to repolarization. EPA-E completely reversed these changes Verapamil partially inhibited these changes. Beneficial effect of EPA-E may be due to its effect on cardiac electrical properties and myocardial metabolism. Verapamil might have shown its effect through calcium handling.

These studies suggest that improvements in diabetic cardiomyopathy are associated with restoration of distinct metabolic abnormalities induced by the diabetic state. The results of this study indicate that cardiomyopathy of diabetic rats can be improved despite the diabetic state. Because glycemic and lipid parameters of the EPA-E treated diabetic rats was not parallel to that of the nondiabetic control animals, this may indicate that EPA-E treatment affects some other mechanism that is responsible for the development of diabetic cardiomyopathy. Although several biochemical and morphological alterations have been identified that may contribute to the diabetic cardiomyopathy, clinical and experimental studies have demonstrated elevated tissue collagen levels in diabetic heart muscle in the absence of coronary vascular changes [128]. In the diabetic rat, cardiac membrane calcium transport activities are attenuated: sarcoplasmic reticulum (SR) calcium transport and calcium ATP^{ase} activities are reduced [129,130] and sarcolemmal calcium-pump activity [121]. In addition, reduced oxygen delivery [131] and reduced levels of cellular ATP [132] may contribute to the impaired heart function. However, the etiology of the complex pathological alterations of diabetic cardiomyopathy remains incompletely defined. Recently, we have demonstrated that positive beneficial effect of Omega-3 PUFA on PAS-positive material accumulation in the diabetic myocardium [30], the most probable etiology proposed for the development of diabetic cardiomyopathy [133]. Hence we are hypothesizing that this may be the major mechanism by which EPA-E completely blocks the development of experimental diabetic cardiomyopathy.

5. Summary

We studied the beneficial effect of EPA-E treatment on diabetic cardiomyopathy rat in comparison with the verapamil, a known beneficial calcium channel blocker. The EPA-E preparation used was highly purified eicosapentaenoic acid ethyl ester. Male Wistar rats (180-200 g) were rendered diabetic by alloxan (ALL; 55 mg/kg). Nondiabetic control rats received the vehicle alone. Four weeks after ALL or vehicle injection, control and diabetic rats were randomly divided into four groups. 1. Normal control, 2. Diabetic control, 3. EPA-E treated diabetic rats and 4. Verapamil treated diabetic rats. EPA-E (90 mg/kg) and Verapamil

(25 mg/kg) were administered to the diabetic rats daily by oral gavage for three months. During this study, plasma glucose, glycosylated hemoglobin, plasma triglycerides, cholesterol, LDL and HDL cholesterol. A significant increase in the plasma glucose, glycosylated hemoglobin, plasma triglycerides, and cholesterol, LDL and HDL ratio in diabetic control over normal control were noticed. All the above parameters were significantly improved ($P < 0.01$) in the EPA-E treated diabetic rats compared with untreated diabetic rats and verapamil treated diabetic rats, although these parameters did not improve to the nondiabetic level. At the end of experiment, ECG, gravimetric ratio and myocardial enzyme markers were studied. In diabetic control group, diabetic cardiomyopathy was characterized by elevated CPK, gravimetric ratio, ST/R ratio in the ECG and bradycardia. EPA-E treatment completely abolishes the development of experimental diabetic cardiomyopathy where as verapamil partially abolishes the development of experimental diabetic cardiomyopathy. These data suggest that EPA-E treatment completely blocks the development of experimental diabetic cardiomyopathy, possibly by multiple target mechanism apart from affecting SR calcium transport activity.

The multiple mechanisms may be through nitric oxide production [134], improvement in Na/K-ATP^{ase} isoenzymes system in the myocardium [135], improvement of cardiac mitochondrial function [136] and the inhibition of PAS positive material accumulation in the myocardium [30], a main etiology proposed for diabetic cardiomyopathy [133]

6. Conclusion

This study has demonstrated that in the alloxan diabetic rat, treatment with EPA-E can ameliorate the cardiac complications better than Verapamil. This clearly indicates that EPA-E acting through multiple mechanisms apart from improving cardiac SR calcium transport activity. Since calcium handling is the major mechanism of action by Verapamil, verapamil treatment partially blocks the development of experimental diabetic cardiomyopathy in this animal model. These studies suggest that EPA-E therapy may be effective in preventing some of the adverse consequences of diabetes. We have demonstrated in this study that EPA-E supplementation is effective in preventing cardio vascular complications associated with experimental diabetes and could be suitable for clinical study with two advantages, harmlessness and low cost.

7. Acknowledgements

This work is dedicated to the memory of C. Edward Paul Christopher. The first author is grateful to his Father Dr. E. Chandra Christopher, Mother F. Celine Mary and family members especially his daughter Ebisha Pauline and son Donald Christopher for their love and affection. We are very grateful to the research scholars of CBMR, SGPGIMS especially Somasekhar, Omkar, Jadesh, Niraj, Naved and Ashish for their invaluable support in the preparation of this chapter

8. References

[1] American Diabetes Association. Diagnosis and classification of diabetes mellitus. *Diabetes Care.* 2004 Jan; 27 Suppl 1:S5-S10.

[2] Saltiel AR. New perspectives into the molecular pathogenesis and treatment of type 2 diabetes. *Cell* 2001; 104: 517–529.

[3] King H, Aubert RE, Herman WH. Global burden of diabetes, 1995–2025: prevalence, numerical estimates, and projections. *Diabetes Care* 1998; 21: 1414–1431

[4] Beller GA. Coronary heart disease in the first 30 years of the 21st century: challenges and opportunities. The 33rd Annual James B. Herrick Lecture of the Council on Clinical Cardiology of the American Heart Association. *Circulation* 2001; 103: 2428–2435.

[5] Taegtmeyer H, McNulty P, Young ME. Adaptation and maladaptation of the heart in diabetes. *Circulation* 2002; 105(14):1727-33

[6] Tahiliani AG and McNeill JH. Diabetes induced abnormalities in the myocardium. *Life Sci.* 1986; 38: 959–974.

[7] McNeill JH and Tahiliani AG. Diabetes induced cardiac changes. *Trends Pharmacol. Sci.* 1986; 7: 364–367.

[8] Starling EH, Lovatt Evans C. The respiratory exchanges of the heart in the diabetic animal. *J. Physiol.* (Lond). 1914; 49: 67–88.

[9] McGarry JD. What if Minkowski had been ageusic? An alternative angle on diabetes. *Science.* 1992; 258: 766–770.

[10] Stanley WC, Lopaschuk GD, McCormack JG. Regulation of energy substrate metabolism in the diabetic heart. *Cardiovasc. Res.* 1997; 34: 25–33.

[11] Burr ML, Fehily AM, Gilbert JF, et al. Effect of changes in fat, fish and fiber intakes on death and myocardial reinfarction: diet and reinfarction trial (DART). *Lancet* 1989; 2: 757–61.

[12] de Lorgeril M, Renaud S, Mamelle N, et al. Mediterranean α-linolenic acid–rich diet in secondary prevention of coronary heart disease. *Lancet* 1994; 343:1454–9.

[13] Morris MC, Sacks F, Rosner B. Fish oil to reduce blood pressure: a meta-analysis. *Ann. Intern. Med.* 1994; 120(suppl):10.

[14] Appel LJ, Miller ER, Seidler AJ, Whelton PK. Does supplementation of diet with "fish oil" reduce blood pressure? A meta-analysis of controlled clinical trials. *Arch. Intern. Med.* 1993; 153:1429–38.

[15] Appel LF, Miller ED, Seidler AJ, Whelton PK. Diet supplementation with fish oils and blood pressure reduction: a meta-analysis. *Ann. Intern. Med.* 1994; 120(suppl):9.

[16] Raheja BS, Sadikot SM, Phatak RB, Rao MB. Significance of the n-6/n-3 ratio for insulin action in diabetes. *Ann. N. Y. Acad. Sci.* 1993; 683:258–71.

[17] Connor WE, Prince MJ, Ullmann D, et al. The hypotriglyceridemic effect of fish oil in adult-onset diabetes without adverse glucose control. *Ann. N. Y. Acad. Sci.* 1993; 683:337–40.

[18] De Caterina R, Caprioli R, Giannessi D, et al. N-3 Fatty acids reduce proteinuria in patients with chronic glomerular disease. *Kidney Int.* 1993; 44:843–50.

[19] Donadio JV Jr, Bergstralh EJ, Offord KP, Spencer DC, Holley KE. A controlled trial of fish oil in IgA nephropathy. Mayo Nephrology Collaborative Group. *N. Engl. J. Med.* 1994; 331:1194–9.

[20] Kremer JM. Effects of modulation of inflammatory and immune parameters in patients with rheumatic and inflammatory disease receiving dietary supplementation of n-3 and n-6 fatty acids. *Lipids* 1996; 31(suppl):S243–7.

[21] Stenson WF, Cort D, Rodgers J, et al. Dietary supplementation with fish oil in ulcerative colitis. *Ann. Intern. Med.* 1992; 116:609–14.

[22] Belluzzi A, Brignola C, Campieri M, Pera A, Boschi S, Miglioli M. Effect of an enteric-coated fish-oil preparation on relapses in Crohn's disease. *N. Engl. J. Med.* 1996; 334:1557–60.

[23] Shahar E, Folsom AR, Melnick SL, et al. Dietary n-3 polyunsaturated fatty acids and smoking-related chronic obstructive pulmonary disease. Atherosclerosis Risk in Communities Study Investigators. *N. Engl. J. Med.* 1994; 331:228–33.

[24] Eaton SB, Konner M. Paleolithic nutrition. A consideration of its nature and current implications. *N. Engl. J. Med.* 1985; 312:283–9.

[25] Simopoulos AP. Evolutionary aspects of diet: fatty acids, insulin resistance and obesity. In: VanItallie TB, Simopoulos AP, eds. *Obesity*: new directions in assessment and management. Philadelphia: Charles Press, 1995:241–61.

[26] Horrobin DF. The roles of essential fatty acids in the development of diabetic neuropathy and other complications of diabetes mellitus. *Prostaglandins Leukot Essent Fatty Acids* 1988; 31:181 –197.

[27] Ruiz-Gutierrez V, Stiefel P, Villar J, Garcia-Donas MA, Acosta D, Carneado J. Cell membrane fatty acid composition in type 1 (insulin-dependent) diabetic patients: relationship with sodium transport abnormalities and metabolic control. *Diabetologia* 1993; 36:850 –856.

[28] Huang YS, Horrobin DF, Manku MS, Mitchell J, Ryan MA. Tissue phospholipid fatty acid composition in the diabetic rat. *Lipids* 1984; 19:367 –370.

[29] Chattopadhyay J, Thompson EW, Schmid HH. Nonesterified fatty acids in normal and diabetic rat sciatic nerve. *Lipids* 1992; 27:513 –517.

[30] Lawrance Christopher C, Mathuram LN, Genitta G, Cyrus I and Jayasundar S. Omega-3-Fatty acids inhibit the accumulation of PAS positive material in the myocardium of STZ diabetic Wistar rats. *Int. J. Cardiol.* 2003; 88(2-3):183-90.

[31] Lawrance Christopher C, Mathuram LN, Genitta G and S. Jayasundar. Lack of synergistic effect of Omega-3-Fatty acid and glibenclamide combination in STZ diabetic Wistar rats. *J. Vet. Pharmacol. and Toxicol.* 2001; 1&2: 57-63.

[32] Bell RH Jr, Hye RJ. Animal models of diabetes mellitus: physiology and pathology. *J. Surg. Res.* 1983 Nov;35(5):433-60

[33] Minami A, Ishimura N, Sakamoto S, Takishita E, Mawatari K, Okada K, Nakaya Y. Effect of eicosapentaenoic acid ethyl ester v. oleic acid-rich safflower oil on insulin resistance in type 2 diabetic model rats with hypertriacylglycerolaemia. *Br. J. Nutr.* 2002 Feb; 87(2):157-62.

[34] Kaymaz AA, Tan H, Altug T, Buyukdevrim AS. The effects of calcium channel blockers, verapamil, nifedipine and diltiazem, on metabolic control in diabetic rats. *Diabetes Res. Clin. Pract.* 1995 Jun; 28(3):201-5.

[35] Sugiura M, Hirano K. A new colorimetric method for determination of serum glucose. *Clin. Chim. Acta.* 1977 Mar 15; 75(3):387-91.

[36] Wybenga DR, Pileggi VJ, Dirstine PH et al. Direct manual determination of serum total cholesterol with a single stable reagent. *Clin. Chem.* 1970; 16: 980–984.

[37] Fossati P and Prencipe L. Serum triglycerides determined colorimetrically with an enzyme that produces hydrogen peroxide. *Clin. Chem.* 1982; 28:2077–2080.

[38] Burstein M, Scholnick HR and Morfin R. Rapid method for the isolation of lipoprotein from human serum by precipitation with polyanions. *J. Lipid Res.* 1970; 19:583.

[39] Cohen MP, Witt J, Wu VY. Purified haemoglobin preparations in the evaluation of HbA1c determination by ion exchange chromatography. *Ann. Clin. Biochem.* 1993 May; 30:265-71.

[40] Hughes BP. A method for the estimation of serum creatine kinase and its use in comparing creatine kinase and aldolase activity in normal and pathological sera. *Clin Chim Acta.* 1962 Sep;7:597-603

[41] Howell BF, Margolis S, Schaffer R. Detection of inhibitors in reduced nicotinamide adenine dinucleotide by kinetic methods. *Clin Chem.* 1976 Oct; 22(10):1648-54.

[42] Pierce GN and Dhalla NS. Sarcolemmal Na+–K+–ATP ^{ase} activity in diabetic rat heart. *Am. J. Physiol.* 1983; 245:C241–C247.

[43] Snedecor, G W and Cochran, W G. *Statistical methods.* 7th edition. Ames, Iowa: Iowa State University Press; 1980.

[44] Cheta D. Animal models of type I (insulin-dependent) diabetes mellitus. *J. Pediatr. Endocrinol. Metab.* 1998 Jan-Feb; 11(1):11-9.

[45] Ozturk Y, Altan VM, and Yildizoglu-Ari N. Effects of experimental diabetes and insulin on smooth muscle functions. *Pharmacol. Rev.* 1996; 48: 69-112.

[46] Lenzen S, Panten U. Alloxan: history and mechanism of action. *Diabetologia* 1988; 31:337–342.

[47] Oberley LW. Free radicals and diabetes. *Free Rad. Biol. Med.* 1988; 5:113–124.

[48] Jörns A, Munday R, Tiedge M, Lenzen S. Comparative toxicity of alloxan, N-alkyl-alloxans and ninhydrin to isolated pancreatic islets in vitro. *J. Endocrinol.* 1997;155:283–293

[49] Szkudelski T. The mechanism of Alloxan and Streptozotocin action in B cells of the rat pancreas. *Physiol. Res.* 2001; 50:537–546.

[50] Holzgreve H, Nakov R, Beck K, Janka HU.Antihypertensive therapy with verapamil SR plus trandolapril versus atenolol plus chlorthalidone on glycemic control. *Am. J. Hypertens.* 2003 May; 16:381-6.

[51] Glauber H, Wallace P, Griver K, Brechtel G. Adverse metabolic effect of omega-3 fatty acids in non-insulin-dependent diabetes mellitus. *Ann. Intern. Med.* 1988; 108:663-8.

[52] Friday KE, Childs MT, Tsunehara CH, Fujimoto WY, Bierman EL, Ensinck JW. Elevated plasma glucose and lowered triglyceride levels from omega-3 fatty acid supplementation in type II diabetes. *Diabetes Care.* 1989; 12:276-81.

[53] Vessby B, Karlstrom B, Boberg M, Lithell H, Berne C. Polyunsaturated fatty acids may impair blood glucose control in type 2 diabetic patients. *Diabet Med.* 1992; 9:126-33.

[54] Connor WE, Prince MJ, Ullmann D, Riddle M, Hatcher L, Smith FE, et al. The hypotriglyceridemic effect of fish oil in adult-onset diabetes without adverse glucose control. *Ann. N. Y. Acad. Sci.* 1993; 683:337-40.

[55] Westerveld HT, de Graaf JC, van Breugel HH, Akkerman JW, Sixma JJ, Erkelens DW, et al. Effects of low-dose EPA-E on glycemic control, lipid profile, lipoprotein(a), platelet aggregation, viscosity, and platelet and vessel wall interaction in NIDDM. *Diabetes Care*. 1993; 16:683-8.

[56] Woodman RJ, Mori TA, Burke V, Puddey IB, Watts GF, Beilin LJ. Effects of purified eicosapentaenoic and docosahexaenoic acids on glycemic control, blood pressure, and serum lipids in type 2 diabetic patients with treated hypertension. *Am. J. Clin. Nutr.* 2002 Nov; 76(5):1007-15.

[57] Nosari I, Cortinovis F, Lepore G, Maglio ML, Pagani G. Use of omega-3 in diabetic patients *Clin. Ter.* 1994 Mar;144(3):213-21.

[58] Lawrance Christopher C, Maturam LN and Sriram P. Effect of eicosapentaenoic acid on biochemical parameters in experimental diabetic rat. *Ind. Vet. Journal*. 2003; 80(1): 1350-54.

[59] Storlien LH, Kraegen EW, Chisholm DJ, Ford GL, Bruce DG, Pascoe WS. Fish oil prevents insulin resistance induced by high-fat feeding in rats. *Science*. 1987; 237:885-8.

[60] Xu HE, Lambert MH, Montana VG, Parks DJ, Blanchard SG, Brown PJ, Sternbach DD, Lehmann JM, Wisely GB, Willson TM, Kliewer SA, Milburn MV. Molecular recognition of fatty acids by peroxisome proliferator-activated receptors. *Mol. Cell.* 1999 Mar; 3(3):397-403.

[61] Giron MD, Salto R, Hortelano P et al. Increased diaphragm expression of GLUT4 in control and streptozotocin–diabetic rats by fish oil-supplemented diets. *Lipids* 1999; 34: 801–807.

[62] Gabby KH, Hasty K, Breslow JL, Ellison RL, Bunn HF, Gallop PM. Glycosylated hemoglobin and long term blood glucose control in diabetes mellitus. *J. Clin. Endocrinol. Metab.,* 1977 ; 44: 859-64

[63] Manley S. Haemoglobin A1c--a marker for complications of type 2 diabetes: the experience from the UK Prospective Diabetes Study (UKPDS). *Clin. Chem. Lab. Med.* 2003 Sep; 41(9):1182-90.

[64] Rodrigues B, Grassby PF, Battell ML, Lee SY, McNeill JH. Hypertriglyceridemia in experimental diabetes: relationship to cardiac dysfunction. *Can. J. Physiol. Pharmacol.* 1994 May; 72(5):447-55.

[65] Phillipson BE, Rothrock DW, Connor WE, Harris WS, Illingworth DR. Reduction of plasma lipids, lipoproteins, and apoproteins by dietary fish oils in patients with hypertriglyceridemia. *N. Engl. J. Med.* 1985; 312:1210–6.

[66] Nestel PJ. Fish oil attenuates the cholesterol-induced rise in lipoprotein cholesterol. *Am. J. Clin. Nutr.* 1986; 43:752–7.

[67] Nestel PJ. Effects of n-3 fatty acids on lipid metabolism. *Annu. Rev. Nutr.* 1990; 10:149–67.

[68] Parks JS, Crouse JR. Reduction of cholesterol absorption by dietary oleinate and fish oil in African green monkeys. *J. Lipid. Res.* 1992; 33:559–68.

[69] Murthy S, Albright E, Mathur SN, Field FJ. Modification of CaCo-2 cell membrane fatty acid composition by eicosapentaenoic acid and palmitic acid: effect on cholesterol metabolism. *J. Lipid. Res.* 1988; 29:773–80.

[70] Pauletto P, Puato M, Angeli MT, et al. Blood pressure, serum lipids, and fatty acids in populations on a lake-fish diet or on a vegetarian diet in Tanzania. *Lipids* 1996; 31(suppl):S309–12.

[71] Connor WE. Hypolipidemic effects of dietary omega-3 fatty acids in normal and hyperlipidemic humans: effectiveness and mechanisms. In: Simopoulos AP, Kifer RR, Martin RE, eds. Health effects of polyunsaturated fatty acids in sea foods. Orlando, FL: Academic Press, 1986:173–210.

[72] Harris WS, Connor WE, Inkeles SB, Illingworth DR. Omega-3 fatty acids prevent carbohydrate-induced hypertriglyceridemia. *Metabolism* 1984; 33:1016–9.

[73] Nestel PJ, Connor WE, Reardon MR, Connor S, Wong S, Boston R. Suppression by diets rich in fish oil of very low density lipoprotein production in man. *J. Clin. Invest.* 1984; 74:72–89.

[74] Sanders TAB, Sullivan DR, Reeve J, Thompson GR. Triglyceride-lowering effect of marine polyunsaturates in patients with hypertriglyceridemia. *Arteriosclerosis* 1985; 5:459–65.

[75] Harris WS, Connor WE, Illingworth RD, Rothrock DW, Foster DM. Effects of fish oil on VLDL triglyceride kinetics in humans. *J. Lipid. Res.* 1990; 31:1549–58.

[76] Goldberg IJ. Lipoprotein lipase and lipolysis: central roles in lipoprotein metabolism and atherogenesis. *J Lipid Res* 1996; 37:693–707.

[77] Weintraub MS, Zechner R, Brown A, Eisenberg S, Breslow JL. Dietary polyunsaturated fats of the W-6 and W-3 series reduce postprandial lipoprotein levels. *J. Clin. Invest.* 1988; 82:1884–93.

[78] Zampelas A, Murphy M, Morgan LM, Williams CM. Postprandial lipoprotein lipase, insulin and gastric inhibitory polypeptide responses to test meals of different fatty acid composition: comparison of saturated, n-6 and n-3 polyunsaturated fatty acids. *Eur J Clin Nutr* 1994; 48:849–58.

[79] Murphy MC, Zampelas A, Puddicombe SM, Furlonger NP, Morgan LM, Williams CM. Pretranslational regulation of the expression of lipoprotien lipase gene by dietary fatty acids in the rat. *Br. J. Nutr.* 1993; 70:727–36.

[80] Rustan AC, Christiansen EN, Drevon CA. Serum lipids, hepatic glycerolipid metabolism and peroxisomal fatty acid oxidation in rats fed omega-6 and omega-3 fatty acids. *Biochem. J.* 1992; 283:333–8.

[81] Barrans A, Jaspard B, Barbaras R, Chap H, Perret B, Collet X. Pre-ßHDL: structure and metabolism. *Biochim. Biophys. Acta.* 1996; 1300:73–85.

[82] Marsh JB, Topping DL, Nestel PJ. Comparative effects of dietary fish oil and carbohydrate on plasma lipids and hepatic activities of phosphatidate phosphohydrolase, diacyglycerol acyltransferase and neutral lipase activities in the rat. *Biochim. Biophys. Acta.* 1987; 922:239–43.

[83] Krauss RM. Atherogenicity of triglyceride-rich lipoproteins. *Am. J. Cardiol.* 1998; 81:13B–17B.

[84] Krauss RM. Triglycerides and atherogenic lipoproteins: rationale for lipid management. *Am. J. Med.* 1998; 105 (Suppl. 1A):58S–62S.

[85] Berneis KK, Krauss RM. Metabolic origins and clinical significance of LDL heterogeneity. *J. Lipid. Res.* 2002; 43:1363–1379.

[86] McNamara JR, Campos H, Ordovas JM, Peterson J, Wilson PW, Schaefer EJ. Effect of gender, age, and lipid status on low density lipoprotein subfraction distribution: results from the Framingham Offspring Study. *Arteriosclerosis* 1987; 7:483–490.

[87] McNamara JR, Jenner JL, Li Z, Wilson PW, Schaefer EJ. Change in LDL particle size is associated with change in plasma triglyceride concentration. *Arterioscler. Thromb. Vasc. Biol.*1992; 12:1284–1290.

[88] Krauss RM, Williams PT, Lindgren FT, Wood PD. Coordinate changes in levels of human serum low and high density lipoprotein subclasses in healthy men. *Arteriosclerosis* 1988; 8:155–162.

[89] Hopkins GJ, Barter PJ. Role of triglyceride-rich lipoproteins and hepatic lipase in determining the particle size and composition of high density lipoproteins. *J. Lipid. Res.* 1986; 27:1265–1277.

[90] Blanche PJ, Gong EL, Forte TM, Nichols AV. Characterization of human high-density lipoproteins by gradient gel electrophoresis. *Biochim. Biophys. Acta.* 1981; 665:408–419.

[91] Roach PD, Kambouris AM, Trimble RP, Topping DL, Nestel PJ. The effects of dietary fish oil on hepatic high density and low density lipoprotein receptor activities in the rat. *FEBS Lett* 1987; 222:159–62.

[92] Lindsey S, Pronczuk A, Hayes KC. Low density lipoprotein from humans supplemented with n-3 fatty acids depresses both LDL receptor activity and LDLr mRNA abundance in HepG2 cells. *J. Lipid Res.* 1992; 33:647–58.

[93] Linga V, Leight MA, Curtiss LK, Marcel YL, Richard W, et al. Dietary fish oil-induced decrease in low density lipoprotein binding to fibroblasts is mediated by apolipoprotein *E. J. Lipid Res.* 1994;35:491–500.

[94] Abbey M, Clifton P, Kestin M, Belling B, Nestel PJ. Effect of fish oil on lipoproteins, lecithin:cholesterol acyltransferase, and lipid transfer protein activity in humans. *Arteriosclerosis* 1990; 10:85–94.

[95] Suzukawa M, Abbey M, Howe PRC, Nestel PJ. Effects of fish oil fatty acids on low density lipoprotein size, oxidizability, and uptake by macrophages. *J. Lipid Res.* 1995; 36:437–84.

[96] Illingworth DR, Harris WS, Connor WE. Inhibition of low density lipoprotein synthesis by dietary omega-3 fatty acids in humans. *Arteriosclerosis* 1984; 4:270–5.

[97] Fein FS, Kornstein LB, Strobeck JE et al. Altered myocardial mechanics in diabetic rats. *Circ. Res.* 1980; 47:922–933.

[98] Jaffe AS, Spadaro JJ, Schechtman K, et al. Increased congestive heart failure after myocardial infarction of modest extent in patients with diabetes mellitus. *Am. Heart J.* 1984; 108:31–37.

[99] Fein FS, Cho S, Zola BE, et al. Cardiac pathology in the hypertensive diabetic rat. Biventricular damage with right ventricular predominance. *Am. J. Pathol.* 1989; 134:1159–1166.

[100] Fang ZY, Prins JB, Marwick TH. Diabetic cardiomyopathy: evidence, mechanisms, and therapeutic implications. *Endocr Rev*. 2004 Aug; 25(4):543-67.

[101] Ganguly PK, Pierce GN, Dhalla KS, Dhalla NS. Defective sarcoplasmic reticular calcium transport in diabetic cardiomyopathy. *Am. J. Physiol.* 1983; 244:E528-E535.

[102] Giacomelli F, Wiener J. Primary myocardial disease in the diabetic mouse. An ultrastructural study. *Lab. Invest.* 1979; 40:460-473.

[103] Regan TJ, Wu CF, Yeh CK, Oldewurtel HA, Haider B. Myocardial composition and function in diabetes. The effects of chronic insulin use. *Circ. Res.* 1981; 49:1268-1277.

[104] Singh K, Xiao L, Remondino A, Sawyer DB, Colucci WS. Adrenergic regulation of cardiac myocyte apoptosis. *J. Cell Physiol.* 2001189:257-265.

[105] Bisognano JD, Weinberger HD, Bohlmeyer TJ, Pende A, Raynolds MV, Sastravaha A, Roden R, Asano K, Blaxall BC, Wu SC, Communal C, Singh K, Colucci W, Bristow MR, Port DJ. Myocardial-directed overexpression of the human ß(1)-adrenergic receptor in transgenic mice. *J. Mol. Cell Cardiol.* 2000; 32:817-830.

[106] Irlbeck M, Zimmer HG. Functional responses of the left and right heart of diabetic rats to α and ß-adrenergic receptor stimulation. *Diabetes. Res. Clin. Pract.* 1996; 31 Suppl: S79-S86.

[107] Lawrance Christopher C. Effect of eicosapentaenoic acid on experimental diabetic cardiomyopathy. M.V.Sc., thesis submitted to the Tamil Nadu Veterinary and Animal Sciences University. 1998.

[108] Afzal N, Ganguly PK, Dhalla KS, Pierce GN, Singal PK, Dhalla NS. Beneficial effects of verapamil in diabetic cardiomyopathy. *Diabetes* 1988; 37:936-942.

[109] Afzal N, Pierce GN, Elimban V, Beamish RE, Dhalla NS. Influence of verapamil on some sub cellular defects in diabetic cardiomyopathy. *Am. J. Physiol.* 1989; 256:E453-E458.

[110] Shah TS, Satia MC, Gandhi TP, Bangaru RA, Goyal RK. Effects of chronic nifedipine treatment on streptozotocin-induced diabetic rats. *J. Cardiovasc. Pharmacol.* 1995; 26:6-12.

[111] Shimada T. Correlation between metabolic and histopathological changes in the myocardium of the KK mouse. Effect of diltiazem on the diabetic heart. *Jpn. Heart J.* 1993; 34:617-626.

[112] Squadrito F, Altavilla D, Squadrito G and Campo GM. 17 b-Oestradiol reduces cardiac leukocyte accumulation in myocardial ischaemia reperfusion injury in rat. *Eur. J. Pharmacol.* 1997; 335:185-192.

[113] Cubria JC, Regwera R, Balana-Fouce R, Ordonez C and Ordonez D. Polyamine-mediated heart hypertrophy-induced by clenbuterol in the mouse. *J. Pharm. Pharmacol.* 1998; 50:91-96.

[114] Hock CE, Holahan MA and Reibel DK. Effect of dietary fish oil on myocardial phospholipids and myocardial ischemic damage. *Am. J. Physiol.* 1987; 252:H554-H560.

[115] Tanaka Y, Kashiwagi A, Saeki Y, Takagi Y, Asahina T, Kikkawa R, Shigeta Y. Effects of verapamil on the cardiac alpha 1-adrenoceptor signalling system in diabetic rats. *Eur J Pharmacol.* 1993 Jan 15; 244(2):105-9.

[116] Wexler C. Myocardial Infarction in young vs. old male rats. Pathophysiological changes. *Am. Heart. J.* 1978; 96:70-80.

[117] Rodrigues B, Goyal RK and McNeill JH. Effects of hydralazine on streptozotocin-induced diabetic rats: prevention of hyperlipidemia and improvement of cardiac function. *J. Pharmacol. Exp. Ther.*, 1986; 237:292-299.

[118] Hebden RA, Bennett T. and Gardiner SM. Abnormal blood pressure recovery during ganglionic blockade in diabetic rats. *Am. J. Physiol.*, 1987; 252: R102-R108.

[119] Nordin C, Gilat E. and Aronson RS. Delayed after depolarization and triggered activity in ventricular muscle from rats with streptozotocin-induced diabetes. *Circ. Res.*, 1985; 57:28-34.

[120] Legaye F, Beigelman P, Deroubaix E. and Coraboeuf E. Effect of 3-5-3'triiodothyronin treatment on cardiac action potential of streptozotocin-induced diabetic rat. *Life Sci.*, 1988 42:2269-2274.

[121] Heyliger CE, Prakash, A. and McNeill JH. Alterations in cardiac sarcolemmal Ca2+ pump activity during diabetes mellitus. *Am. J. Physiol.* 1987; 252: H540-H544.

[122] Makino N, Dhalla, KS, Elimban, V. and Dhalla NS. Sarcolemmal Ca2+ transport in streptozotocin-induced diabetic cardimyopathy in rats. *Am. J. Physiol.*, 1987 253, E202-E207.

[123] Nicholl, TA, Lopaschuk, GD. and McNeill JH. Effects of free fatty acids and dichloroacetate on isolated working diabetic rat heart. *Am. J. Physiol.*, 1991; 261: H1053-H1059.

[124] Sundaresan, P.R., Sharma, V.K., Gingold, S.I. and Banerjee, S.P. Decreased b-adrenergic receptors in rat heart in streptozotocin-induced diabetes: role of thyroid hormones. *Endocrinology*, 1984; 114:1358-1363.

[125] Kahn, J.H., Sisson, J.C. and Vinik, A.I.QT interval prolongation and sudden cardiac death in diabetic autonomic neuropathy. *J. Clin. Endocrinol. Metab*, 1987; 64: 751-754.

[126] Tong, N.W., Yang, T.G. and Lliang, J.Z. Ventricular late potentials in patients with diabetes mellitus. *Chung. Hua. Nei. Ko. Tsa. Chih.*, 1993; 32: 464-466.

[127] Ueno Y, Koike H, Nishio S. Beneficial effects of beraprost sodium, a stable prostacyclin analogue, in diabetic cardiomyopathy. *J Cardiovasc Pharmacol.* 1995: Oct; 26(4):603-7.

[128] Ledet T, Gottzche O, Heickendorff L: Diabetes and Heart Disease. New York, Elsevier, 1984, p. 25-26

[129] Penpargkul S, Fein F, Sonnenblick EH, Scheuer J. Depressed cardiac sarcoplasmic reticular function from diabetic rats. *J. Mol. Cell Cardiol.* 1981; 13:303-309.

[130] Lopaschuk GD, Katz S, McNeil JH. The effect of alloxan- and streptozotocin-induced diabetes on calcium transport in rat cardiac sarcoplasmic reticulum: the possible involvement of long chain acylcarnitines. *Can. J. Physiol. Pharmacol.* 1983; 61:439-48.

[131] Dillmann WH. Diabetes mellitus induces changes in cardiac myosin of the rat. *Diabetes* 1980; 29:579-82.

[132] Jenkins RL, McDaniel HG, Digerness S, Parrish SW, Ong RL. Adenine nucleotide metabolism in hearts of diabetic rats: comparison to diaphragm, liver, and kidney. *Diabetes* 1988 37:629-36.

[133] Spector KS, Diabetic cardiomyopathy. *Clin. Cardiol.* 1998; 21:885–887.

[134] Nishimura M, Nanbu A, Komori T, Ohtsuka K, Takahashi H, Yoshimura M. Eicosapentaenoic acid stimulates nitric oxide production and decreases cardiac noradrenaline in diabetic rats. *Clin. Exp. Pharmacol. Physiol.* 2000 Aug; 27(8):618-24.

[135] Gerbi A, Barbey O, Raccah D, Coste T, Jamme I, Nouvelot A, Ouafik L, Levy S, Vague P, Maixent JM. Alteration of Na,K-ATPase isoenzymes in diabetic cardiomyopathy: effect of dietary supplementation with fish oil (n-3 fatty acids) in rats. *Diabetologia.* 1997 May; 40(5):496-505.

[136] Ovide-Bordeaux S, Grynberg A. Docosahexaenoic acid affects insulin deficiency- and insulin resistance-induced alterations in cardiac mitochondria. *Am. J. Physiol. Regul. Integr. Comp. Physiol.* 2004 Mar; 286 (3):R519-27. Epub 2003 Nov 06.

Index

A

B

C

D

I

K

L

M

N

Q

R

S

T

U

V

W

X

Y